THE DOCTOR DISSECTED

The Doctor Dissected

A CULTURAL AUTOPSY OF THE BURKE
AND HARE MURDERS

Caroline McCracken-Flesher

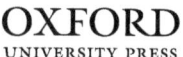

OXFORD
UNIVERSITY PRESS

Oxford University Press, Inc., publishes works that further
Oxford University's objective of excellence
in research, scholarship, and education.

Oxford   New York
Auckland   Cape Town   Dar es Salaam   Hong Kong   Karachi
Kuala Lumpur   Madrid   Melbourne   Mexico City   Nairobi
New Delhi   Shanghai   Taipei   Toronto

With offices in
Argentina   Austria   Brazil   Chile   Czech Republic   France   Greece
Guatemala   Hungary   Italy   Japan   Poland   Portugal   Singapore
South Korea   Switzerland   Thailand   Turkey   Ukraine   Vietnam

Copyright © 2012 by Oxford University Press, Inc.

Published by Oxford University Press, Inc.
198 Madison Avenue, New York, New York 10016

www.oup.com

Oxford is a registered trademark of Oxford University Press

All rights reserved. No part of this publication may be reproduced,
stored in a retrieval system, or transmitted, in any form or by any means,
electronic, mechanical, photocopying, recording, or otherwise,
without the prior permission of Oxford University Press.

Library of Congress Cataloging-in-Publication Data
McCracken-Flesher, Caroline.
  The doctor dissected : a cultural autopsy of the Burke and Hare murders / Caroline McCracken-Flesher.
    p. cm.
  Includes bibliographical references and index.
  ISBN 978-0-19-976682-6 (cloth : acid-free paper)   1. Literature and history—Scotland.   2. Crime in popular culture—Scotland.   3. English literature—Scottish authors—History and criticism.   4. Murder in mass media—Scotland.   5. National characteristics, Scottish, in literature.   6. Burke, William, 1792–1829.   7. Hare, William, 1792?–1870?   I. Title.
  PR8518.M33 2012
  820.9'3556—dc23   2011041415

1 3 5 7 9 8 6 4 2

Printed in the United States of America
on acid-free paper

*Dedicated to
Paul and Conor,
who delight in horrible histories
and in memory of
Craig Arnold and Douglas S. Mack,
who loved all strange stories*

People remember badly. But *societies* remember well....
Sometimes the truth keeps itself alive in devious ways
despite the best efforts of the official keepers of information.
TERRY PRATCHETT, *Lords and Ladies*

Up the close and doon the stair,
But an' ben wi' Burke and Hare.
Burke's the butcher, Hare's the thief,
Knox the boy that buys the beef.

Contents

Acknowledgments   ix
Abbreviations   xiii

1. *Medicine, Murder, and Scottish Story: Doctor Knox and Burke and Hare*   3

2. *The Story Begins: The Law versus the Press, and the Doctor versus Walter Scott*   28

3. *Enlightened System versus Religious Sympathy: The Sensational Tales of Alexander Leighton and David Pae*   56

4. *Dissecting the Doctor:* Mr. *Jekyll,* Dr. *Hyde, and Robert Knox*   89

5. *Anatomizing the Audience: James Bridie, Melodrama, and the Movies*   118

6. *Bringing Out the Dead: Silent Victims Speak in Alasdair Gray's* Poor Things   155

7. *Resting in Pieces? Present Comforts or Restless Futures in Ian Rankin's Scotland*   193

Notes   233
Bibliography   243
Index   263

Acknowledgments

A BOOK SUCH as this owes debts to many fields, archives, places, and persons. My first thanks, as always, go to Paul Flesher and Conor McCracken-Flesher, and to stalwart friends and colleagues Valerie and Oli Ludlow, Penny Fielding, Pippa Berry, Pete and Lynne Simpson, Christine Stebbins, Donna Bagby, Ian Duncan, Robert Crawford, and Murray Pittock.

My debts to librarians, curators, and archivists now map the United States and Britain. I am grateful for help from the National Library of Scotland, especially Iain Brown, Graham Hogg, Eoin Shalloo, Sheila Mackenzie, Anette Hagan, and George Stanley; the University of Glasgow Special Collections, Sharon Lawler, and Niki Pollock; the University of Stirling Library and Helen Beardsley; Dundee Central Library, Eileen Moran, Carol Lamb, Deidre Sweeney, and David Kett; Edinburgh Central Library's Edinburgh Room and Anne Morrison; the Mitchell Library, Glasgow; the University of Edinburgh Centre for Research Collections and Tricia Boyd; the British Library, and the Newspaper Collection at Colindale; the Bristol Theatre Collection and Heather Romaine; the Rylands Library, Manchester; the National Archives of Scotland; the Museum of Fine Arts, Boston, and Marta Fodor; the Thomas Cooper Library at the University of South Carolina; the New York Public Library; the Library of Congress; and as always, the American Heritage Center, the Interlibrary Loan office, and the Ellbogen Center for Teaching and Learning at the University of Wyoming, with their staff Anne Marie Lane, Dee Salo, and Andy Bryson.

Colleagues in medicine and medical archives were invaluable, given my foray into this new field. I here thank Tony Payne, Professor of Anatomy at the University of Glasgow; Jamie Davies, Professor of Experimental Anatomy, University of Edinburgh; the Royal College of Surgeons of Edinburgh, especially Dawn Kemp, Steven Kerr, and Marianne Smith; the Royal College of Physicians of Edinburgh, notably John Dallas and Iain Milne; the Royal Society of Edinburgh and Journals and Archive Officer Vicki M. Hammond; Surgeons' Hall Museum, Edinburgh; the Hunterian Museum, Glasgow; the Hunterian Museum, London; the Wellcome Institute and Library; Professor Roger Cooter; Bob Stevenson, RLS's dental historian; and Lisa Rosner.

Special thanks to Judith and Anthony Cooke for access to Pae family materials in their private collection, and for their hospitality.

Given the topicality of this book as it moves up to the present, I have depended on the generosity of numerous authors and artists to discuss their work or share it in manuscript. Thanks and admiration to: Alasdair Gray, Jonny Berliner, Fintan O'Higgins, Robert Stocks, Dan Bianchi, Richard Crane, Chris Ballance, Peter Robinson, Irvine Welsh, Owen Dudley Edwards, George Young, Elizabeth Bagby, Douglas McNaughton, Rob Crouch, Martin Conaghan, Will Pickering, and Gary Erskine. And sadly posthumous appreciation to Edwin Morgan, with thanks, too, to Carcanet Press.

Colleagues have thrown their energy into the search for a Burke and Hare melodrama. I hope one of them will yet find and enjoy it. My thanks to Ann Featherstone, University of Manchester; Vanessa Toulmin, Director of the National Fairground Archive, Sheffield; Barbara Bell; Ian Brown; Graham Topping; and Stephen Arata. Michael S. Sims proved indefatigable in tracking connections to Sherlock Holmes.

I have presented elements of my argument at many places. Everywhere I received helpful feedback, and I owe a great debt to those who made this possible: Edinburgh University's Department of English and the Centre for Scottish Writing in the Nineteenth Century, especially Penny Fielding and Alex Thomson; Edinburgh's Institute for Advanced Study in the Humanities, and Susan Manning; the University of Oxford and the Romantic Realignments Seminar, especially Anna Camillieri, Kate Barush, James Grande, and Georgina Green; the University of Glasgow Scottish Literature faculty, especially Gerry Carruthers, Alan Riach, John Corbett, Kirsteen McCue, Duncan Jones, Donald Mackenzie, and Margery Palmer McCulloch; the University of Stirling Department of English Studies, Scott Hames, Suzanne Gilbert, Stephen Penn, Ruth Evans, and David Richards; Hastings College Department of History, Robert Babcock, and Antje Anderson; the University of Leeds, Julia Reid, and Matt Rubery; the Edinburgh Sir Walter Scott Club, Paul Henderson Scott, Fraser Elgin, Dairmid Gunn, Sheriff Isobel Poole, and Lee Simpson; the University of Wyoming Faculty Senate, Phil Holt, and Amy Kopp; the University of Wyoming/Casper College and Bruce Richardson; the University

Acknowledgments xi

of Wyoming Office of the President and Office for Research, Bill Gern, and Angela Faxon; the 2001 Robert Louis Stevenson conference, Richard Dury, and Richard Ambrosini; the Walter Scott Conference, Sylvia Mergenthal (2003), and Caroline Jackson-Houlston (2007); and additional friends, hosts, and advisers without number: Janette Currie, Eric Massie, the sadly missed Douglas S. Mack, Alison Lumsden, Jane Millgate, Catherine Jones, Faith Pullin, Viccy Coltman, Matt Wickman, Gwen Enstam, Fiona Wilson, Ken McNeill, Aileen Christianson, Jenni Calder, Micah Gilbert, Peter Garside, and Gill Hughes.

My research and its presentation have been supported by the Huntington Library and British Academy (special thanks to Sharon Strange); the City of Literature, Edinburgh; and the Royal Society of Edinburgh. At the University of Wyoming, I thank the Faculty Senate (Faculty Senate Speaker Award); the Kaiser Ethics Foundation and Jane Nelson (Kaiser Ethics Grant for teaching); International Programs and Ann Alexander (International Travel Grant); the Research Office and Vice President Bill Gern (Faculty Grant-in-Aid); the Faculty Development Committee (Flittie Award); President Tom Buchanan (Presidential Speaker Award); the Office of the Provost and Myron Allen; and, prominent for the Humanities, the College of Arts and Sciences and Dean Oliver Walter.

Sincere thanks are always owed to colleagues at home, in this case Janice Harris, Craig Arnold (deceased), Barbara Chatton, Susan Aronstein, Susan Frye, Sandra Clark, Bob Torry, Ric Reverand, Bunny Logan, Jeanne Holland, Peter Parolin, and Carolyn Young.

I'd also like to thank the following individuals and organizations for their generous help, and for giving permission to reproduce materials: Alasdair Gray; Anthony and Judith Cooke; British Library Board; Douglas McNaughton; Dundee Central Library; Edinburgh City Libraries and Information Services; Edinburgh University Library, Centre for Research Collections; Edwin Morgan and Carcanet Press; Jonny Berliner and Fintan O'Higgins; Martin Conaghan, Will Pickering, and Gary Erskine; Museum of Fine Arts, Boston; National Library of Scotland, the Trustees; New York Public Library General Research Division, Astor, Lenox, and Tilden Foundations; Royal College of Physicians of Edinburgh; Royal College of Surgeons of Edinburgh; Royal Society of Edinburgh; University of Bristol Theatre Collection; University of Glasgow Library, Department of Special Collections; University of South Carolina Libraries, Irvin Department of Rare Books and Special Collections; University of St. Andrews; and Wellcome Library, London.

And of course, there would be no book without supportive editors Shannon McLachlan and Brendan O'Neill at Oxford.

A book so well assisted should have no errors, but those that surely remain must be my own. My apologies for any mistakes or omissions in this list or the book—they testify, once again, to the extent of my debts.

Abbreviations

APJ	*Aberdeen Press and Journal*
BL	British Library
Blackwood's	*Blackwood's Edinburgh Magazine*
BTC	University of Bristol Theatre Collection
Courant	*Edinburgh Evening Courant*
Curtain	*Curtain*
DCL	Dundee Central Library (Local History Centre)
DNB	*Dictionary of National Biography*
DPJ	*Dundee... People's Journal*
DT	*Daily Telegraph*
ECL	Edinburgh Central Library
EdEDis	*Edinburgh Evening Dispatch*
EdENews	*Edinburgh Evening News*
EN	*Evening News*
Era	*Era*
ES	*Evening Standard*
EWC	*Edinburgh Weekly Chronicle*
EWJ	*Edinburgh Weekly Journal*

GBulletin	*Glasgow Bulletin*
GEN	*Glasgow Evening News*
GH	*Glasgow Herald*
ISDN	*Illustrated Sporting and Dramatic News*
Lady	*The Lady*
Lancet	*Lancet*
LP	*Liverpool Post*
Medical Times	*Medical Times and Gazette*
Mercury	*Caledonian Mercury*
MG	*Manchester Guardian*
Mitchell	Mitchell Library, Glasgow
MP	*Morning Post*
NLS	National Library of Scotland
NSN	*New Statesman and Nation*
Pae papers	Pae family papers (Judith and Anthony Cooke)
NW	*News of the World*
NYWT	*New York World Telegraph*
PMG	*Pall Mall Gazette*
RCPEd	Royal College of Physicians of Edinburgh
RCSEd	Royal College of Surgeons of Edinburgh
RSE	Royal Society of Edinburgh
Rylands	Rylands Library Manchester
Scotsman	*Scotsman*
SDT	*Sheffield Daily Telegraph*
Sphere	*The Sphere*
SR	*Saturday Review*
Stage	*Stage*
Star	*Star*
STimes	*Sunday Times*
Times	*Times*
T&T	*Time and Tide*
UE	University of Edinburgh Centre for Research Collections
UGla	University of Glasgow (Bridie)
USL	University of Stirling Library
Wellcome	Wellcome Library, Wellcome Institute London
WF	*World's Fair*

THE DOCTOR DISSECTED

His life was a failure until he died.

—Lecture on the centenary of Robert Burns's birth, by Henry Ward Beecher.

1

Medicine, Murder, and Scottish Story

DOCTOR KNOX AND BURKE AND HARE

IN "MARY'S GHOST" the hapless Mary, torn from her grave by bodysnatchers, haunts her lover.[1] She wails: "My rest eternal ceases; / Alas! my everlasting peace / Is broken into pieces" (v. 2). What worries Thomas Hood's character most, however, is not the breaking of her eternal rest, but that of her body. She laments to her William:

> The arm that used to take your arm
> Is took to Dr. Vyse;
> And both my legs are gone to walk
> The hospital at Guy's. (v. 6)
>
> I can't tell where my head is gone,
> But Doctor Carpue can:
> As for my trunk, it's all pack'd up
> To go by Pickford's van. (v. 9)

Mary has been sold to the doctors, and the cutting-edge science of the day has sliced her into pieces in pursuit of the secrets of disease and on behalf of health. So as Mary fades into the sunrise, she can only promise William partial commitment:

> The cock it crows—I must begone!
> My William we must part!
> But I'll be yours in death, altho'
> Sir Astley has my heart. (v. 11)

Mary's tale, then, is one of loss—but it is not quite one of absence. She concludes:

> Don't go to weep upon my grave,
> And think that there I be;
> I haven't left an atom there
> Of my anatomie. (v. 12)

If Mary's body has been obliterated through the anatomists' depredations, she still speaks. In the process of her thorough dissection, she has achieved a strange new poetic—and in her case punningly playful—life.

In fact, Mary becomes more lively because she has died and been passed around. Uncanny postmortem mobility affects the dissecting doctors, too—or one doctor in particular. In 1828, Robert Knox was Edinburgh's most charismatic anatomist. By 1829, however, he was the most reviled, and today, while his colleagues lie forgotten, he and his murderous associates Burke and Hare continue to cut a gash in Scottish literature. This book tracks the cadaverous culture of Burke and Hare and Doctor Knox from the dark beginnings of their tale, in Enlightenment science matched with nineteenth-century commerce, through to our present moment. Their deathly exploits animate tales and tellers all over the world—as I write, John Landis's movie prepares for release. And they dominate in Scotland. Although Walter Scott refused to tell his contemporaries' sordid tale, later authors have been haunted by their memory: Robert Louis Stevenson's elegant Henry Jekyll and the proclivities of Mr. Hyde descend from Doctor Knox; Alasdair Gray's "Poor Things" are kin to his dissected subjects; Ian Rankin's Inspector Rebus fights crime in an Edinburgh resonant with the evil deeds of Burke and Hare; and Irvine Welsh imagines them still at work, hacking away at "the Meat Trade." It is our task to wonder why—why the world seeks out this tale, and why Scots cannot leave it behind.

DOCTOR ROBERT KNOX—AND BURKE AND HARE

Who was Doctor Knox, and what did he do that was so important, so strange, or so wrong it could dig its way into a culture's narrative? An Edinburgh boy who excelled in high school, Knox went on to study anatomy at the university, taking his degree in 1814. Knox thereby joined an elite group, for "by 1800 study at the University of Edinburgh was widely acknowledged to be the most prestigious medical training" (Digby, 54). In June 1815 he served as a Hospital Assistant in the aftermath of Waterloo, and for the next two years he dealt with injuries and illnesses sustained at war and in service of the British Empire at the depot hospital near Portsmouth. At Waterloo, with one surgeon and one assistant per regiment, he must have learned surgery hard and fast, and his work with returning troops unfortunately allowed considerable practice in dissection (Youngquist, 175–76, 178; Bates, 30–32). From 1817 to 1820, he was at the African Cape, with light medical duties and able to explore other branches of science such as meteorology and comparative anatomy. There, he began to develop his complex theories of race (Bates, 32–38 and 52; Rosner *Anatomy Murders*, 84–86). Finally, he rounded out his studies in Paris with the great Cuvier (Bates, ch. 5).[2]

When Knox returned to Edinburgh, his abilities allowed him to join the Royal Society of Edinburgh (1823), establish a museum of comparative anatomy for the Royal College of Surgeons, and take over Professor John Barclay's private school of anatomy. Now established alongside the university, Knox rapidly became its successful rival. The university professor Alexander Monro *tertius* was rumored to read out his grandfather's notes and suffer mayhem among his disaffected students. In 1825, the young Charles Darwin was revolted, finding him "so dirty in person and actions."[3] By contrast Knox, with his blind eye, frilled cuffs, and inspiring talks emerged as a compelling figure (see figure 1.1). This doctor "courted popularity, and it [came] as a flood," says Henry Lonsdale, who studied and worked with Knox after the scandal (Lonsdale, 130; Bates, 96). But as Lonsdale himself may have experienced when they parted company in 1842, never one to shirk an invidious comparison, Knox's "sharp, pithy sentences...came like sparks from a furnace...igniting by their satire, [and creating] sad havoc among doubtful medical reputations" (Bates, 9; Lonsdale, 151). Knox took no prisoners, reportedly denouncing Monro for having "inherited his anatomical genius from his ancestors," and vilifying Monro's student, the famed surgeon Robert Liston, as "a professional celebrity" whose carelessness killed patients on the operating table (MacGregor, 237, 236). Still Knox was generous to his students: he entertained them to dinner, and visited them when they were sick—Thomas Giordani Wright appreciated Knox coming "four or five times a day" to check on him (Johnson, 408). So whether berating the inadequacies of his competition or laying out a complex dissection, to the young men who ventured to his messy but fascinating anatomy classes, by 1828 Knox stood as *"primus et incomparabilis"* (Lonsdale, 46).

A year later, in 1829, however, Knox was known differently. What had happened? After all, Knox was a gifted and successful teacher. The sympathetic Lonsdale

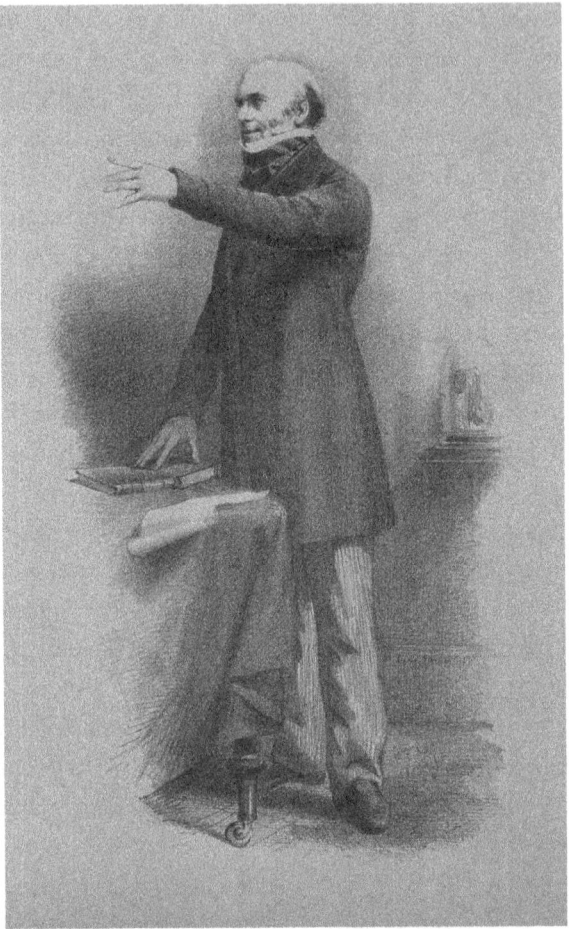

FIGURE 1.1 Robert Knox. Lithograph. Courtesy of the Wellcome Library, London.

remembered him as "a luminary to the [students].... [H]e had two-thirds of the [University] medical school in his class rooms"—for which, we might note, they had to pay (Lonsdale, 90). By October 1828, in only his third year of teaching independently, according to Knox's own report he had boosted his classes to an unparalleled 504 students, and was obliged to teach the same lesson three times daily. Certainly, his ads for 1828 promise two courses of lectures and two demonstrations running concurrently (Rosner *Anatomy Murders*, 80; Knox *Letter*, 7 n.1).[4] The reason for Knox's fall lay in his success. From 1826 to 1827, dissection became compulsory first for diploma candidates with the Royal College of Surgeons of Edinburgh, and then for Edinburgh University medical students (Bates, 61). Knox's classes overflowed. A dedicated teacher, Knox required good materials for all these students, and ads for his 1828 lectures promised that "Each of these Courses will as usual comprise a full

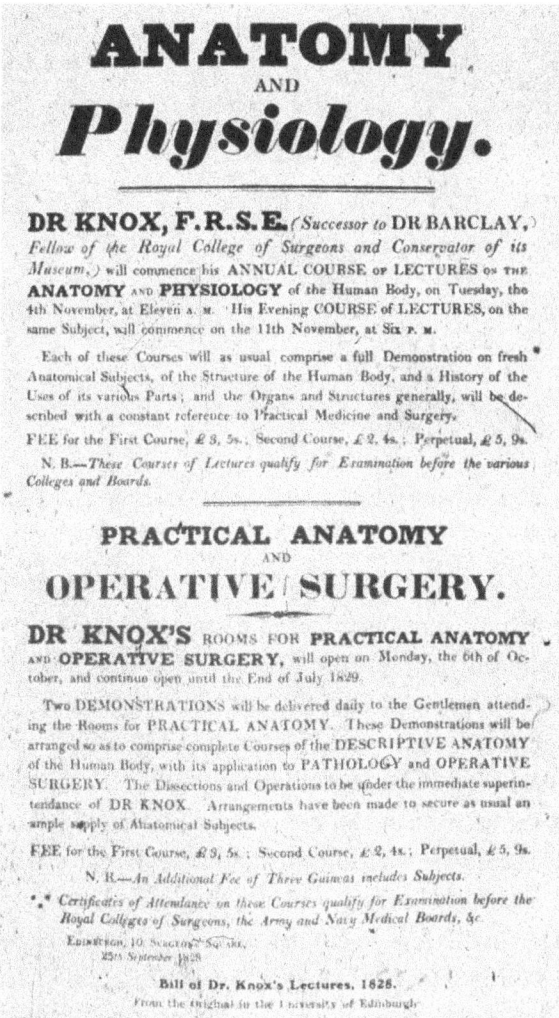

FIGURE 1.2 Bill of Dr. Knox's Lectures, 1828. Courtesy of the Royal College of Surgeons of Edinburgh.

Demonstration on fresh Anatomical Subjects" (see figure 1.2). Knox assured students that "Arrangements have been made to secure as usual an ample supply." But where did those subjects come from—"as usual"? In November 1828 Edinburgh learned that William Burke and William Hare, lured by the fees dictated by high demand and scarce supply, had taken to manufacturing the commodity.

After discovering the retail value of an unfortunate indigent, who had died owing rent to Hare, these enterprising Irish immigrants sought to speed production. In less than a year, perhaps assisted by their women folk Margaret Hare and Helen McDougal, they murdered at least sixteen people (see figure 1.3). There were rumors of more. The drunk, and those who could be lured and subdued by alcohol,

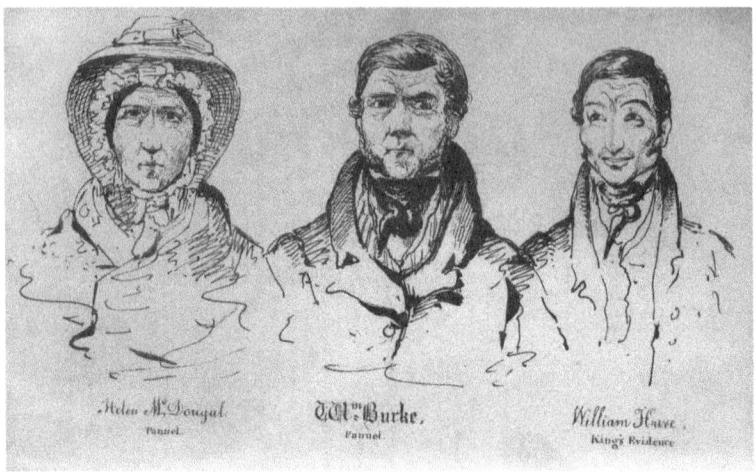

FIGURE 1.3 McDougal, Burke, and Hare. Contemporary print. Courtesy of the Royal College of Physicians of Edinburgh.

succumbed one by one, and sometimes in pairs. Seduced by offers of hospitality, the wandering Irish and impoverished Scots fell either to the suffocating pillow or to Burke and Hare's improved technique: the two held the nose, and leaned on the chest until a victim's resistance ceased ("Confessions of Burke" in *Trial*, published by Buchanan). Old Mrs. Haldane, and then the fallen daughter who sought her; Mary Paterson; an old woman and her dumb grandson together; the neighbor's washerwoman; "Daft Jamie," well known in Edinburgh for his deformed figure and harmless nature, all died. On and on until Mrs. Docherty, a confused old Irishwoman looking for her son in this foreign city, had the misfortune to be found by William Burke. The jovial Burke claimed kin and led her to drink and to death. Next morning the Grays, recent guests at Burke's and relatives of Helen McDougal, his mistress, found her, unexpectedly naked and dead, under a heap of straw in Burke's house. The honest Grays, though offered ridiculous bribes, brought the police. Mrs. Docherty, however, had moved on. Edinburgh's finest found her, not yet unpacked, awaiting dissection at Surgeons' Square. Burke and Hare had crammed their sixteen victims into tea chests and barrels and sold them to Doctor Knox. The encouraging doctor congratulated them that their supply was "fresh" (*Authentic Confessions*, 231–32).

THE SCOTTISH DILEMMA

What did Robert Knox know? Enquiring Edinburgh hoped to clarify and thus mitigate the relationship between the doctor, a prominent representative of Scottish progress, and the murderers—between society and a rather gothic criminality. Yet the story fought resolution. Worse, over time Scottish writers have proved unable to resolve it—to heal this wound opened by Knox, Burke, and Hare in the body politic. Often, they have done more damage. The papers immediately worried the story into mountains of newsprint, and later generations have proved just as fascinated by it. The nineteenth century saw the story move through melodrama and novel; today, it dominates as a theme for Edinburgh Festival plays and the "Edinburgh Dungeon" is developing their Burke and Hare exhibit. Still, no telling seems enough: the story is retold from generation to generation, and a perplexing number of authors seem compelled to tell it twice—including Stevenson, who led with "The Body Snatcher." Outside Scotland, too, this past attracts major authors and repeat customers. Hitchcock embraced its horrors, and it figures in two BBC audiodramas of *Doctor Who*. The story seems crucial to tell, but impossible to finish off. Or perhaps this is a wound that Scots and their surrogates refuse to let heal—after all, generation after generation, they probe it.

Through to our twenty-first century, no tale of medical horror other than *Frankenstein*, and no true tale of the doctors, maintains such ongoing power. Especially in Scotland. Here, we focus on the Scottish aspect of this phenomenon. Although the story multiplies elsewhere, Scotland provides oddity enough for one book. Nonetheless, *The Doctor Dissected* invokes examples of this Scottish tale from other places, for they highlight the peculiar difference it manifests and perhaps makes for Scots. This book hopes along the way to encourage others to explore not just the Scottish case, with its obsessive retellings, but also why outsiders are drawn to tortured tales not their own, and this one in particular.

So why do Scots choose to pick at their own horrible past—an old injury that should long ago have healed itself? We consider, to begin with, the way that the scandal surrounding Doctor Knox trenched its way into the national psyche, cutting a wound so damaging it continues to weep within Scottish culture. This strange case remains open because in 1828, patient and physician and life and death came disturbingly close at the point of the anatomist's knife. Through his many Marys and their worrisome provenance, Doctor Knox made public all the anxieties about health and mortality, self and other, killing and curing that weigh on the point of the deftest scalpel. Thereby, Knox opened a wound that resisted closure; worse, its closure might actually knit Edinburgh and these dark medical worries together. Such a story, freighted with anxiety, over time aligns itself with and exacerbates the divisions of a culture vexed by its dual role as Scottish and British, by the unpredictability of the early press, by religion, commerce, medicine, professionalism, local politics, and now globalism. Focusing on moments when, driven by contemporary anxieties, Knox's story intensifies, *The Doctor Dissected* argues that it recurs as a symptom of cultural disease but becomes the irritant that stimulates healing. In recent days, Scots aiming for the grand political narratives of Western culture (self-government, for instance) provoke the pains of this distressing memory and compromised identity as a counter-anesthetic. Fearing that their long-desired inclusion in the parade of nations might deaden their cultural difference, Scots with their own Parliament now activate their unpleasant history and compromised identity to know themselves. By the deathly Doctor Knox, it seems, Scottish culture lives.

WAS THERE A TALE TO TELL? MEDICINE AS USUAL FOR BODYSNATCHERS, BURKERS, AND DOCTOR KNOX

The Doctor Dissected grounds itself in the notion that the Burke and Hare scandal has proved a lasting distress for Scotland. We begin by asking how the events of 1828 carved themselves into Scottish culture such that in years to come they are wrestled with as, alternately, the tale of Knox's blame, of Burke and Hare's underclass inevitability, a community's guilt, a victim's need, or a society's self-critique, but always as a story of Scotland.

Yet at the start, murders notwithstanding, we might say there was no necessary connection between the activities of Burke and Hare and Scottish trauma. The affair began almost casually, with an act not unusual anywhere in Britain—the presentation of a corpse at an anatomist's door. When Knox tactlessly declared that his just "happened to be the establishment with which Burke and Hare chiefly dealt," and implied the disaster that was Burke and Hare could have befallen any of his colleagues, he was right (*Caledonian Mercury* March 21, 1829: 4). It nearly happened to Knox's rival, Monro: when Burke and Hare sought to dispose of their first body—a lodger who died a natural death but who, owing money, could repay his debt by being sold to the anatomists—they approached a student in Surgeons' Square. The two inquired "if there were any of Dr Monro's men about, because [Burke] did not know there was any other way of disposing of a dead body—nor did Hare. The young man...referred [them] to Dr Knox" (*Edinburgh Weekly Journal* February 11, 1829: 45).

Moreover, resurrection of the dead for the purposes of dissection had been going on for centuries all over Britain—a 1711 Edinburgh poem anticipates Mary's lament as the corpse wonders "What kind of resurrection this may be. / I thought God had reserved this power alone / Unto himself [*sic*], till he erect'd his throne" (*Trial*, xi). Indeed, bodysnatching was quite an industry in the early nineteenth century, as Thomas Hood knew when he wrote "Mary's Ghost." Hood had lived in Dundee from 1815 to 1817, but significantly, the surgeons to blame for Mary's untimely resurrection all work around London.[5] Graves lay empty anywhere within reach of a major anatomical center, and even as far afield as Ireland (Ruth Richardson, 83). There was an equal and visible industry to frustrate the bodysnatchers, involving metal coffins, watch houses and, in Scotland, communal "mort safes" (large iron cages) designed to keep a body snug until putrefaction would devalue it for the doctors (Adams *Scottish*, illus. 59–68; Moir *Life of Mansie Wauch* for a fictive description in 1828).[6] There was nothing new about the inappropriate circulation of the corpse in the services of dissection.

Scandals were legion—upturned graves and boxes of corpses lost and unfortunately found in transit maintained public disgust (Cole, 12–15, 84, 94–106). In Glasgow, "militant opposition of citizens versus surgeons and students produced a series of clashes...[leading] to the storm that raged through 1813 and 1814" when unclaimed rag bales at the docks emitted a stench and revealed "the putrefying bodies of men, women, and children" (97–98). And there had been a recent spate of scandals that kept the bodysnatchers unpleasantly in the public eye up to the moment of Burke and Hare (see *Spoliation*). In 1825 "the Portsmouth police arrested a London gang that had been robbing the Royal Naval Hospital burial ground at Haslar. [In 1826] William Clarke...was indicted for stealing four bodies from the churchyard at Walcott, near Bath" (79). That same year in Liverpool, three casks bound for Leith (Edinburgh's port) were found to contain human bodies (84). The next year, a Dublin smack was delayed on its way to Liverpool, and arrived so aromatic that "it was almost unnecessary for the customs officers to open [a] box and declare that it contained a body of a man" (85); Great Yarmouth found numerous graves empty (Ruth Richardson, 83–84). In Aberdeen even after the Burke and Hare scandal, "a dog [unearthed] a human limb [at the back of the anatomical theater]. The dog went on digging...and it was soon apparent that the left-overs from the dissecting-room had been buried on this piece of waste land in a much too casual fashion" (Cole, 96; Richardson, 91). The Report from the Select Committee on Anatomy (1828) summarized similar exploits, just less colorfully (Report, 5). And bodysnatchers caught in the act suffered rough justice (Richardson, 87–90). Among this plenitude of ripening bodies, how noxious could one more scandal be?

Amazingly, too, bodysnatchers were so bold as to court the public gaze: London resurrectionists, seeking to put pressure on their recalcitrant customer Joshua Brookes, unloaded rotting corpses at either side of his anatomy school. Their protection racket was duly rewarded when two young women stumbled hysterically over first one and then the other reeking subject (Report, 83). Notably, the surgeons often joined in the frolics. Robert Liston, practicing in Edinburgh from 1818, was legendary both as a speedy surgeon and for his exploits after dark. Once, when digging for corpses with his students, Liston was discovered; the doctor hoisted a corpse under each arm and made off with both (Lonsdale, 66; Cole, 100). An 1827 article in the *Monthly Magazine* rejoiced in the title "On the Pleasures of 'Body-Snatching,'" and detailed the writer's career from surgeon's apprentice through various (we might hope fictional) resurrecting and dissecting exploits. In a discourse that bemoaned how, for the good of humanity, "the teachers of anatomy should be brought into contact with [degraded people like bodysnatchers]," doctors advertised their prowess as heroes of medicine willing to flout death even in the graveyard (Thomas Southwood Smith *Use of the Dead*, 45). Aiming at an Anatomy Act and an increased supply of cadavers (as in *Use of the Dead to the Living*), they often placed themselves at the center of a tale that was gory but good. Doctors, snatchers, and death could be heroically aligned, however scandalous their exploits.

The meaning of the scandals certainly varied according to whether one was a noble doctor or a relative outraged by the "spoliation" of a loved-one's grave. Yet if it is tempting to assume that the general public resisted dissection, this was not necessarily the case. For the ostentatiously enlightened or even the commonsensical among the middle class, though no one wanted to be dug up by vulgar bodysnatchers, medical science was both exciting and necessary. It was a mark of status after death to have the dissection of your brain, at least, announced in the paper: the *Examiner* for January 24, 1825 advertised *The Oracle of Health, Economy, and Good Living* containing "Dissection of the Body of Lord Byron, and State of His Brain" (63; also Dickey). Thus Granville Sharp Pattison thought there were perfectly logical and easily addressed reasons for the shortage in bodies, arising from the circumstances leading to dissection, not from dissection itself. Pattison had given up his school in Glasgow after various bodysnatching scandals. Nonetheless, in dispassionate testimony to the Select Committee on Anatomy, he argued that dislike of dissection reached across Britain because of bodysnatching (not the other way around). He argued further that class-conscious Britons avoided dissection because they didn't want to be associated with criminals—murderers were dissected. And he suggested things would go better if there was simply less mystery (Report, 84).

Pattison was sure that even "the prejudice which existed in the minds of the lower orders" was removed when they actually saw dissection performed (Report, 84). In fact, he made his case against the hint that "particular circumstances"—code for religion in notoriously Calvinist Scotland—might be to blame for public unease. Although some later critics have argued as a matter of course that religious sensibilities dominated against dissection (MacGregor, 14), the discourse of the times does not insist that the resurrection of the body was at stake. Doctor Barclay, who would later teach and be succeeded by Knox, in 1819 issued a pamphlet applauding Scots for their liberal religious attitudes to dissection:

they are better informed, and have fewer prejudices against the opening of dead bodies, than the populace either of London or Dublin.

It is well known, that the generality freely permit, and sometimes request that the bodies of their deceased relatives should be inspected by the medical attendant, and that should he meet with any appearances calculated to illustrate the nature of disease, and improve his art, he is made welcome to carry them away and to preserve them.

... [T]hey have no tendency to that gross species of idolatry that induces the savage and the superstitious to undertake regular pilgrimages to the graves of their friends.... They still less understand the application of a scriptural expression ... that the dead shall be raised incorruptible. They have all been told, on Divine authority, and are all convinced, that not a particle of flesh or blood is ever to enter the kingdom of heaven. (Barclay, 8–9)

The "Haddington Shoemaker," strong against grave robbing in three poems, dwells only upon the lasting peace in "this resting bed," not upon expected resurrection of the body upon the Last Trump (William Smith, 111–16). Today, A. W. Bates makes a good case that for Edinburgh's poor Irish Catholics, economic need bore down religious sentiment when their relatives died (Bates, 69). So even given the possibility of special pleading by doctors like Barclay or Pattison, it seems that alongside local scandals and medical heroics, thoughtful and practical debate murmured on about the uses of the dead.

Maybe we should not be surprised, then, that across the country, there was quite open discussion concerning the lack of supplies to maintain a high-quality medical education. The *Examiner* actually parodied well-meaning attempts to substitute for anatomical training and supposedly self-interested doctors by "Gratuitous Surgery"—no, the paper joked, having publicly minded citizens operate in place of doctors trained on cadavers would not aid the public good (January 17, 1825: 44). Clearly, bodysnatching, dissection, and surgery were linked, and no matter how much officials hinted that it was best to keep such mysteries close, they were an open secret.

In Edinburgh, as the city's medical reputation grew, need for cadavers increased. Thus in 1822, the Royal College of Surgeons of Edinburgh sent William Cullen to France (where bodies were plentiful and available) to improve their museum (RCSEd Records 1822–28, Sederunt June 21, 1822: 13). They advertised their continuing plight to Home Secretary Robert Peel in 1828, complaining that "from the present state of the Law [restricting anatomical supply to executed criminals], and from the prejudices which exist against the practice of Anatomical Dissection it is impossible to obtain the necessary opportunities of studying or teaching Anatomy without being directly or indirectly engaged in the Commission of crime" (Records 1828–32, Sederunt April 1, 1828: 4). In 1824, "Use of the Dead to the Living" by Thomas Southwood Smith, onetime medical student in Edinburgh, appeared in the *Westminster Review*. Smith baldly—yet not shockingly—argued on the Scottish doctors' behalf for a supply direct from hospital mortuaries to cut out the body-snatching middle man.[7] His argument circulated widely in pamphlet form over the next few years.

The pervasiveness, but also the relative calmness, of this debate in Scotland might be reckoned by the turn to comic doggerel on either side. When the "Shoemaker, Haddington," spoke against the doctors, it invited some poetaster to carve "the Cobbler" up in print:

> How could we know that you'd a brain,
> (It shames thee, faith, but that's no matter,)
> Heart, and lungs, and bladder strain,
> If all, like you, had made such a clatter?
>
> 'Tis *we*, those midnight robbers! *We*,
> Vile spoilers of the silent grave!
> It is from *us* those comforts be,
> 'Tis *ours* the noble task, "to save."
> ("The Haddington Cobbler Dissected Alive," v. 17 and 27)

Then the cobbler was defended, and the doctors dissected, by an "East Linton Gravedigger":

> Why thus:—Form a corps, which perhaps we may dub
> By prophetical license, "the Skeleton Club";
> And let it embrace the whole medical tribe,
> Be Barclay the preses, and Hudibras scribe.
>
> And be this of your system the first standing rule,
> That each leave his bones to the Medical School:
> O think of the honour—O think with what grace
> Your bleach'd bones will stand in their crystalline case.
> ("The Haddington Cobbler Defended")

There were so many such exchanges among "cobblers" and "gravediggers," in fact, that they themselves became the target of humorists. "The Sadducee" remarked:

> The good people of Edinburgh have for some time been amused with various Pamphlets distributed amongst them, calling their attention, with the help of their unbiassed and most unbigoted judgments, to an affair of a most serious and alarming nature....
>
> ...we find that the windows of our Librarians, from the vender of the Regent's Classics, to the petty retailer of Tom Thumb, are crowded, gorged, and glutted with these ingenious productions....
>
> An epidemic has of late visited this town...we mean the writing epidemic. (*Sadducee*, 1, 4, 6)

Inevitably, the Sadducee had his own, tongue-in-cheek observation to make: "The difference is very great no doubt, in being dissected by worms and in being dissected by men" (14–15). The subjects of bodysnatching and dissection were at once the stuff of good story, serious debate, and humor—at least in Scotland and among the literate. Even if we count in the riots, before Doctor Knox and his associates became involved, they did not amount to a lasting scandal that could resonate in literature. In Scotland, dissection and its issues were no secret, and in that respect, Burke and Hare would come as no shock.

Surely, we might presume, Burke and Hare's innovation on their trade made the difference. They killed people. In fact, murder was not unsuspected as a mode of medical supply. Popular stories abounded. A London retelling of Edinburgh's scandal, *Murderers of the Close*, made its argument in support of the Anatomy Act and for a regulated way of providing doctors with subjects by playing upon readers' feelings: it claimed a recent Newcastle case where a hamper delivered from York contained a "fresh" child, with "a wound in the side as if it had been stabbed"; in North Shields, "about two years since," the locals concluded a missing man must have been done away with for the doctors—as if that were not unusual; in Liverpool, a "warehouse used for *pickling* bodies" for Edinburgh contained a young woman "never...interred, and of whom no knowledge was ever obtained" (*Murderers*, 171–72). Similarly, the words of famed London surgeon Astley Cooper, again on behalf of regulation, already echoed round Britain. He had told a House of Commons committee: "if [the resurrectionists] would imagine that I should make a good subject, they really would not have the slightest scruple, if they could do the thing undiscovered, to make a subject of me" (Report, 18). In the moment of Burke and Hare, the Professor of Anatomy and Surgery to the Royal College of Surgeons in London agreed with him, and with popular fear, that murder for the purposes of medicine was widespread. Worse, G. J. Guthrie declared in his *Remarks on the Anatomy Bill*: "It is not to London or Edinburgh that these murders are confined.... [I]n other towns and places in England...they can be perpetrated with even greater security" (1; also *Reflections*).

Historically, both rumor and informed opinion were correct. The *Caledonian Mercury* retrieved from its archives the 1752 case of Helen Torrence and Jean Waldie. They had waylaid a mother. While she was drinking with one, the other abducted and murdered her child; they then sold him to a surgeon for two shillings plus tenpence for drink (*Mercury* January 10, 1829: 3). London hinted that Guthrie had it right for the present moment: Thomas Wakley editorialized in the *Lancet* that "We have ourselves, within a recent period, seen bodies brought into dissecting-rooms in this metropolis...with all the indications...of men who had died within a few hours, and in a state of perfect health" (*EWJ* January 7, 1829: 13; Packard, 70). Then in 1831, the capital saw two such crimes up close. Bishop and Williams turned to drugs and drowning among other methods; Elizabeth Ross was presumed to have "burked" a woman by sitting on her chest and holding her nose (see Wise, ch. 9; Cecil Howard Turner, 165–76). Both passed their victims to the doctors. But Edinburgh had been so unimpressed by Torrence and Waldie that they had been forgotten. And in London, the murders did not demonize the doctors (though they put paid to the killers, who were executed). Rather, they speeded the Anatomy Act and got turned into comedy—through Dickens's Jerry Cruncher, the good-hearted bodysnatcher of *A Tale of Two Cities* (1859), and Mr. Weg in *Our Mutual Friend* (1864–65), with his leg residing in a jar on his mantelpiece. Burke and Hare themselves featured in the *New Monthly Magazine's* parody review of *The Newgate Calendar*: "The Newgate Annual; or, The Guide to the Gallows"—"A Medley of Frolick, Fun, and Filching; Sentimentality and Swindling; Bon-Mots and Burglary; Pathos and Profligacy; Banter, Blasphemy, Laughter, Larceny, Love, and Murder" (58.229: [January 1840]: 112–25). Alternately, we get full-on grotesquery, as in Bulwer Lytton's *Lucretia* (1846). In Edinburgh alone did the scandal run out of control. Only in Scottish culture, and in this case, were doctor and criminals anatomized in the public press, becoming a tale and a wonder that would not die.

A SCOTTISH STORY: 1828–2010

What kinds of stories get told about the murderers and the doctor in Scotland? They are different over time, arising from Scotland's shifting responses to and uses for the trauma that was Burke and Hare from 1828 to the present day. *The Doctor Dissected* will focus on instances when the scandal seems particularly prominent, or to be taking a new turn in story, and from that consider its work as a national metaphor.

We must recognize first how pervasive the story has proved in Scottish culture. Between the murder of the pathetic Mrs. Docherty, which exposed Burke and Hare on November 1, 1828, and Burke's execution on January 28, 1829, the papers fulminated about events, personalities, and medical and legal practices. Upon the conclusion of Burke's trial, publishers rushed wads of legal and newly historical documents into print (*Trial* [publ. Buchanan]; also the less reliable *West Port Murders* [publ. Ireland]).[8] The story continues to motivate histories poised between the academic and the sensational—from Lonsdale's defense of his teacher (1870) and MacGregor's thoughtful response (1884), to reconsideration of the Irish context by Edinburgh academic Owen Dudley Edwards (1980, 1994) and the recent blood-spattered "archive" by Scottish crime writer Alanna Knight (2007).

This nasty story has resonated wildly in Scotland's popular culture. Ballad sheets and broadsides immediately abounded, with preference given to the story of poor Daft Jamie (see figure 1.4), and Burke's confession. One ballad delights in the epigraph "Alas! Jamie's Pickled," inscribed on a barrel, and continues in dialect rhyme: "Attendance give, whilst I relate / How poor Daft Jamie met his fate; / 'Twill make your hair stand on your head, / As I unfold the horrid deed." Knox figured in contemporary caricature such as *Noxiana*, and *Wretch's Illustrations of Shakespeare* "intended rather for the cottage than the cabinet" (advertisement). In one cartoon he apostrophizes a tea chest, presumably with a murder victim inside, in the words of Macbeth: "Is this the Tea-chest which I see before me?" (*Wretch's*, IV). Apparently, he is about to fail Macbeth's test and take up not the dagger, but first the crowbar to unpack Mrs. Docherty, and then his surgeon's lancet. And interest has never waned. Today, the past lives on in the memories of many Scots. Edinburgh University's folk archive overflows with retellings (*Tobar an Dualchais*); Edinburgh schoolchildren gleefully echo their predecessors:

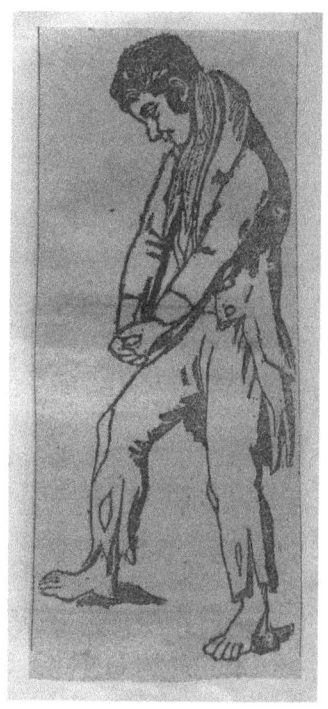

FIGURE 1.4 Daft Jamie. Contemporary woodcut. Courtesy of the Royal College of Physicians of Edinburgh.

Up the close and doon the stair,
But an' ben wi' Burke and Hare.
Burke's the butcher, Hare's the thief,
Knox the boy that buys the beef.

From 1828 until today, the story has driven Scottish authors as much as the myths of Jacobitism and swathes of tartan that more gaudily speak Scottishness along

Edinburgh's Princes Street. To cite but a few cases: David Pae novelized the past in a newspaper serial of 1858–59 (*Lucy*); Alexander Leighton produced *The Court of Cacus* in 1861. Oddly, and initiating a pervasive practice, Pae gave the Edinburgh of 1828 a return telling in *Mary Paterson* (1864). Events were converted into a short story by Stevenson in 1884 ("The Body Snatcher"), then immediately retold by him as *Strange Case of Dr Jekyll and Mr Hyde* (1886). Sherlock Holmes's experimental forensics developed from the case ("A Study in Scarlet," 1887). There appear to have been many, unfortunately untraceable, regional melodramas through the nineteenth century. Then in 1930, James Bridie resurrected Burke and Hare and Doctor Knox for respectable theater in *The Anatomist*. In Scotland's depressed years surrounding votes related to devolution (1979 and 1997), the tale of Doctor Knox and his associates bled into novels of victimization by the handful, some centering women, others considering the Irish. This moment climaxes in Alasdair Gray's inventive *Poor Things* (1992). Plays abound, and the Edinburgh Festival manifests what amounts to a subgenre of Fringe theater—the year 2009 actually featured two high school musicals on the theme. These performances merit treatment as a group, whoever produced them, given their predominant Edinburgh ethos. In today's Scotland, the story battles it out between the Festival, a strange new phenomenon of versions for children, and darker, more overtly political tales such as Paul Johnston's *Body Politic* (1997) and Ian Rankin's progression *Set in Darkness* (2000), *The Falls* (2000), and *Resurrection Men* (2001). Many of these retellings, too, gain color from other literary and cinematic imaginings.

TELLING TALES OUT OF SCOTLAND? FICTION AND FILM, THE STAGE AND THE SMALLEST SCREEN

The lines of influence between Scotland and elsewhere can get complicated. Through Stevenson and Bridie, our horrible threesome of Burke and Hare and Doctor Knox took to film. They resonate in England and America through *The Body Snatcher* (RKO 1945, from Stevenson) and *The Anatomist* (British International Pictures 1961, from Bridie). The lost melodramas from the nineteenth century morph into *Horror Maniacs*, aka *The Greed of William Hart* (Bushey Studios 1948); *The Flesh and the Fiends* (Independent International Pictures 1960, starring Peter Cushing and rereleased over time as *Mania* [USA], *Psychokillers*, and *The Fiendish Ghouls*); *The Horrors of Burke and Hare* (Kenneth Shipman 1971); and *The Doctor and the Devils* (Brooksfilms 1985, from a Dylan Thomas screenplay). These also did well in translation.[9] The story inflects numerous additional movies, including in America *Corridors of Blood* (1958, with Boris Karloff), *Nightmare in Blood* (1976), and

Extreme Measures (1996); and in Britain *Doctor Jekyll and Sister Hyde* (1971) and even the comedy *Doctor in Love* (1960). It has inspired television shows: Bridie's play came to the BBC in 1939, then Alfred Hitchcock took up the story as "The McGregor Affair" (1964), and it echoes in a 2007 episode of *Smallville* ("The Cure"). On the American stage this story appears as Dan Bianchi's *The Burke and Hare Company* (1981, The Threepenny Theatre Company, New York), and Elizabeth Bagby's *Practical Anatomy* (2006, Chicago). Increasingly, to suit today's diverse international audience, there are novels as well, including at their best American Sheri Holman's *The Dress Lodger* (2000) and Englishman Matthew Kneale's *English Passengers* (2000). Children beyond Scotland quake to the story of Burke and Hare in books for early readers. Our villains made it into the comics quite early, featuring as *Ghoul's Gold* in the series *Crime Does NOT Pay* (1946). Now they show up with Doctor Who in audiodramas. Not surprisingly, they enjoy a lively career in video games. Doctor Knox actually lurks in a Japanese manga, now an anime: *Fullmetal Alchemist*. These retellings color the story as it is retold in Scotland—although sometimes the Scottish story goes beyond providing fodder for the wider market and taints the commercial practices of other times and places with its traumatic local concerns.

Importantly for this book, however, Scottish and other retellings of Doctor Knox's story are similar by their number, and sometimes by their story, but generally not by their cultural role. Before we turn fully to the Scottish tradition of Burke and Hare, three recent movie projects indicate the difference between Hollywood and homegrown representations and point to the peculiar significances generated through Scotland's use of her untellable tale. Owen Dudley Edwards has declared that "The real reason for the terror inspired by Burke and Hare is that they invited people to parties in their houses and if they had had too much to drink and they fell asleep well then they might never wake up.... The murderous host is the most terrifying tale there is."[10] As a tale of betrayal, or about respectable society stalked by its others—the doctor himself as a disease—this story speaks to deep human anxieties. For this reason, outside Scotland it serves conventional genres in predictable ways. Notably, it translates easily into gothic horror. *I Sell the Dead* (2008), which carries the tagline "Never Trust a Corpse," deploys the tale as a standard sensation vehicle for a star. Filmstalker.co.uk characterizes the American film (with its Irish writer) as "about 18th century grave diggers.... Monaghan and Fessenden play the gravediggers and Perlman is lining up to play the priest who takes Monaghan's confession. The two diggers perform certain services for a strange doctor."[11] Filmstalker contextualizes the film: "Burke and Hare anyone?" It thereby hints at glib historicism for an unwitting mass audience looking for a thrill. John Landis's *Burke and Hare* [2010], simply by casting Simon Pegg, hints at the same, but with a laugh a minute. Significantly, the American Landis asserts the Britishness of his film—"in the Ealing tradition"; made "entirely by Brits"—but does not think to link it to Scottishness. Although "British," it is still an outsider tale.[12] In the absence of cultural memory and with no direct line to trauma, whether for Perlman or Pegg, the story serves as a generic token. By contrast, Irvine Welsh's putative version easily evokes context and more challenging possibilities. IMDb gives the plot synopsis: "Edinburgh, Scotland 2007 and there are body snatchers on the streets."[13] With a script by Welsh and featuring Robert Carlyle—who played the psychopath Begbie in Danny Boyle's production of Welsh's *Trainspotting*—this project presumes on an ability to tap a Scottish cultural complex by the slightest mention of place and persons. Edinburgh and bodysnatchers; bodysnatchers and Begbie. "The Meat Trade," scripted and intended to be acted by Scots, triangulates anxieties across 180 years. Moreover, if anything, Scotland's texts are remarkable for their lack of interest in the story's obvious horror and gothic potential. Typically, they don't find it too funny, either—except in rather disturbing ways. In Welsh's imagining, the incisions of Doctor Knox and the scarifications of Edinburgh's drug-taking underclass promise to align in a play of memory and trauma as distinctively Scottish—the sign of Burke and Hare.[14]

A THEORY OF SCOTTISH TRAUMA

This strange case of Doctor Knox, and its even stranger use in Scottish literature, together pose questions about the "imagined community" (see Anderson, Ashcroft). Scotland is known for its energetic rendition of cultural distinctiveness: kilts, bagpipes, bonny princes, and caber-tossing warriors provide markers for Scottishness but have been questioned as all too obvious symptoms of imagination that can be co-opted to other and inherently hostile ends—by English usurpers or American romantics (Nairn, "Three Dreams," 34–35). Kilts are fine, we might understand, but only if you choose to don one for yourself. A Scotland bedecked in tartan by a foreign imagination is a limited place. Walter Scott, supposed artificer of this Scotland, has been blamed for pushing his nation out of politics and into the past or some separate (and unfortunately powerless) realm of meaning and action (Craig *Out of History*). Or his readers are held responsible for their naïve and nostalgic response (Craig, "Recovering History"; McCracken-Flesher, *Possible Scotlands*). But Doctor Knox's afterlife in Scottish literature, which will challenge us here, suggests a simultaneous and resistant possibility for reading and writing in a postcolonial space, one more akin to Homi Bhabha's thinking in "DissemiNation." This tale is not nostalgic, nor does it line out an easy opposition between suffering locals and thoughtless usurpers.

Scots shed any tartan-tinted spectacles to tell a dark reality. In so doing, they go far beyond the kicking against the pricks now de rigueur in stories of the postcolonial self. They tell about the horror of home.

To date, criticism of Scottish literature and culture focuses on Scotland's paired Britishness and nostalgia, and it hopes that national difference is protected in secret spaces. Cairns Craig has noted that Scotland is delimited by backward-looking romances of the nation, yet constructs its own space within and beyond them (*Out of History*; *The Modern Scottish Novel*). Robert Crawford suggests that Scotland's narratives drive British culture, but remain self-questioning (*Devolving*). I have argued that Scott renegotiates his country's value through the canny use of story, turning apparent predictability into open-ended possibility (*Possible Scotlands*). In *The Doctor Dissected*, we consider a more assertively negative option. Scott figures in the early transformation of a medical scandal into a national metaphor, and self-aware compatriots like Pae, Stevenson, Bridie, Gray, and Rankin, all successful writers grounded in questions of community and nation, leap to follow his lead. For us, the unlikelihood of any culture, in the process of reimagining itself, embracing the home-grown horror of Doctor Knox, points to the uses of the *un*imaginable in the construction of community.

Thus the story of Doctor Knox and his criminal companions may help us to understand how the world's smaller cultures maintain their distinctiveness—or it may provide a model for resistance, encouraging other peoples and places to recognize, for better and for worse, the otherness of their inner Doctor.

An argument with such a disciplinary and historical reach, and such wide potential application, necessarily co-opts many types of information and modes of analysis. In what follows, we will dwell in literary, political, and medical archives. To understand only the moment that incised a medical scandal into Scottish awareness we will draw on the history, politics, and ethics of the period's medicine, the nature of the contemporary press, the strategies of national authorship, and the emphases of cultural metaphor. We will be most interested not in facts, but in how they are remade.

One perspective brings these diffuse materials into focus for our question. This book thinks through ideas of cultural memory, trauma, and an opportunistic use of history that critiques both present annoyances and the process of writing about the past itself.[15] Let me sketch this context.

In cultures that have "little or no historical capital" (like Scotland after the Union), says Pierre Nora, memory flourishes (Rossington, 145–46). "Our" memory is "nothing more...than sifted and sorted historical traces"; nonetheless there resonates "a memory...that ceaselessly reinvents tradition." Such a memory "remains in permanent evolution, open to the dialectic of remembering and forgetting, unconscious of its successive deformations." In other words, we make up the past as it suits us. This is the powerful nostalgia attributed to Walter Scott in his British context. We might agree, here, that a Scotland lacking politics has managed to persist through its memories of Jacobitism and the myth of other brave hearts and British betrayals (see Craig, *Out of History*, and McCracken-Flesher, *Possible Scotlands*, for two variations on this theme).

What, then, do we make of less romantic, more disruptive memories? Why does Scotland repeat the tale of Burke and Hare, which can only undermine nostalgic imaginings of the nation's past? A shocking experience can trench its way into memory. As Cathy Caruth explains: "the event is not assimilated or experienced fully at the time, but only belatedly" (Caruth ed., 4). Impossible to grasp, the traumatizing event continues to dominate in the present, forcing itself once more upon its victim. Reexperiencing this past only increases the horror, for we are compelled to repeat, but can never resolve it. Dori Laub concludes: "no amount of telling seems ever to do justice to this inner compulsion" (Caruth ed., 63). Trauma thus scars a pathway for future experience and is in turn cut deeper by new anxieties (Caruth ed., 8 and 9).

The moment of Burke and Hare might be considered adequately traumatic. Impossible to understand at the time, it persists into the future where it provides a template for new anxieties. But Burke and Hare's victims are dead. So who remembers? Who bears the trauma? Kai Erikson posits that "the tissues of community can be damaged in much the same way as the tissues of [individual] mind and body" (Caruth ed., 185). Trauma, he argues, "can create community." Moreover, for Shoshana Felman, "one does not have to *possess*, or *own* the truth, in order to effectively *bear witness* to it" (Caruth ed., 24). In this book, we will see how the moment of Burke and Hare resisted integration for an entire community, and cut its way into cultural memory such that Scottish society continues to wrestle with it, and to share its trauma with the world, today.

The phenomenon is grounded in the fact that our memories are stories, and in the case of trauma, they are stories we tell ourselves in hope of resolution. Caruth observes that traumatic events "cannot be placed within the schemes of prior knowledge.... Not having been fully integrated as it occurred, the event cannot become, as [Pierre] Janet says, a 'narrative memory' that is integrated into a completed story of the past" (Caruth ed., 153). Because we cannot integrate these pasts, our desire for their completion through story only increases. Caruth says: "the pathology" that is trauma "consists... in the *structure of its experience* or reception" (4). Traumatic events must be repeated. Through repetition, they take predictable shapes, and themselves become "cultural" forms. Trauma, by definition something we cannot describe, redirects our stories, how we tell them, and what they mean.

In the social trauma derived from Doctor Knox and his associates Burke and Hare, the struggle between the compulsions inherent in narrative and the disruptions caused by unnarratable events have bred an edgy literature. Shoshana Felman argues that the traumatic event compels repetition, nonetheless "the witness [victim]...*pursues the accident*...because the witness...has understood that from the accident a *liberation* can proceed" (Caruth ed., 30). If we can come to terms with it, we can move through and beyond this past. That is, although the trauma is untellable, it nonetheless suggests narrative opportunities against the grain. So, even as Scots deploy nostalgia to alleviate past events, the Burke and Hare story disrupts the very possibility. It exposes nostalgia as generic, naïve, and unfulfillable desire. Scots, moreover, "pursue the accident," in Felman's terms, that is Burke and Hare. Creatures of desire but subject to trauma, as agents within narrative Scots have learned to have their nostalgia, and through the cross-referencing ironies of narrative repetition, to critique it, too.

Irony exposes the structures by which historical meaning is made, says Michael S. Roth (*The Ironist's Cage*). It is inherently deconstructive. Therein he sees a problem. How do ironists critique their own position (148, 160)? I suggest that in a context full of worry about whether story can integrate trauma or, unfortunately, separate us from its lessons (Caruth ed., 153–54), the act of retelling the past can deliberately and liberatingly question what is told, and critique us for our choices as we tell it. Out of Scotland's trauma comes a productive irony that resists the lure of coherent memory and manages to critique the very notion of remembering. The story of Burke and Hare has taught Scots to privilege not just the memories by which we live, but the disruptive experiences that undermine meaning. Scots demonstrate that through the combined challenge of memory and impossibility—because we can never really remember—we can resist. We can have our nostalgia, but it cannot have us.

RESURRECTING SCOTLAND: A NASTY NATIONAL TALE

This book explores just why and how our terrible trio enjoys such a substantial cultural afterlife. Here, it is important to note medical biographies such as Isobel Rae's *Knox the Anatomist*, and particularly Ruth Richardson's magisterial *Death, Dissection and the Destitute*, which locates the threesome within medical history. Recently, Lisa Rosner and A. W. Bates have retraced Rae's steps. Yet *The Doctor Dissected* generally sets these aside, for its interest lies with the shape, uses, and energy of a tale told many times.

Burke and Hare's long career in Scottish story has been largely popular and not much analyzed. In Scotland, from November 1828, when newspapers rushed to articulate the horrors, through the moment of the trial when publishers fought to print its documents for a clamoring public, and on to today, historians, like other writers, typically supply a market eager for gory detail. The antiquarian Charles Kirkpatrick Sharpe met Walter Scott's expectations for him as "curious after Scandal…[yet loving] it fresh…always master of the reigning report and…telling the anecdote with…gusto" (Scott *Journal*, 5). Sharpe luxuriated in his preface to Buchanan's *Trial*: "The tragedy is now growing to a close; but it is very likely *from strong presumptions* that many more of the same horrid kind may ensue. Let the lower classes, then, 'be sober, be vigilant'" (9). In 1861 Alexander Leighton turned to sensation in the title for his novelized history: *The Court of Cacus* (iii). Choosing to forgo direct reference to Virgil's *Aeneid*, he evoked a ghastly epigraph:

> The *monster Cacus*, more than half a beast,
> This hold, impervious to the sun, possess'd.
> The pavement ever foul with human gore;
> Heads and their mangled members, hung the door.
> (Book 6, trans. John Dryden)

William Roughead's descriptive *Burke and Hare* (1921) veers toward the popular as "The Wolves of the West Port: A Tale of Terror" (1938), in his *The Murderer's Companion* (1941). Alanna Knight, then President of the Edinburgh Writer's Club, contributed a "Crime Archive," complete with blood-spattered cover, for the National Archives (2007).

Yet Scottish historians who review this past wrestle so between history and sensation because something lurks for them beyond. Leighton writes under a religious imperative that "what has really occurred on the stage of the world…must and will be known" (Leighton *Court*, iii). Criminologist Roughead vividly describes an inch-square bit of brown leather that sits on his desk as he writes—a family heirloom from the tanned hide of William Burke (Roughead *Knave*, 292). As for Knox's Scottish-based biographers, in the course of their descriptions they reveal their own perplexed relation to this past by turning into apologists and crusaders (Lonsdale, Knox's student, in 1870; Rae, who eventually returned from England to her family's native Nairn, as late as 1964). Lonsdale and Rae actually use the same imperious portrait of Knox as their frontspiece (see figure 1.1). That is, in different ways, even Scottish books that aim to describe the scandal of Burke and Hare and Doctor Knox objectively still refract its trauma.

The Doctor Dissected owes a debt to many of these histories while recognizing them, too, as participants in the ongoing problem that is Burke and Hare and Doctor Knox. Thus, unlike its predecessors, it focuses not on the events of 1828, but on moments when the story comes particularly alive in Scotland—in academic and popular histories such as these, and in literature and culture in general. This book tracks the ways in which the facts require yet nonetheless resist integration, and it considers the cultural anxieties that express themselves through the story, or that embrace the tale as an impetus for critique. Of course, no book can include every text, or track every nuance of the tale. Rather, I hope to invite a broader, more analytic discussion of the uses of Burke and Hare and Doctor Knox in Scottish culture. That, in turn, might imply how a negative story can contribute to a developing cultural dynamic in this and equivalent imagined communities.

Consequently, now that events themselves have been established, chapter 2 will consider just how, exactly, our local crime enters national culture as trauma. Facts seemed unexplainable, but worse, they remained unexplained by those who alone could know them. Indeed, the most authoritative participant, Doctor Knox, refused to speak. Both the perpetrators and the nation were keen to close this story down— to integrate it in narrative and stop its turn toward the lasting damage that is trauma. Yet as Walter Scott realized, no one else could tell the story adequately. In this context, trauma might not simply be inevitable, but also necessary. In fact, the horrific tale of the West Port murders might helpfully connect with a body politic already productively metaphorized through the uncertainties that made up contemporary medicine.

Chapter 3 looks at the first moment in which it seemed possible really to get to grips with the tale. In the late 1850s to 1860s the imperatives of a burgeoning newspaper culture and a popular literature, together with the religious tone of the times, demanded materials. To David Pae (the most published serial writer in the north during the Victorian era) and Alexander Leighton, the West Port murders seemed to provide grist for moral tales as sensational fact and fiction both (Law, 48; *Lucy* xi). Pae produced *Lucy, the Factory Girl; or, The Secrets of the Tontine Close* (1858), and *Mary Paterson; or, The Fatal Error*, subtitled *A Story of the Burke and Hare Murders* (1864); Leighton offered *The Court of Cacus: The Story of Burke and Hare* (1861), a factual account. But here facts and fictions struggled with one another, making "truth" and genre risky categories. Moreover, for moral arbiters and Knox's now adult students, the authors themselves came into contention for their irresponsible tangling with the past. Symptoms of "the end of times" for Pae, the events of 1828 still marked the limits to civilization in *these* times. Thirty years after the scandal, there was as yet no outside to the trauma that was the West Port.

If the tale seemed to Scott that it should not be told, and proved untellable for Leighton and Pae, chapter 4 shows that Robert Louis Stevenson had no concerns as he composed "The Body Snatcher." Thoroughly subjected by Scotland and by period medicine, Stevenson writes as if he has at last escaped the clutch of both, and thus the traumatizing reach of Doctor Knox. In the Christmas Extra for the *Pall Mall Gazette* of 1884, he purveys this Scottish horror for the British market. England celebrated his winter's tale in screaming advertisements, and gobbled it up through numerous reprintings. Sixty years seemed to have turned scandal into style. But "The Body Snatcher" is only Stevenson's first visit to the doctor. Trauma demands repetition, and in *Strange Case of Dr Jekyll and Mr Hyde* (1886), Stevenson translates the anxieties of 1828 into the era of chemical medicine—and exports them to London. Then in *The Wrong Box* (1889) he displaces them into yet another genre: comedy is the symptom of a broader critique. The Doctor is in—even outside Scotland.

For Scots, Doctor Knox gets a yet more troubled outing in James Bridie's 1930s play, *The Anatomist*. Chapter 5 tracks Bridie [Osborne Henry Mavor]—a doctor, playwright, and later screenwriter (with Hitchcock). Post–World War, this was the era of "Red Clydeside," when Hugh MacDiarmid [Christopher Murray Grieve] proved instrumental in founding the Scottish National Party, yet was equally a member of the Communist Party. Bridie, himself a board member for the Scottish National Players, in this circumstance scripted a Shavian dilemma in direct opposition to the melodramatic discourse that had built over the previous century. He represented the doctor as superman, but society as perplexed, suffering, and responsible. Gerard Carruthers notes that "over sixty per cent of Bridie's work was premiered in England," and thus brought him under attack in Scotland (Carruthers, xi). But Bridie's choice to situate Knox at the center of what was hoped to be Scotland's new, nationalizing discourse, suggests the doctor's developing role within cultural critique. In the moment of Scotland's resistance, Bridie's dominating Knox hinted that supermen, whether medical or national, sat oddly within a life freighted by class and politics, but ever ordinary, and always prone to imagine itself wrongly. And of course from Bridie, with his Hollywood connections, and Stevenson, in his English market, a further, foreign discourse of Burke and Hare developed: film, directed by and aimed at outsiders, would always cast a counter to Scotland's narrative—and imagine perhaps wrongly, but influentially.

The Scottish tale, chapter 6 argues, continues in all its particularity, despite the homogenizing trends of globally distributed cinema. In 1979, Scotland suffered an unsuccessful devolution vote. Then 1997 made a new Parliament possible, and in 1999 the Parliament sat for the first time. From the anxious period around the 1979 vote, through to the moment when a Scottish Parliament actually met in Edinburgh, Doctor Knox led a tortured and torturing life in Scottish literature. The degradations of the present turned the tale inward. Thus—also as the '70s demanded—novels address victimhoods by the handful: for instance a Scottish/Indian professor of medicine in Edinburgh, Hector Bryson, blames and excuses the students (1978); Elizabeth Byrd, an enthusiastic American import to Scotland, questions women as sufferers yet survivors in Maggie Hare and her child (1974; 1976); the Irish Owen Dudley Edwards, teaching in Edinburgh, takes steps to recuperate the Irish and question the upper class (1980; 1994). Bodies of the politic are laid out, scraped and sectioned as anxieties meet. But Alasdair Gray's *Poor Things* (1992) translates past and present anxieties into a more disturbing modern meaning. This novel, with its pieced-together heroine, recalls the "things for the surgeon," but Gray's walking corpse disturbs the living—and the reading. We see now, perhaps, whence comes the agency to haunt *today's* community in the story of Burke and Hare. These dead at last may live as a positive force.

Post-parliamentary retellings of the West Port murders might be expected to turn toward narrative coherence and cultural integration—the politic is once more fully embodied, and the story of Burke and Hare has been told, every victim counted. Comedies at last abound (Robin Mitchell's *Grave Robbers*, 1999); the Edinburgh Festival swells with popular, commercial plays that bond a local tale and an international audience in Scotland's economic narrative; and children's versions of the tale have become oddly prevalent. Chapter 7 argues, however, that the narrative has split. This last chapter considers what drives the intense re-presentation of the scandal of Doctor Knox and Burke and Hare but also its refocusing into something much more rich and strange. Michael Roth notes that "memory, like history, is always constructed in or is a response to the present" (Roth, 9). But who are the Scots in a post-parliamentary world? Christopher Wallace, originally German but now an Edinbourgeois, in his *The Resurrection Club* (1999) queries the dissection and consumption of ourselves through markets of memory like Edinburgh Festivals. Across three novels, Ian Rankin invokes both the market and the memory: Rankin's novels, grand narratives of commerce themselves, foreground trauma as ironic comment on a moment of cultural success that may still turn to failure. Rankin suggests that whether we get profit or loss (whatever those may be) can depend on how we position ourselves between past and present—through stories like that of Burke and Hare.

Yet are these stories still Scotland's to tell? At the time of writing, Burke and Hare are going viral on the Internet, and Irvine Welsh's "The Meat Trade" seems to have been usurped by John Landis's Hollywood comedy *Burke and Hare*.[16] In this context, the Scottish response to Gunther von Hagens's *Bodyworlds* exhibits proves informative: when von Hagens sought to present his work in Edinburgh's civic spaces during the Festival, the town council balked. In Scotland, the trauma of the West Port murders can be resolved or ironized only by Scots, and they are still working on it. The story, in increasingly Pythonesque terms, is "Not Dead Yet!"

2

The Story Begins

THE LAW VERSUS THE PRESS, AND THE DOCTOR VERSUS WALTER SCOTT

BURKE WAS EXECUTED; Hare testified then fled; Knox suffered opprobrium. So why were Burke and Hare not dismissed through their punishment, unlike Torrence and Waldie, Bishop, Williams, and Ross? Why was Knox, of all the doctors, cut from the discourse of heroic medicine and sutured to that of criminality? In important ways, Scotland's problem was not so much scientific as social, and therefore a matter of story. Negotiated through fictions, whether legal or in the popular press, it came alive.

It is worth observing, to begin with, that although the story was horrific, it ran to the point of boredom. *Blackwood's Edinburgh Magazine*, always witty, considered it "too monotonous to impress the imagination" (March 1829: 382). The victims merged as "First ae drunk auld wife, and then anither drunk auld wife—and then a third drunk auld wife—and then a drunk auld or sick man or twa." Hardly the stuff of trauma or even a lasting tale. As for Burke and Hare, in a scenario almost begging for closure in the form of a hostile mob with its flaming torches and lethal pitchforks, they were outsiders and presumably easy to blame and expel from Scottish society. The Irish novelist Maria Edgeworth was concerned that "two of the murderers are Irish—I feel," she wrote to her friend Sir Walter Scott, "the immediate effect must be dreadful for all my poor countrymen now seeking shelter in Scotland—God help them—noone else can—or will I fear."[1] Yet the country did not turn on its Irish immigrants and wrap up events that way. Still, justice promised to do the deed. Burke was thoroughly done to death: executed to cries of "Burke him, Burke him, give him no rope," and "Wash blood from the land!" then dissected in front of large audiences (*Scotsman* January 28, 1829: 62; "Execution of Burke," *Trial*, 45–48). Surely this was closure? And in Knox's case, what was there to close? He had not killed anyone. But the slow dissection in literature was about to begin. Doctor Knox would be first on the slab, with Burke and Hare pickled for later.

What rendered this apparently manageable scandal traumatic, and thus an obsessively retold tale? Trauma is what cannot be assimilated into the world we know and expect. The story of Burke and Hare fell between two ways of enacting the law, and thus not quite within the control of either. Michel Foucault argues that "At the beginning of the nineteenth century...the great spectacle of physical punishment disappeared....The age of sobriety in punishment had begun" (*Discipline*, 14). Elevated above a crowd of twenty thousand, giving "several convulsive heaves...to each of which the spectators responded by another shout of triumph," Burke provided quite the spectacle (see figure 2.1; *Mercury* January 29, 1829: 3). Burke, in the end, was hanged, flayed, dissected, and displayed; his skin tanned, inscribed, and circulated among Edinburgh antiquarians. One contemporary detailed his dissolution into portable property:

Burke was cut up and put in pickle for the lecture-table....the skin of his *neck* and of the right arm....I had *tanned*—the neck brown, and the arm white. The

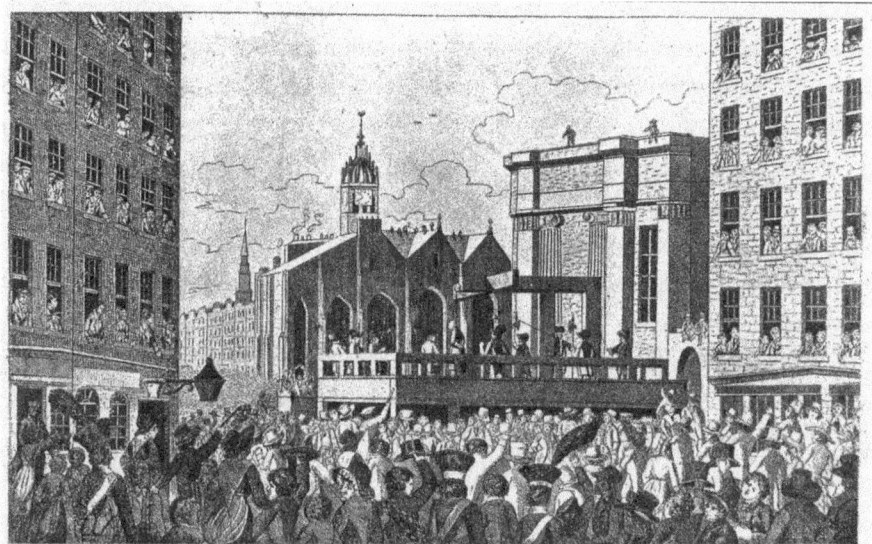

FIGURE 2.1 "Execution of the notorious William Burke." Contemporary print. Courtesy of the Wellcome Library, London.

white was as pure as white kid, but as thick as white sheepskin. It was curious that the mark of the rope remained on the leather after being tanned. Of that neck-leather I had a tobacco-doss made; and on the white leather of the right arm I got Johnston to print the portraits of Burke and his wife, and Hare, which I gave to the noted antiquarian and collector of curiosities, Mr. Fraser. (Leighton *Court*, 279–80, fn.)[2]

Bits of Burke circulate in Edinburgh today—one may be seen in wallet form at the Royal College of Physicians in Edinburgh. So Burke offered a pretty impressive and even a lingering spectacle that represented the purging of criminal otherness. Still, this was a display toned down toward nineteenth-century expectations. In sentencing, even as he insisted on Burke's public dissection, the Lord Justice-Clerk stressed that the murderer's corpse should not hang in chains in the old-fashioned way, since it was offensive to Edinburgh sensibilities (*Trial*, 199). Moreover, of all the available perpetrators, Burke alone died; he was executed for one death that stood for fifteen more; and he was subject to a decidedly modern and classificatory scientific punishment. Thus he represented the return to a social, sober present. Neither spectacle nor sobriety, however, was enough to close the scandal of Burke and Hare and Doctor Knox.

In the new age of sobriety, Foucault tells us, "The art of punishing... [rests] on a whole technology of representation" (*Discipline*, 104). The Lord Advocate appreciated his responsibility, remarking in court: "It is my duty, Gentlemen, to endeavour to remove that alarm which prevails out of doors, and to afford all the protection which the law can give to the community against the perpetration of such crimes.... and I trust [the trial] will tend to tranquillize the public mind" (*Trial*, 134–35). Thus poised between "spectacular" and "sober" judicial eras, Edinburgh's lawyers focused on providing a usable representation of the facts. Their version, therefore, was selective. At a moment when this "most extraordinary and novel [subject] of trial" stimulated "in the public mind the greatest anxiety and alarm," the Lord Advocate congratulated his associates for allowing "[no] improper disclosures" and exercising "secrecy [and] circumspection" (134). Even Henry Cockburn, advocate for the defense, argued behind the scenes that bringing private investigations of Knox to public attention "would do great harm; chiefly because these anatomical mysteries can never be fitted for the public eye" (to John Robison, February 10, 1829, Robison Correspondence NLS Acc. 10000/328). Official Edinburgh aimed to obviate all other stories and bring Scotland's scientific and social anxieties to an end. But the lawyers too obviously focused on excessive punishment of one person, and a reductive representation of the facts, to enforce an end to public anxiety.

Under the pressure of the law, indeed, Burke's story raveled into loose ends. Burke was indicted for only three murders of the sixteen, then tried and sentenced for one;

consequently, the remaining thirteen deaths—perhaps more—were never subject to discussion in court. Hare turned king's evidence and was not prosecuted; he was doubly protected because his common-law wife, Margaret, who also testified for the state, could not testify against him. Burke's mistress, Helen McDougal, was tried with him, but gained the Scots verdict of "not proven" due to the genius of Henry Cockburn (*Trial*, 200). Because Doctor Knox had not unpacked the body on which the case turned, he never even appeared in the dock (Rae, 79). Worse still, these compromises of the law as it strove to manifest "truth" and thus finality—to close the case—revealed the law itself, in Foucault's terms, as mere "strategy" (*Discipline*, 26–27).

The papers, representing public desire, sought closure but (in the early days of the steam press) were eager for copy, and so they obsessively teased out these hanging threads. As the voice of the people, they required complete investigation and justice for all—the *Glasgow Courier* insisted, "There must be nothing left to imagination. The truth, and the whole truth, must be made known, and this in a manner that can neither be suspected nor disputed" (qtd. *Edinburgh Evening Courant* January 1, 1829: 3). Given the compromises of the law, however, the Scottish papers found themselves noting and debating the legal moves that should have terminated all discussion. The *Mercury* complained: "the matter cannot possibly be allowed to rest here. The united voice of society calls loudly for further, deeper, and fuller investigation" (January 3, 1829: 3). A correspondent pointed to the danger of mob justice: "I need not inform you," he writes, "of the state of public feeling in Edinburgh at present, occasioned...by the prevailing rumours that the Crown Counsel do not intend to prosecute any of the other parties implicated." He anticipates—and perhaps hopes for—"tumultuous proceedings against the whole body of Anatomical Teachers" if "the Crown Lawyers [are] left altogether to exercise their own arbitrary power of refusing to bring the parties involved to a trial" (ibid., 3). Unresolved criminality might beget criminal action in the general public. Not capable of narrating a completed tale, the paper breathlessly stands witness to a crime becoming a legal scandal and bending toward trauma in the people.

In such uncomfortable circumstances, the official bodies of law and medicine rushed to explain that they had everything under control. They rehearsed the legal and ethical imperatives that protected Hare as a witness and set the medical community above reproach. Though Hare was involved in many murders, his role as state's witness precluded his being prosecuted even for those not mentioned at Burke's trial (*Mercury* February 5, 1829: 3). Anatomists, fearing that they would all be implicated, "met with the Lord Advocate, at his request"; the Royal College of Physicians published resolutions "to express their deep and sincere regret, that...anatomical instruction...should ever have furnished a temptation to such unexampled atrocities" (*Courant* January 8, 1829: 3). The Lord Advocate himself teetered on shaky ground, and was rumored to have entered the public debate in his own behalf (*Mercury* January 5, 1829: 3). But the papers were not convinced. Rather, they made hay with these clear manifestations of strategy falling into confusion. In successive articles titled "The Public Prosecutor and His Apologists," and "Official Treachery" (followed up in "West Port Murders"), the *Mercury* railed that "the quashing of all investigation," though "calculated to *allay* the excitement of the public mind," was likely to "produce the very opposite effect"; "Mr. Peel [the Home Secretary]," it declared, "is far from being satisfied with what has been done" (January 8, 1829: 3; January 10, 1829: 3). Owen Dudley Edwards rightly smells a "cover up" (Edwards *Burke and Hare*, xi). It was not, however, a very good one.

Moment to moment, meanwhile, the case slid further beyond the possibility of closure. The suspects were getting away. The papers anxiously tracked them as they slipped out of Edinburgh and back into the wider society of Britain. Helen McDougal, Burke's Scottish mistress, was harried from Edinburgh and rumored to be on her way to Stirlingshire (*Courant* December 29, 1829: 3). A few days before Burke's execution, Hare's wife was stoned out of town (January 29: 2); two weeks later the *Glasgow Chronicle* was appalled both to find her lurking in the sister city, and that "The authorities…will probably make arrangements for procuring her a passage [to Ireland]" (qtd. *EWJ* February 11, 1829: 46). Hare himself was spotted at Dumfries, and though he was said to have been killed by a lowland mob at Annan, the latest news placed him beyond Carlisle (ibid., 46). (Within two years, he would be rumored to lurk in New York, still practicing his trade; ["Burkism!"]). Every day, additional crimes were charged against him from near and far. He was hunted "for the murder of a servant of a reverend clergyman in [Edinburgh]," and Inverness sought "some of our poor Highland shearers" (*EWJ* January [7], 1829: 13). "Two gentlemen from Newcastle" anxiously inquired for a young man (*Mercury* February 7: 3). As the law worked to avoid public panic, the newspapers whipped up hysteria. In every dimension and in every new moment, it seemed, the case exceeded containment.

ENLIGHTENED EDINBURGH? THE ROYAL SOCIETY, THE SILENCE OF THE DOCTOR, AND PANIC IN THE STREETS

The case would never be controllable because it was not just about Burke and Hare and Doctor Knox. The *Scotsman* obsessively celebrated the removal of the "pollution" that was Burke and his consort Helen McDougal, but the paper protested too much (January 3, 1829: 6; January 10, 1829: 22). The English *Sun* wryly hinted that the

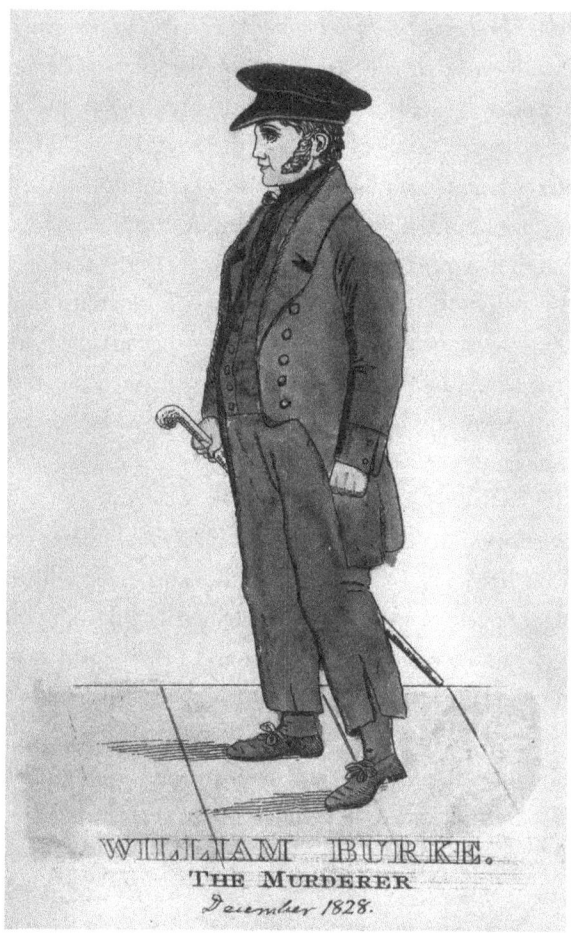

FIGURE 2.2 "William Burke. The Murderer." Contemporary print, tinted. Courtesy of the Royal College of Physicians of Edinburgh.

Scottish papers "[seem] *to think* [their] *own honour implicated in the business*," and certainly, the taint lay close to home (qtd. *Mercury* December 29, 1829: 3). *Blackwood's* was bemused to find Burke "a neat little man of about five feet five...intended by nature for a dancing-master....a pleasant enough companion over a jug of toddy. Nothing repulsive about him...and certainly not deficient in intelligence" (*Blackwood's* March 1829: 383; see figure 2.2). Amateur phrenologists discovered few clues to his actions in the bumps on his head, the *Edinburgh Evening Courant* remarking: "There is nothing in his physiognomy, except perhaps a dark lowering of the brow, to indicate any peculiar harshness or cruelty of disposition" (December 25, 1829: 2). Burke's ordinariness actually prompted Thomas Stone, President of the Royal Medical Society, to use him as an opportunity to demolish a whole field in his

Observations on the Phrenological Development of Burke, Hare, and Other Atrocious Murderers... Presenting an Extensive Series of Facts Subversive of Phrenology, which he presented before the Royal Medical Society of Edinburgh.[3] But traffic to the phrenologists only intensified, as anxious Scots checked their own bumps. Alexander Leighton would recall: "Everywhere there was a measuring of craniums, and even wise people, who never had any doubt of the smallness of their destructiveness, were startled into the conviction that they required not only to take care of themselves, but to be taken care of by others" (Leighton *Court*, 280–81). Burke looked just like everyone else; perhaps everyone else, even in the Athens of the North, could be Burke.

Burke's story, too, could include us, insofar as it remained incomplete and unsettled. Up to the moment of his execution, Burke promised he had more to tell. The *Mercury* claimed he had:

> offered to make important disclosures to an individual he has named.... but, on [that person] applying to the civic authorities...for admission, it was refused, in virtue of positive orders which had been issued from a higher quarter to exclude every one except the Confessor and other spiritual guides of the wretched criminal. (January 17, 1829: 2)

The law was not inclined to let him speak, insisting on the singular story that came out of the trial. When the confession ultimately was recorded, it remained a matter of contention. Mr. J. Smith, S. S. C., tried to stop the *Courant* publishing it, alleging:

> that the document in possession of the Editor of the Courant, and authenticated by Burke's signature, was intended for him (Mr Smith), and was to be conveyed to him by means of a prisoner named Ewart. This document, it was alleged, had been entrusted to Mr Wilson, one of the turnkeys. He disposed of it to the Editor of the Courant, and defeated, as was alleged, the intention of Burke. (*Courant* February 5, 1829: 2)

Debate raged over whether the dead had rights in their last words, whether the papers could publish them, or the law restrict them (ibid. and *Mercury* February 7, 1829: 3). They must belong to the people (*Mercury* January 17, 1829: 2). But how nearly? In the meantime those words were swollen by speculation: were Burke and Hare in a larger way of business (ibid.)? Scots across the country wondered if their missing friends made up the tally in Burke's accounts (*Mercury* January 10, 1829: 3).

In these open-ended circumstances, Edinburgh focused in on Doctor Knox. Surely the enlightened doctor could explain. Lonsdale writes that:

Relying upon his entire innocence in the "Burking business," Knox allowed the winter of a nation's discontent to pass over without making any public declaration that might have appeased the raging clamour. He expected the excitement to subside, and that the better classes would never believe in so dire a motive as his connivance with criminal acts of fearful enormity, much less his associating with monsters of the deepest dye of infamy. (80)

Knox presumed on his alignment with "the better classes." But whether Lonsdale interprets rightly or not, to newspapers and colleagues alike the Doctor appeared to be standing on his dignity rather than sharing his knowledge. He thus proved the case's major loose end. The *Mercury* appreciated that "dissection is an occult operation, the nature of which may be imagined but cannot be known by the public," and medicine was recognized for its twinned discourses of science and secrecy (*Mercury* November 15, 1828: 3). As a scientist, whatever the pressure of events or the truth of the matter, Knox thought his work and its ethic should put him above debate. Lonsdale comments wryly: "He calculated wrongly" (Lonsdale, 81). The orator, "never at a loss for words" in front of a class, and always with a paper at hand for presentation, refused to speak as even his social and intellectual Edinburgh cohort required.[4] His one public comment on the Burke and Hare debacle offered no personal explanations or apologies (*Mercury* March 21: 4). Indeed, Knox did not hesitate to implicate his colleagues. He claimed a group identity: ironically he spoke to defend "the character of the profession to which I have the honour of belonging"; no teacher of anatomy could avoid "being imposed upon by those who furnish the material of their science." At the same time, Knox appropriated all suffering to himself. He did not acknowledge the murder victims, and insisted that he was subject to a witch hunt: "Nobody...requires to be told from what quarter these attacks have proceeded" (Knox implied the university professors and the Tories, but attacks came from all around). And his control erupted in histrionics against his critics: "Scarcely any individual has ever been the object of more systematic or atrocious attacks than I have been." Not surprisingly, Doctor Knox failed to alleviate the problems he had caused for his profession, or for Edinburgh, by posing as victim.

Today's sociology of medicine suggests the recuperative power of explanation and apology from doctor to injured patient (Lazare; "Doctors Say"). Knox's resistant silence increased public anxiety, for it invited speculation not just about details, but about the doctor's responsibility. In court, even as he walled out criticism of the surgeons, Lord Meadowbank stressed: "God forbid...it should ever be conceived, that...the claims of science...should ever give countenance to such awful atrocities as the present" (*Trial*, 198). But as Foucault points out, classificatory medicine—evolved from Enlightenment practices—sometimes requires the doctor to "subtract the [patient].... [T]he individual [is] merely a negative element the accident of the disease" (*Birth*, 14). Might Knox, in the rush to see the disease, have overlooked the recently living body? What could the doctor have intended or allowed when he congratulated Burke and Hare that their supply was "fresh" (*Authentic Confessions*, 232)? "The Echo of Surgeons Square," in reality Knox's disgruntled doorkeeper David Paterson, who had received numerous of the bodies, sought to implicate the doctor on those grounds. "I think it is but natural to infer, that if the Doctor saw these bodies, he is either horribly ignorant of his profession, or he wilfully withheld that information he ought to have given" (Paterson, 14). Paterson hinted that the dissection of "Daft Jamie," a physically recognizable subject well known in Edinburgh, was speeded along to make away with the evidence (16–18). The wider press speculated, too. The *Edinburgh Weekly Journal* hinted broadly:

> We shall not here speak of the impossibility, that [Daft Jamie] could fail to be recognized *as* a murdered man, by a body of scientific individuals, to whose close inspection his corse was subjected by a skilful teacher; but simply ask, what would have been the natural movement of a humane mind, on beholding this wretched creature, who two days before had been seen in health, lying for dissection upon an anatomist's table? Would it not have been to fly to the scene of his haunts, and inquire into the cause of his death? (*EWJ* January 7, 1829: 4)

The *Journal* wondered the more that other doctors, in similar circumstances, claimed to have balked. One, supposedly offered the victim of the final murder, "sternly refused to purchase it at any price" (ibid.) The *Mercury* let public concern echo loudly through its correspondence column: "is not the Anatomist who receives such bodies alike criminal with the murderer, in so far as by purchasing such subjects, knowing them to be murdered, he encourages and participates in this monstrous system of slaughter and bloodshed?" (January 10, 1829: 3). Leading questions to Burke implied the press presumed he had either medical advice or medical implements at his disposal through his murderous career (January 5, 1829: 3, and January 8: 2). Denying such help, Burke himself menaced: "that dissecting-room ought to be better looked after [checked into]!" (*EWJ* January 7, 1829: 13). Even when a supposed January 21 autograph declaration from Burke of Knox's innocence made it posthumously into the *Courant* on February 7, it did not alleviate criticism. Burke was reported as saying: "docter Knox Never incoureged him Nither taught or incoreged him to murder any person" (facsimile in *Courant* February 7, 1829: 2; transcribed in *Trial* as "Confessions of Burke"). But how could a murderer speak for a doctor? The anatomist's absence from public discourse only became the more obvious. By his silence, Knox not only failed to provide an acceptable, integratable tale, he himself became a suspicious gap in public knowledge—a gap filled with speculation.

Knox's efforts to control his own story made things worse. Just before the Burke and Hare disaster, in his role as an enlightened medical man and Edinburgh authority, Knox had drafted a letter to Home Secretary Robert Peel, concerned that his supply of cadavers was uncertain, often interrupted, and subject to law. He wrote with a predictable reservation: "I have ever been an advocate for the making of these matters as little public as possible" (Rae, 62–63). Now, Knox's compulsion to control what people were saying became overwhelming. A committee of what Walter Scott called "Mr. Knox's friends" compiled a mild report on the doctor's involvement in recent events (Scott *Journal*, 571). In public Knox claimed he had no influence on the document: "I took no charge whatever of their proceedings," he temporizes (*Mercury* March 21, 1829: 4). But its preamble declared that the committee served "at the request of Dr Knox" (*Scotsman* March 21, 1829: 183). Moreover, privately Knox promised their report to one Edinburgh paper, not another, and quarreled with editors over who would get to print it and how. Papers of John Robison, the first General Secretary to the Royal Society of Edinburgh, reveal a vicious battle under cover of the Society's respectability (Robison Correspondence). Mr. Allan of the *Mercury* imagined that he had been promised first right of publication by Knox himself, and been scooped by Robison colluding with the *Scotsman*; the Doctor implied he was a liar (Allan to Robison, March 22, 1829; Knox to Robison, March 24, 1829). Knox declared to Robison his "contempt and horror...for the conduct of the Editors of the Scotch papers" and charged that Allan had "allowed, nay dictated the most atrocious & infamous libels daily almost for months (*and for the sake of a little paltry gain*)" (to Robison, March 19, 1829, and "Monday Evening"). The *Scotsman* fared no better: editor Charles Maclaren had to explain to Robison that "The three lines in the Scotsman to which Dr Knox alludes were written by me without the slightest intention either to injure or serve him....I think you will pardon me for expressing the indignation which I feel at the Doctors effrontery in making these three lines a reason for withholding [the Committee's Report] from the Scotsman" (March 20, 1829). And Maclaren points to problems with the range of Edinburgh papers, themselves aligned with elite society as much as with the rapacious public. Maclaren situated himself with the Royal Society, enlightened thinking, and proper behavior, complaining: "The refusal to the Courant...came from the Doctor himself, and since he chooses without any reason to make that paper his enemy, I cannot think it is incumbent on me to screen him from a danger he has gratuitously exposed himself to." Not surprisingly, he concludes, "I confess I feel no desire to oblige Dr Knox." Knox clearly was not winning friends or influencing anybody by his obsessively controlled, stripped-down narrative.

The doctor would take yet one more step too far. At last writing to the papers, supposedly to vindicate his school and its procedures, Knox attacked those who had "[converted] my misfortune into positive and intended personal guilt." He, in fact, converted the report into an attack on his supposed slanderers, claimed it identified their "actionable matter," and implied *his* recourse to the law against *them* (*Mercury* March 21, 1829: 4). *Blackwood's*, losing its sense of humor, challenged: "Does he dare to presume to command all mankind to be mute on such a series of dreadful transactions!" (*Blackwood's* March 1829: 388). Doctor Knox could not silence anyone: "Nae system o' divinity shuts mortal mouths against such enormous monsters," moralized the Ettrick Shepherd (a characterization of James Hogg). "God has given us voices to be lifted up from the dust, when horrid guilt loosens our tongues" (382). But no one else could speak for the doctor either. The students who applauded their master and offered him a piece of celebratory plate exposed themselves to Christopher North/John Wilson through a "savage yell within those blood-stained walls."[5] They accomplished no more than "so much squeaking and grunting in a pig-sty" (388). "Dr Knox," North snapped, "stands arraigned at the bar of the public....He is ordered to open his mouth and speak, or be forever dumb." Small wonder that editors set aside their politics to join in frustration, generating heaps of uninformed and unfocused speculation, and the youth of Edinburgh broke the doctor's windows (*Courant* December 29, 1829: 3).

When justice failed to be publicly done, and guilt remained unacknowledged, rumor became rife. The Ettrick Shepherd remarked "ane likes to hear about monsters" (*Blackwood's* March 1829: 384). Certainly, in London *Murderers of the Close* describes a public anticipating Sweeney Todd, and fearing the sausage maker, or following Polidori and presuming vampires on the loose (*Murderers*, 38). In Scotland, newspapers flew off the shelves, "eagerly sought after," according to the *Aberdeen Journal,* "by people who hardly ever looked into them in their lives before" (qtd. *Scotsman* January 17, 1829: 38). The *Courant* happily reported "the number of extra newspapers" sold around the trial "cannot be fewer than 8000"—on top of the usual 3,000 (*Courant* December 29, 1828: 3). Here, readers found tales of Burke and Hare, and of copycat crimes. An epidemic of "plaistering"—slapping adhesive plasters over the mouths of unsuspecting victims to imply they were off to the dissectionists— reached from Aberdeen to Glasgow. In a Glasgow case, an assailant "suddenly clapped the plaister on [a woman's] mouth, and seized her by the nose"—in the fashion now known as "burking" (*Mercury* January 31, 1829: 3). One plaister "was manufactured of such an adhesive substance, that it could not be got off without taking the skin along with it" (*Scotsman* January 17, 1829: 38). The *Scotsman* railed against "Wretches who can behave thus at any time, and more especially in the present state of public feeling" (ibid.). Among Aberdonians, as a result, "the credulity of the younger classes [was] at such a height, that those of them who [had] to go out early or late [would] not venture without a convoy. As may be expected," the *Mercury* remarked, "several people are stated to be amissing" (*Mercury* February 7, 1829: 3). Even in the calm Scottish borders, panic reigned: Walter Scott's "next neighbour shot a man [one] night, thinking him a robber or a Doctor."[6] And those seeking an added frisson could read a letter to the editor of the *Mercury*. The writer claimed to recount being kidnapped and awakening in a cold room with "a nasty smell like putrified butcher meat," then hearing three men, one with "a long knife," praise him as a "great catch…for to-morrow's demonstration of the abdominal viscera" (*Mercury* December 15, 1828: 3). The story was made for a career as horror, and we should not forget that Burke and Hare met the gothic moment in literature, although Scottish responses turned to sensation, and later to confusion and complexity. In the meantime, Scots fought confusedly back: rural Haddington proposed "houses of refuge" to protect the indigent from the doctors; an itinerant flute player, minus his right hand, was nonetheless taken for Hare and wounded by "ill-directed popular fury" (RCPEd, STR-SM 5.22). The representation of punishment clearly had not contained anxiety; that was running rampant, taking on a new life in legend across the country. Scotland was well into the compulsion of repetition that is both symptom and site of trauma.

Of course, Knox did not escape unscathed. Even loyal doctors such as the American James Moores Ball who—at a comfortable distance in time—considered Knox "a great, strong, outstanding, and valiant character; the most eloquent, the most versatile, and the most thorough teacher of anatomy that Scotland…ever has produced," and who thought Knox's encounter with Burke and Hare merely "fortuitous," agree that from now on the anatomist's life was "wrecked" (Ball, 96). The orator who insisted his brief statement would vindicate him, and that the law *could* vindicate him against slander, lost control of his own story. In what might have been Knox's worst prognosis for himself, as his reputation died that hidden story, much like Mary under dissection, gained independent life. Whence might enlightenment come?

A TALE THAT TELLS ITSELF: THE SILENCE OF SIR WALTER SCOTT

If Knox would not speak, and no one could speak for him, nonetheless Scotland needed its trauma to be told. Yet it would be no easy task to shut down the discussion left open by the failures of Doctor Knox, the compromises of the law, the speculations of the newspapers, and the distress of the populace. A great deal of ink had already been spilt in the cause. Among the press of journalists and historians, Charles Kirkpatrick Sharpe struggled to get a foot in the door at Burke's trial and a place at a window for the execution (ECL West Port Murders, MS letters to and from J. Stevenson, editor). Buchanan's edition (*Trial*), for which Sharpe provided the preface, entered a market chockablock with competition (most notably, publisher Thomas Ireland's *West Port Murders*). But no amount of "full accounts," with their legal transcripts and reprinted newspaper stories, could provide the narrative coherence to resolve the scandal that was Burke and Hare and Doctor Knox.

The scandal needed the more urgently to be shut down because all recognized this was a moment of national embarrassment. *Murderers of the Close*, rushed into publication in London, had no difficulty with providing the resolutions of storytelling—its London perspective triangulated "civilized England," the ruffianly "Irish," and "Scotch surgeons" (*Murderers*, 2, 7, 263). The *Sun*, an English paper, mocked that the West Port murders were of "*decidedly…Scotch origin*. There is a cool, methodical, business-like air about [them], a scientific tact in the conception, and a practised ease in the execution, *which no* IRISHMAN *could ever yet attain!*" (qtd. *Mercury* December 29, 1828: 3).[7] The *Morning Chronicle* in all seriousness drew the same national distinction: "Let Edinburgh…talk no more about civilizing and evangelizing distant and barbarous nations, until she civilize and evangelize all her own citizens, and wipe off from her name such a foul reproach for ignorance, brutality, and savage barbarity" (qtd. *Mercury* December 18, 1828: 4). The *Times* devastatingly stated: "the capital of the Scottish nation has been disgraced" (qtd. *EWJ* January 7, 1829: 5). Who could speak with enough authority to confine the burgeoning discourse and tell Scotland's tale aright? The compiler of *West Port Murders* thought the scandal never would be resolved except when "some future Sir Walter Scott grubs it out" (*West Port*, 215). But Edinburgh could not wait; a worsening trauma needed instant retelling if it was to be integrated in Scottish culture and the nation to be healed.

With so much at stake, Edinburgh looked to the author himself (see figure 2.3). Scott was a lawyer, President of the Royal Society of Edinburgh, and the acknowledged novelist of the nation. His stories had recuperated Jacobitism, transformed it into nostalgia, and bonded Scotland in Britishness (consider *Waverley*, 1814). In 1822, Scott had choreographed a royal visit that made an unpromising king look monarchical—he turned portly George IV into a romantic Scot, and gave Scots value in England because they were recognized by the monarch.[8] Better yet, Scott compelled an English market. To top it all, after his financial collapse in 1826, he had shown how to regain reputation by composing and living the right kind of story (McCracken-Flesher *Possible*, 143–63). Surely this general comptroller of Scottish culture could write Edinburgh's dreadful events and their riotous popular retelling into one manageable history, and bring all speculation to an end.

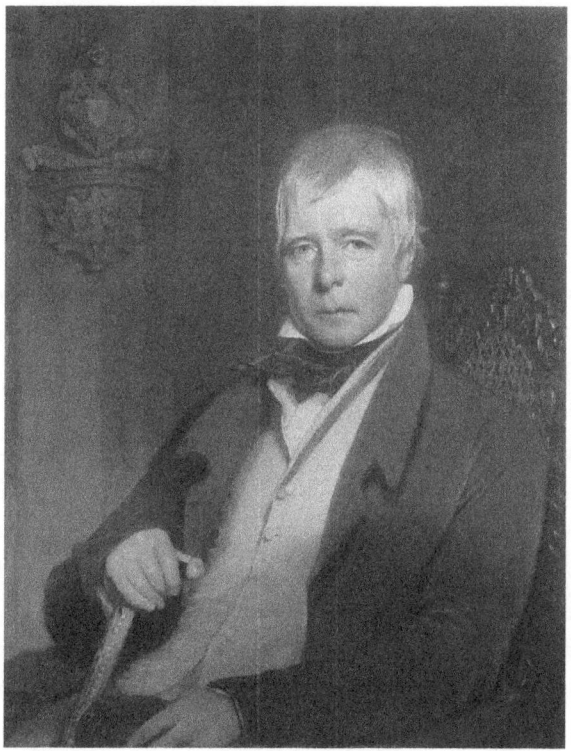

FIGURE 2.3 *Sir Walter Scott*, 1824. By Charles Robert Leslie, English, 1794–1859. Oil on canvas 36 x 28 in. Museum of Fine Arts, Boston. Bequest of Miss Anna Eliot Ticknor. 96.945. Photograph 2010. Courtesy of the Museum of Fine Arts Boston.

Maria Edgeworth feared that a "systematized practice of murder has been carried on not only with the knowledge but with the sanction...with the assistance, under the tutoring of scientific, highly educated men, of persons whose profession it is to save human life" (to Scott, NLS MS3908: 19–22). She anguished: "Is it possible that this can be true?" In the crisis, she turned to Scott: "It would be...friendly [to] your fellow creatures of you who can moralise without *prosing* to produce some explanation of these moral paradoxes." Charles Mackay the actor went further. He wrote in his character of Nicoll Jarvie (from Scott's *Rob Roy*) to complain, "What's a this in the gude Town of Edinburgh!—naething but murder and cruelty—downright barbarity!" He summed up the general feeling: "none but you Sir Walter can give a finishing blow and wipe away the otherwise lasting stain upon our Country—and if ever a man should glory in being instrumental to the act surely—surely it is this" (to Scott, January 19, 1829, NLS MS3908: 31–32). MacKay joked that Scott should play executioner! Scott alone could cut away disease, stanch the wound, and retell Scotland as truth.

Ironically—but predictably—each party to the case also tried to enlist Scott to tell their tale and make them respectable once more. Knox's porter and receiver of bodies fell under suspicion. In heated exchanges with the *Mercury* and in that long, anonymous, third-person and possibly ghostwritten publication from "The Echo of Surgeons Square," Paterson had attempted his own defense.[9] But the *Mercury* pelted him with skeptical questions—so he turned to Sir Walter. Scott recorded in his journal for April 4, 1829: "I have a letter from one David Paterson, a fellow who was Dr. Knox's jackall for buying murdered bodies, suggesting that I should write on the subject of Burke and Hare and offering me his invaluable collection of anecdotes" (*Journal*, 608). Knox, although refusing to speak for himself, nonetheless wanted the Royal Society to speak for him, and Scott was approached to serve on the investigative committee (571). To the porter, Scott denied any response. "Curse him's imperance and him's damn insurance," he expostulated angrily: "Did ever one hear the like?" (608–9; Scott quotes the stagey black servant in *The Padlock* [1792]). And though Scott's grandfather Rutherford had been a noted doctor and member of the Edinburgh medical faculty, the author was no partisan of Knox, either. He refused to sit as "one of... Mr. Knox's friends," or in any way to "whitewash this much to be suspected individual" (571). Scott parodied the proclivities of the bodysnatchers to snort: "he shall ride off on no back of mine."

Why did Scott refuse to speak? He was invested in the nation, and he usually had plenty to say. Moreover, he did have an interest in the story. Charles Kirkpatrick Sharpe procured a "share of a window" for him at Burke's hanging (though it is unclear whether Scott attended).[10] And Scott certainly had opinions. But Scott's opinions pointed away from the reconstructive narratives sought by the worthies of Edinburgh and the associates of Burke and Hare. Knox had distanced himself from criticism because he considered it fomented by the mob (Lonsdale, 110–11). Indeed, the whiggish Knox was a bit of an inverted snob—in his quarrel with Allan, Knox boasted that he enjoyed better social connections than the editor (to Robison, Monday Evening, Robison Correspondence). Scott found one spring for the horrors of Burke and Hare in precisely such a separation between classes. To Maria Edgeworth he emphasized the steadiness of most immigrants, but also the poverty of this underclass and thus the logic behind Burke and Hare's crimes: "Our canals, our railroads, our various public works, are all wrought by Irish.... But most unhappily for all parties they work at far too low a rate... [T]hey become reckless, of course.... Extreme poverty brings ignorance and vice, and these are the mothers of crime" (*Letters*, 11:123–29). Burke and Hare revealed Edinburgh's suspect class dynamic. They also connected the doctor and the lawyer—even all of Edinburgh's vaunted professions. Scott associated the doctor and the murderers with "The state of high civilization to which we have arrived" that allowed "the *few* [to be] improved to the highest point" but "the *many* [to be] in proportion brutalized and degraded" (128). Knox offered a "horrid example of how men may stumble and fall in the full march of Intellect" (72). "*Here* is a doctor who is able to take down the whole clock-work of the human frame, and may in time find some way of repairing and putting it together again; and *there* is Burke with the body [of his] murdered countrywoman on his back, and her blood on his hands, asking his price from the learned carcass-butcher" (128). "I cannot imagine," Scott determined, "that this same Doctor who paid a high price to the most wretched & desperate of men for the bodies of his fellow creatures with marks of violence on them which intimated the manner of their death can be exculpated" (93). Knox's case is exceptional—how could he not have known? But it is familiar, too: he fell in the march of superior Edinburgh intellect.

Scott, in fact, recognized the proximity between all sides to the case. President of a Royal Society a good half of whom were medical men, and himself a determinedly enlightened man, he claimed, "I should...be willing that I myself should be dissected in publick if doing so could produce any advantage to Society"—and his brain actually was removed and examined after his death (*Journal*, 567). He understood public feeling, too. Scott's wife had recently died, and though he seems to have taken no steps to preserve her grave from bodysnatchers, he looked back in gratitude to the "servants and dependants who had been attached to her during life" and who had quietly guarded the cemetery (*Letters*, 11:125). Scott understood that though he took a scientific perspective for himself, "when I think on relations and friends being rent from the grave the case is very different" (*Journal*, 567). He was capable of turning that observation toward self-criticism, concluding "So inconsistent we are." In general, too, Scott declared his suspicion of a science divorced from humane values, saying: "I am no great believer in the extreme degree of improvement to be derived from the advancement of science; for every pursuit of that nature tends, when pushed to a certain extent, to harden the heart, and render the philosopher reckless of everything save the objects of his own pursuit" (*Letters*, 11:127). He questioned his similar dedication to the courts, for "I have myself often wondered how I became so indifferent to the horrors of a criminal trial, if it involved a point of law" (ibid.). Scott recognized himself as caught between science and society, with all the attendant responsibilities and worries. From this perspective, could Edinburgh's anxieties be brought home to Burke and Hare and Doctor Knox, and thereby allayed? Presuming they might be constricted by the author's powerful creative memory, should they be?

Significantly, Scott did nothing to close down this terrible tale. Rather, he caught its lure. His son-in-law, John Gibson Lockhart, gleefully recounted to his wife that "Margaret...went into convulsions at hearing yr papa expatiate, as is his custom, on the minutiae [about] Daft Jamies Murder" (NLS MS1553: 34). Scott's son Charles also experienced the author's vivid turn of phrase. Scott wrote to him: "Any person with the ordinary number of limbs was exposed to be kidnapd for Dr Knox's purposes—or indeed if he had more or less than the usual share his risque was only the greater" (*Letters*, 11:89). This, the author winked, was "a dainty piece of news for a long night and a dying candle" (72). By gossiping with Charles in lively, storytelling fashion, Scott passed the tale to someone else (see Benjamin). He told his daughter Sophia: "Charles will tell you about these shocking matters as I have wrote him at length to put him in force [?] to spin a tough and terrible Story at Christmas eve" (68). Scott would not resolve this tale for Scotland. Rather, he worked to multiply it through other tellers, spurring it into the obsessive repetition that is the pathway for trauma.

Scott worked particularly against Robert Knox. *Blackwood's* insisted that Knox should explain; Scott, the sophisticated author, was equally concerned that Knox should not distract with any different tale. Dori Laub, discussing the massive trauma of the Holocaust, observes that "The perpetrators, in their attempt to rationalize...brutally imposed upon their victims a delusional ideology" (Caruth ed., 66). In his local circumstances, Knox may have betokened the same when he tried to cast medicine as victim of ignorance, and to forge ahead in professional Edinburgh as its hero. Nothing was his fault. Scott, however, insisted that the story should tell itself fully. So when Knox sensed someone was blocking him within that engine of scientific and cultural authority, the Royal Society of Edinburgh, he was right. That someone was Walter Scott. If Scott held back from any role in official narratives of Knox's scandal, he was busy behind the scenes. In a flurry of activity, he:

> calld on Mr. Robison and instructed him to call a meeting of the Council of the Royal Society as Mr. Knox proposes to read an essay on some dissections [midway between the trial and the execution]. A bold proposal truly from one who has had so lately the boldness of trading so deep in human flesh. I will oppose his reading in the present circumstances if I should stand alone....It is very bad taste to push himself forward just now. (*Journal*, 565)

Scott was sure that "hearing [this paper] before Mr. Knox has made any defence (as he is stated to have in view) would be an intimation of our preference of the cause of Science to those of Morality and Common Humanity" (566). The author was daring Knox to express the complexity of the situation, not to maintain what the doctor's biographer would later call his "noli me tangere" relationship to Burke and Hare,

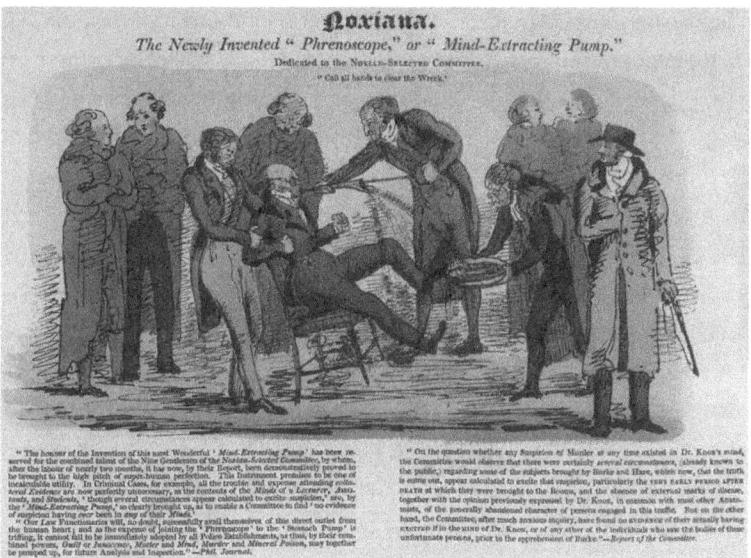

FIGURE 2.4 "The Newly Invented 'Phrenoscope,'" *Noxiana* No. VI. Courtesy of the National Library of Scotland.

which Knox extended with regard to his subjects, their sources, and public opinion (Lonsdale, 102). Knox, however, was not up to the challenge. He clung to the idea of himself as scientific hero, doggedly trying to give his paper and fulminating to Robison: "The advice [to defer delivery of a paper from] the persons you speak of in your note as friends, is extremely suspicious. Will you have the kindness to let me know who they are?" (January 15, 1829, Robison Correspondence). "They," of course, were Walter Scott. And for Scott, if Knox did not tell his own implicated tale, the story would remain open, alive, and capable of producing fascinated and horrified cultural debate.

A contemporary cartoon sought to redirect society's pains through the body of Doctor Knox (see figure 2.4). It showed Knox as a patient, subject to "The Newly Invented 'Phrenoscope,' or 'Mind-Extracting Pump.'" This medico-legal apparatus supposedly assisted Knox's investigatory committee. "In Criminal Cases," the "Phrenoscope" avoided "all the trouble and expense attending *collateral Evidence*": it would simply suck out what witnesses knew. In the case of Doctor Knox, however, the "Phrenoscope" found nothing. It implied innocence. But was the committee, whatever its methods, a scam, only faking Knox's pristine memory and clean conscience? The text comments acerbically: "the contents of the *Minds* of a

Lecturer, *Assistants*, and *Students*, 'though several circumstances appear calculated to excite suspicion,' are, by the '*Mind-Extracting Pump*,' so clearly brought up, as to enable a Committee to find 'no evidence of suspicion having *ever* been in *any* of their *Minds*.'" The committee's investigations found an exculpatory vacancy within the surgeon and his assistants. Knox and his students were thus more than innocent of guilt. Although the doctors had received remarkably fresh corpses, dissected them, and in some cases speedily carved away their distinguishing features, "enlightened" procedures found these innocents simply not connected to the case which could, as Knox implied, have happened to anyone (*Mercury* March 21, 1829: 4). But the cartoonist found the doctors' minds suspiciously empty of curiosity about their cadavers' origins—given that they should have been full of medical knowledge. Scott, though he may well have thought Knox's students empty-headed, also saw an excess behind this apparent absence. The national author who was supposed to bury the tale's unpleasant parts deep in acceptable story instead kept exposed the tissue of memory that (should) interconnect doctor, students, and society across the bodies lying on Doctor Knox's dissecting slabs. Doing nothing, Scott exhumed and disturbed everything. It was he who animated a local trauma to walk down the years in Scottish culture and even beyond.

MORBID ANATOMY AND METAPHORIC LIFE

We have seen how the story of Burke and Hare and Doctor Knox caught contemporary attention, and we know why it remained unintegrated. Dreadful events scar deeply, cutting a pathway for their obsessive retelling—a symptom of trauma. This gives shape to later anxieties: future and quite different distresses can fall into that same line (and cut the pathway deeper again). The first stage of this dynamic was well under way in newspaper stories about suspected "burkings" but also in obsessive and unsuccessful attempts to tell a different official tale. To add to Doctor Knox's woes, however, although his story eventually gave shape to later problems, in 1828 it cut so deep because it was already a twice-told tale, taking a pathway marked by previous distresses. Doubling between past and present allows cross-reference between cultural moments, and opens the possibility of critique of each by the other, even in the midst of new horrors. The ironies that result offer enlivening comment on the coherence traumatized societies desire. Indeed, they frustrate the turn toward a comfortable end to any story. Here, they deny an end to Doctor Knox.

Knox had the misfortune to practice his dissections within a theater of metaphor. The word "autopsy," which we might think separates the surgeon and the subject—the one cutting up the other—also connects them. It implies seeing oneself with one's own eyes. As he systematically picks apart what lies before him, the doctor should understand the other in, and thus the reality of, himself (Helen Deutsch in Rosenthal, 112; Wootton, 106). As the famous (Scottish) obstetrician and anatomist William Hunter observed, "nothing can give more pleasing Ideas than the knowledge of Oneself" (qtd. Allard, 22). What is more, aligned with himself as he performs an autopsy, the doctor should understand his implicated role as "author" of what he sees. Unluckily for Knox, though he resisted such connections, Walter Scott recognized his own inner doctor. A sympathetic anatomist of culture, this national author understood that in any social pathology, every emphasis on separation—every cut of the knife—implied a disturbing consanguinity between self and other.

Even more unluckily for Knox, Scott the master of metaphor held this in mind. Post-Union Scotland manifested an uneasy body politic—British yet Scottish and partly Highland, to name but a few of its warring members.[11] Scotland needed to be mended in its metaphor. And in recent years the nation had invoked the bodies of the past to heal the present. In 1815 and 1818, Robert Burns and Robert the Bruce were exhumed then reinterred, re-embodying Scotland and being reburied as singular story put appropriately to rest (McGuirk, 48–50; Douglas S. Mack, 72–73). Literature, however, expressed such enactments of proto-Scottishness as problematic. James Hogg's *Private Memoirs and Confessions of a Justified Sinner* (1824), with its preserved corpse and the perplexing tale retrieved from the grave, suggests that digging up the past is tantamount to bodysnatching, dissecting that past yields no answers, and what we unearth may walk disturbingly through Scottish culture.

Walter Scott embraced this possibility. In 1826 he deliberately connected Scotland's anxieties to the uncertainties of dissection. Scott's "Malachi Malagrowther" letters fought a national cause to animate Scottish society against the Westminster government's depredations on Scotland's independent rights (McCracken-Flesher, "Speaking"). Britain sought to absorb Scotland's banks within one grand economic design. Keen to benefit from Britishness, yet not to lose Scottish identity and powers, Scott pondered how to rouse his countrymen to a sense of their danger. His strategy was to represent his country under England's legislation as "a subject in a common dissecting-room, left to the scalpel of the junior students, with the degrading inscription,—*Fiat experimentum in corpore vili* [Experiment on this vile body/body of little worth]" ("Malachi" 1:10–11). Under the knife of the author's invasive English anatomist, Scotland came alive (which is why Scott features on Scottish currency today—in thanks). Scott's image was so painfully ugly that it shocked his nation back into political consciousness, and also into an embarrassing and enlivening self-consciousness. Pain had sutured the life and death of a culture at the point of the metaphorical anatomist's knife. Through Scott, then, the events of 1828 collided with a metaphor around which many Scottish discourses already swirled. And Scott, recognizing that every cut of Knox's scalpel only appeared to separate surgeon and subject—indeed, it potentially connected surgeon and subject in an excruciatingly awakened society—also understood the moment's opportunity for creative irony.

Of course, despite the appeal of an impressive image (the anatomist cuts a corpse and it sits up and yells), we might assume that one medical truth undermines this grisly scenario: what is dead is dead and cannot speak back. More, what is anatomized must be double-dead and should not concern us. However, Knox's dissections and Scott's metaphorics of anatomy resonated according to a science much different from that of today. In medical terms, the dead certainly seem different from the living. The 1824 pamphlet "Use of the Dead to the Living" situates death and life as clearly opposed, with life subordinating the dead (Thomas Southwood Smith). But were death and life so distinct? In fact, the dead, in medical experience, were not far removed from the living. To begin with, whereas today's medicine separates out the roles of pathologist and surgeon, in Scott's day anatomists were often surgeons.[12] (Knox, we know, did attend sick students, and in his final years he set up a private practice in the London borough of Hackney; he fought, too, for pathological anatomy to remain central in the medical curriculum [Johnson; Rae, 159; Knox, *Letter*].) Because of their dual role, doctors of the early nineteenth century saw life and death more nearly bonded in the physiology of a disease. As an anatomist, the doctor mapped the illness that terminated life across the bodies of the dead; as a surgeon, he extracted disease and death from life—though sometimes the quickest way to die was to visit the doctor. Moreover, given the primitiveness of contemporary medicine, the modes of dissection and surgery intersected on the slab. In an operation, speed and precision were equally important—as a student of Liston's was rumored to know to his cost, having supposedly lost some fingers to the scalpel as he assisted the master.[13] William Blake memorably satirized the work of surgeon-anatomist John Hunter, whom he called "Tearguts":

> he'll plunge his knife up to the hilt in a single drive, and thrust his fist in, and all in the space of a Quarter of an hour. He does not mind their crying, tho' they cry ever so. He'll Swear at them & keep them down with his fist, & tell them that he'll scrape their bones if they don't lay still. (Blake, 50)

In these circumstances, what marked the difference between surgery and anatomy? Before the use of anesthetics, the patient's crying gave the sign of life at the moment of apparent destruction.

Even more interestingly, according to the period's physiology, the dead themselves might cry out. In the eighteenth and nineteenth centuries, the signs of death were uncertain and much debated. J. B. Winslow's 1740 volume on *The Uncertainty of the Signs of Death and the Danger of Precipitate Interments and Dissections* ran into numerous editions and was supplemented and extended through the nineteenth century (see MacKay for the later period). It was replete with tales of belated revivals, and revivals recognized too late as manifested by contorted bodies whose owners had apparently eaten their own fingers to sustain themselves in the grave (65 and 90, 58; also Taylor, in 1816). While such stories echo more as folklore than as truth, we might note that in an age of poor medical equipment and the early use of narcotics, the diagnosis of death might, in Mark Twain's phrase, be "greatly exaggerated." It might even, if the patient was lucky, produce the effect of resurrection in *this* life, rather than in the life to come (see figure 2.5).

Uncertainty was exacerbated by the early practice of artificial respiration and the emergent science of cryogenics. Martin S. Pernick notes that "Beginning in 1767, physicians and reformers across Europe and the Americas organized what they called 'humane societies' to teach artificial respiration, resuscitate victims of drowning and suffocation, and promote research on new life-restoring techniques. The London

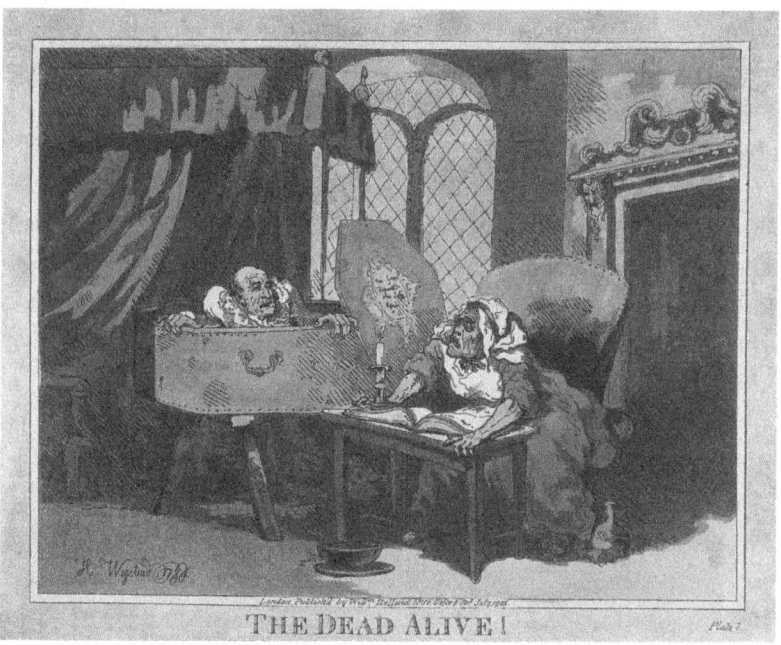

FIGURE 2.5 *The Dead Alive!* 1805. Colored aquatint after a drawing by Henry Wigstead, 1784. Courtesy of the Wellcome Library, London.

Society alone claimed to have revived over 2,000 people by 1796" (Pernick, 22). Tales of revival included many drowning victims who had supposedly survived under ice for weeks at a time. Winslow's Contents include "A Person recovered to Life after having been sixteen Hours in the Water," and "Another who had been under Water no less than seven Weeks." John Hunter consequently experimented on frozen dormice—though eventually he conceded that his idea of "[prolonging] life to any period by freezing a person" failed in its application (Moore, 242). The arts, however, could pursue such possibilities.

Visual arts that situated themselves at the very instant of death—at the crux of possibility either way—bonded intensely felt life to the phenomenon of death. Madame Tussaud's waxworks supposedly were produced at the drop of a guillotine, and for Marat, killed in his bath by Charlotte Corday, Madame "rushed to the scene to take a death mask...arriving so quickly that the murderer was just being taken away" (Pilbeam, 50).[14] Frederick Ruysch's embalmed bodies remained so fresh and alive that Peter the Great was moved to kiss one infant—at least that was the story (Hansen, 673–74). De Fontenelle wrote of his colleague's achievement: "One would have taken [Ruysch's preparations] for living persons in profound repose.... Ruysch had discovered the secret of resuscitating the dead. His mummies were a revelation of life" (Hansen, 673).

Modern medicine, indeed, was a spectacle that expressed itself as gothically animated display. Luigi Galvani's nephew brought Galvanism to Britain in 1803, experimenting on the body of a murderer. Then in 1818, Andrew Ure described similar experiments in Glasgow (see figure 2.6). When stimulated:

> every muscle in [the corpse's] countenance was simultaneously thrown into fearful action; rage, horror, despair, anguish, and ghastly smiles, united their hideous expression in the murderer's face, surpassing far the wildest representations of a Fuseli or a Kean. At this period several of the spectators were forced to leave the apartment from terror or sickness, and one gentleman fainted. (Ure, 290)

Medicine was itself such an art that as recently as 1819, the Reverend Walter Whiter suggested in his *Dissertation on the Disorder of Death* that apparent death might actually manifest the crisis—in the sense of the turning point—in a disease. He was not alone, for he quoted Erasmus Darwin: "*Death* will operate as the *cure of...Disorder*, and as the means of possessing Life in an improved and ameliorated condition" (Whiter, 129). "*Death*," to Whiter—who has to go down in history as one of the world's great optimists—was "sometimes not a *Disorder* but a *Remedy*, not merely capable of being cured, but itself potent even to cure" (130–31).

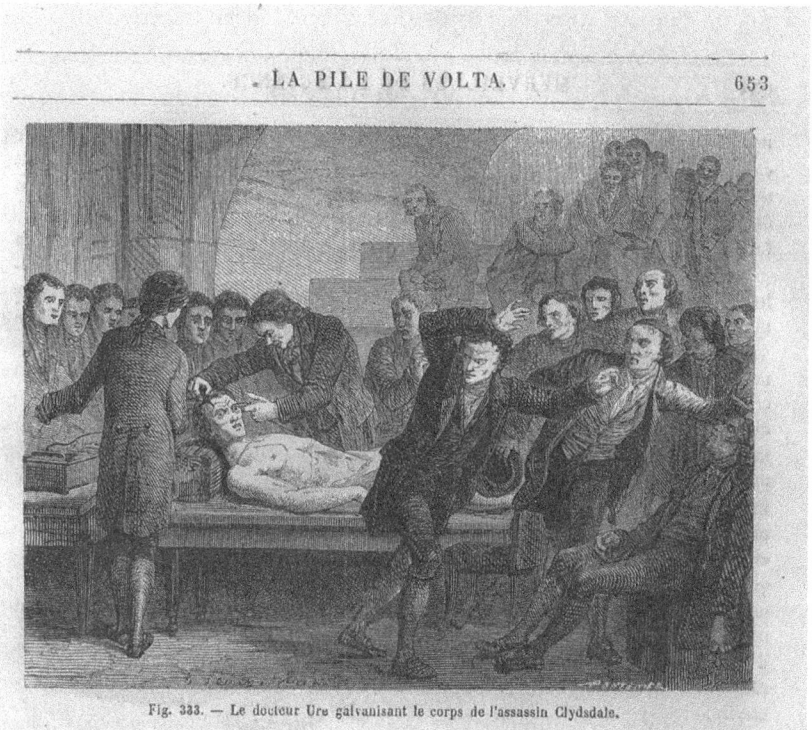

FIGURE 2.6 "Le docteur Ure galvanisant le corps de l'assassin Clydsdale." Louis Figuier, *Les Merveilles de la Science*, vol. 1 (Paris: Fourne, Jouvet, 1891), 653.

In this context, the anatomist's knife and Scott's national metaphor of the body on the dissecting table cut both ways. Winslow and his successors, concerned about premature burial, had recommended a regime of pokings, proddings, and scrapings to be practiced on the corpse to diagnose life in death:

> we ought to irritate [the corpse's] Nostrils by introducing into them Sternutatories [to induce sneezing], Errhines [to make the nose run], Salts, stimulating Liquors, Synapisms [mustard powders], the Juice of Onions, Garlic, and Horse-radish, or the feathered End of a Quill, or the point of a Pencil.... stimulate his Organs of Touch with Whips and Nettles; irritate his Intestines by Means of Clysters [enemas] and Injections of Air or Smoke; agitate his Limbs by violent Extensions and Inflexions; and if possible shock his Ears by hideous Shrieks and excessive Noises. (Winslow, 21)

If all else failed, Winslow recommended "Wounds made either with pricking or cutting Instruments, or by Means of Fire" (22). And Pernick tells of equally invasive tests reaching through to the late nineteenth century, such as "jabbing a long needle with a flag on one end directly into the heart," and "'deep insertion' of a heated cautery"—which Roy Porter translates as a hot poker up the rear (Pernick, 39; Porter *Flesh*, 215). Particularly fearful patients—perhaps hoping to avoid these tests—from the 1790s trusted to "safety" or "security" coffins, with their apparatus of breathing tubes and alarm bells, not to be caught napping under ground (Bondeson, ch. 6). In Europe, from 1823 and increasingly through the century, public mortuaries developed wherein, in a perverse manifestation of the panopticon, slowly sweetening corpses lay under the anticipating eye of a central guard (Pernick, 31). But those not content to rely on such equipment or services turned, again, to the anatomist. Pernick sums up their options: they "demanded bloodletting, embalming, autopsy, cremation, even decapitation...to guarantee that they would not be alive when buried" (35). In 1846, *Hogg's Instructor* tried to correct the general fear: "One capital fact has been discovered, which serves at once to distinguish apparent from real death...the pulses of the heart" ("Apparent," 308). William See insisted on "The Extreme Rarity of Premature Burials" in 1880. Still, as late as 1904, Francis Power Cobbe "left a neighboring physician twenty guineas 'to perform on my body the operation of completely and thoroughly severing the arteries of the neck & windpipe (nearly severing the head altogether) so as to render my revival in the grave absolutely impossible'" (Behlmer, 222). Weirdly, the dissectionist proved—or perhaps made sure—you were really dead.

But the anatomist might also imply that you were not dead yet. Treatises on the uncertainty of death and on premature burial heave with tales of revival upon the cut of the dissector's knife. Winslow lists: "A pregnant Woman, thought to be dead, discovers Signs of Life as the Surgeon was cutting the Child out of her Womb," and "A Man of Quality" who "comes to Life whilst the Surgeon was laying open his Body, twenty-four Hours after his suppos'd Death" (Winslow, Contents). The apocryphal story of Vesalius, subject to the Inquisition after a corpse started to life at the touch of his scalpel, resonated up through the nineteenth century—Lonsdale named it one of Knox's favorites as he paralleled his own martyrdom with noble predecessors (Lonsdale, 111–12 and n.). There were less suspect cases, too. Wendy Moore cites the 1587 experience of a hanged man who "sprang to life on the dissecting table just as a knife was plunged into his chest, providing the gathered audience with more than the usual public spectacle" (Moore, 81). In 1650, another hanging victim, Anne Greene, revived under the scalpel. In 1740, William Duell came back to life in the laboratory even though he had swung from the scaffold for thirty minutes. And Edinburgh had its own tale of postmortem vitality at the hands of the surgeon. In a story of the 1720s confused by its folk transmission, Margaret Dickson was hanged only to revive either when the cart carrying her bumped over the cobbled streets, or—and tellingly as legend if not as fact—because the surgeons' apprentices had tussled over her body as it was cut from the scaffold.[15] Simply the idea of the knife was enough to recall "half-hangit Maggie Dickson" to the disturbance that is life.

Not surprisingly, such stories enjoyed a vital career in gothic literature—and not just in *Frankenstein* (1818). They seem almost common: "On the Pleasures of 'Body-Snatching'" (1827) reprises a rumor from Ure's dissection of the murderer Clydesdale:

> a sudden inflation of the subject's chest 'gave us pause.'—'O Jasus!' cried Malony—who was not a man to stick at trifles, when the interests of science were concerned—'is it after chating the law he is?' and immediately thrust a probe into the temple far enough to set the question of vitality at rest. (361)

Scottish author John Galt told of "The Buried Alive" in 1821. Significantly, for a sick young man, "One day towards evening, the crisis took place," and he is appropriately interred (Galt, 262). But as we might expect in the Reverend Walter Whiter's universe, snatched from the grave and being prepared for dissection: "I felt a dreadful crackling, as it were, throughout my whole frame... and a shriek of horror rose from all present. The ice of death was broken up" (264). At the crux of medicine as metaphor, these dead walk.

THE AUTHOR DISSECTS THE DOCTOR

In part, this explains why Doctor Knox, at the hands of Walter Scott, cannot die. The doctors testifying at Burke's trial acknowledged the difficulty of determining cause of death, even in a subject showing signs of violence: Doctor Black "Examined [Mrs. Docherty] externally. No marks or blemishes of any consequence. There was some blood about her mouth and nose.... The eyes and face were much swollen, and the latter of a blackish hue. In a medical point of view he could give no opinion as to the cause of death" (*Mercury* December 25, 1828: 3). Doctor Christison, who inspected internal injuries, did "not consider that the contusions could be produced after death, but the injury of the spine... might have been caused as well after death as before it. An injury properly applied 18 hours after death would cause the same appearances" (ibid.). Thus Cockburn could sum up in McDougal's defense: "The appearances found in the body justify only a suspicion, and... they amount only to a probability" (ibid.). Still, attempting to distinguish themselves from Knox, in the press doctors asserted "they would have infallibly detected and as certainly refused every such subject" (*Mercury* January 1, 1829). And as the better anatomist, perhaps Knox should have been surer than they. Knox's 1814 thesis: "De Viribus

Stimulantium et Narcoticorum in corpore sano"—on the effect of stimulants and narcotics on the healthy body—might have pointed to a better than average understanding of the margins between life and death (Rae, 8). Further, in 1824 Knox noted the distinctive postmortem effects of the eye. "He had examined the eyes of an executed criminal eight hours after death, and found the *foramen* of Soemmering 'remarkably distinct, and of a deep yellow tinge; *there was no fold*, a fact which proves the appearance to be a *post-mortem* one'" (Lonsdale, 31; Knox, "Inquiry"). Was Knox poised to detect the signs of murder in the subjects delivered by Burke and Hare? Did he bother to look? Whatever the realities of the case, most unfortunately for him, Knox as dubious dissector embodied contemporary anxieties and tapped national metaphor about the reversible polarities of death. In 1828, surgeons worked to divorce death from life (cutting away disease), and anatomists served to enforce death (making sure you did not come back), but dissections were liable to produce life (you might come back). At this moment Knox, whose suppliers Burke and Hare sped the living across the boundaries of death in order to serve the cause of health, evoked the uncanny liveliness that lurked at the bounds of Scott's metaphorized national identity.

Walter Scott was just the man to take advantage of this coincidence, spinning new Scottish life out of the apparent death of ethics, responsibility, and reason in the pathology of Doctor Knox. *Blackwood's* circulated a rumor that Scott had declared "with all his wonderful imagination, he could picture to himself nothing so hideous" (*Blackwood's* March 1829: 384–85). Not in the details, perhaps, but Scott was well acquainted with the operations of this dreadful tale. The author had a thesis, too: for his admission to the Faculty of Advocates in 1792 he had produced *Disputatio Juridica... de Cadaveribus Damnatorum*—on the bodies of condemned criminals. Furthermore, Knox's was a type of tale and a story function he appreciated and practiced. When Edinburgh wished Scott to provide a definitive resolution to national anxiety, it was confusing Scott's authority with his role as author. Scott, in fact, was well known for his huddled up endings, which he repeated unrepentantly from book to book despite criticism from critics and friends (McCracken-Flesher *Possible*, 55–57). The author was more interested in stealthy beginnings that never finished, particularly in prefaces that posed questions to animate but not conclude a text. And in his texts, Scott was always raising the dead, to make them walk with a difference in Scottish culture—he was a historical novelist after all, but one with an interest in a revivified future. For him, the long gone Thomas the Rhymer returned from early poem to late novel, showing up at the point of crisis in moments scattered across history to imply a meaning and a nation yet in production (*Minstrelsy of the Scottish Border*, 1802; *Castle Dangerous*, 1832). The wizard Michael Scott, exposed in his grave, glowers and grasps, disturbing the present (*Lay of the Last Minstrel*, 1805). He is not dead yet, and others must therefore live a more anxious, more lively life. Nostalgia notwithstanding, Scott situated himself at the crisis of culture—that moment of apparent death that ironically produced and critiqued life. He was always doing it.

Scott, then, had no interest in closing down Doctor Knox's tale into the reductive narratives of official and rather deathly Edinburgh. Instead, by not speaking of Knox's case, Scott maintained the doctor as the upright corpse. In Scottish culture, Knox, Burke, and Hare remain ever subject to Scottish resurrection—whether in times of trauma or when Scotland requires the enlivening clutch of grinning irony from its own memento mori. Under the care of Scott the national pathologist, in Michel Foucault's phrase, "Death left its old tragic heaven and became the lyrical core of man: his invisible truth, his visible secret" (*Birth*, 172). Thereby, through the ongoing embarrassment of Doctor Knox, again and again—and again—Scottish culture starts painfully back to life, consciousness, and meaning.

3

Enlightened System versus Religious Sympathy

THE SENSATIONAL TALES OF ALEXANDER LEIGHTON
AND DAVID PAE

IN 1827, ROBERT KNOX represented the "march of intellect" in Edinburgh. An anatomist, he figured prominently in a leading science of the time, for which Edinburgh itself enjoyed a substantial reputation, but Knox was also a "transcendental anatomist." To him, for all his achievements in anatomy, that science was "a means towards an end." He would declare in 1852: "It is pursued by the physician and surgeon for the detection of disease, and the performance of operations; by both to discover the functions of the organs; and by the philosopher with the hope of detecting the laws of organic life, the origin of living beings, and the transcendental laws regulating the living world in time and space" (Knox *Great Artists*, 141–42). For Knox, everything was connected to everything else. Anatomy supported the "systematic" thinking by which, according to David Hume, the "[a]ccurate and regular argument...such as is now expected of philosophical inquirers" proceeds (Hume, 6).

By 1828, however, Knox had marched right up to the intellectual borders of Enlightenment. Edinburgh learned that systematic medicine based on experiment and exploration depended on Burke and Hare, who had assisted the pursuit of medicine and its transcendental philosophy by murdering sixteen people and selling them, freshly dead, at Doctor Knox's door. The doctor and his pupils, eager for enlightenment, apparently never shone the lamp of their flaring intellect over the corpses. This led Edinburgh to question their competence, suspect their complicity, and imagine dark possibilities. Lord Meadowbank recognized the issue as one of enlightened methodology—of "system" pursued beyond reason. Speaking from the bench at Burke's trial, he thought it:

> impossible... not to advert... to that most extraordinary,—that most sanguinary and atrocious system, which... has been developed and established....
> ...in the history of this country,—nay, in the whole history of civilized society,—there never has been exhibited such a system of barbarous and savage iniquity.... that there should, at this time of day,—in this country... have been found to be regularly organized and established a system of cold and premeditated murder.... It would be in vain that I should search for words to express the ideas which the general announcement of such a system of horrible atrocity, must necessarily create. (*Trial*, 195–96)

Popular writers north and south shared his concern and worried about the full extent of the problem. The *Edinburgh Evening Courant* imagined "systematic murder," even as it anxiously intoned that "the medical faculty, generally, are above all suspicion" (*Courant*, December 29, 1828: 3; January 1, 1829: 3). *Murderers of the Close*, from the comfortable distance of London, connected criminals and doctors in one "system."[1] This book's author obsessed about the "organized system in [Burke's] operations, and those of his associates which shewed that 'science' had, somehow or other, mixed itself with the most dreadful criminality that ever disgraced the name of man"; "the infernal system which [Burke] and his associates had matured for the interests of 'science'" in the persons of "the Scotch surgeons" (*Murderers*, 262, 265, 263). And he swayed between satisfaction that justice had been done and the impossibility of knowing and expressing the alternatives had Burke and Hare not been exposed and punished. Again and again he falls into incoherence: "It is not to be credited"; "It is impossible to say" (262, 263). Lord Meadowbank had done no better: the case was "inexpressibly horrible"; "It would be in vain that I should search for words" (*Trial*, 196). That is, together, Burke and Hare and Doctor Knox disturbingly manifested the end—both the logical outcome and the inevitable collapse—of systematic thinking in Scotland. As Meadowbank found, by their alignment and enactment of medical and commercial systems, they had stepped beyond the law's powers of explanation, and even expression.

To David Hume, the methodical and didactic expression through which system emerges stands against its opposite: dialogue. System and dialogue seem mutually exclusive. System aims (at least) at clarity; to formulate a system in dialogue is to lose the point in process, for the author risks wandering off through the distractions of conversation. Dialogue, then, is for matters so sure they can use the entertainment value of a conversational style, or those so obscure they can be enjoyed simply as discursive opportunity. Notably, Hume suggests: "Reasonable men may be allowed to differ, where no one can reasonably be positive: Opposite sentiments, even without any decision, afford an agreeable amusement: and if the subject be curious and interesting, [dialogue] carries us, in a manner, into company" (*Dialogues*, 8). Through Doctor Knox, I suggest, where facts are unclear, and systems suspect, dialogue is the only form of expression available. However dialogue, because it carries us "into company," multiplies conversation and mingles perspectives. Terms clash, meld, transpose and transform; all systems collapse as expression burgeons. Thus the cultural distress initiated by medicine and its murders cut ever deeper.

Edinburgh, feeling traumatized, was of course keen to locate the horrors of 1828 within knowable systems—to assemble data, order it, analyze it, categorize events, and thus reduce the scandal into a manageable space. But day by day, this proved a more difficult task: the trial depended on dubious witnesses—Hare and his wife testified against Burke and McDougal; the principals told tales that conflicted not just in their analyses of blame, but in their assemblage of facts; though Hare looked ferrety enough for criminality (see figure 3.1), Burke was the typical neighbor no one suspects. Worse still, justice proved merely representative: only Burke died, and the doctors did not even testify. Confused and anxious, Edinburgh fought to make its systems work once more. Daft Jamie's mother brought a civil suit against Hare, but the law allowed her no day in court—though Hare had admitted to crimes not charged against Burke, he had done so as king's evidence and could not be tried. The *Caledonian Mercury* declined from optimism that "The public, with their usual generosity, will [sponsor Mrs. Wilson's suit]," to assurances that her case will stand, to frustration that the crown refused to hear the case (*Mercury*, January 8, 1829: 3; January 17: 2; January 22: 3). So Edinburgh rowdies challenged the systematic indifference of Doctor Knox—and perhaps that of the law—by rioting. A broadsheet reports with some satisfaction:

> an Effigy of a certain Doctor, who has been rendered very obnoxious to the public by recent events. The figure...bore a tolerable resemblance....the appearance of the crowd was very threatening, the whole flower-plot and railing in front of the Doctor's house being literally packed with people, who were shouting in a wrathful manner—blending the names of the West Port murderers with that of the medical gentleman....Another mob...[broke College windows]. A third crowd....again attacked the house of Dr Knox...when a great number of windows were broken. ("Full and Particular Account")

The failure to contain the offending doctor and his devils threatened the end of judicial system and social order, both in court and on the street (see figure 3.2).

Enlightened System versus Religious Sympathy 59

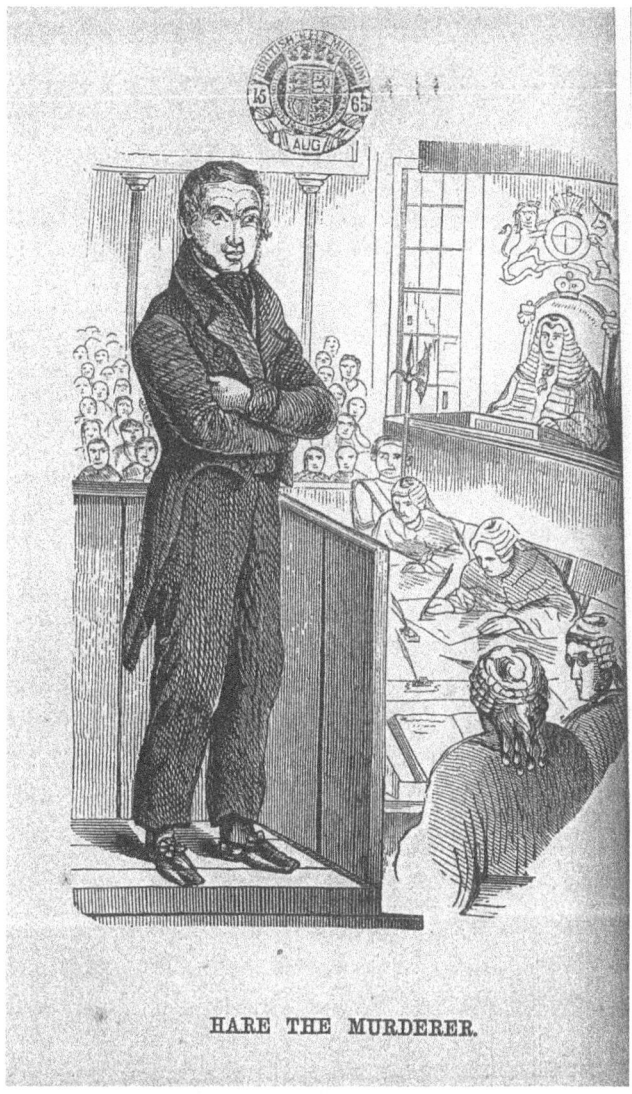

FIGURE 3.1 "Hare the Murderer." From David Pae, *Mary Paterson* (London: Fred Farrah, 1866). Courtesy of the British Library.

Increasingly then, Edinburgh needed the doctor to speak. He alone (one might presume), held the information, boasted the intellect, and could claim the authority to explain events and reorder society. After the unsatisfactory trial of Burke and McDougal, a broadside appropriately titled "An Expostulation" resonated with the city's growing desperation. It begged, challenged, coerced and exhorted Knox to explain to enquiring Edinburgh, on the assumption that if the doctor would only respond, all could be resolved:

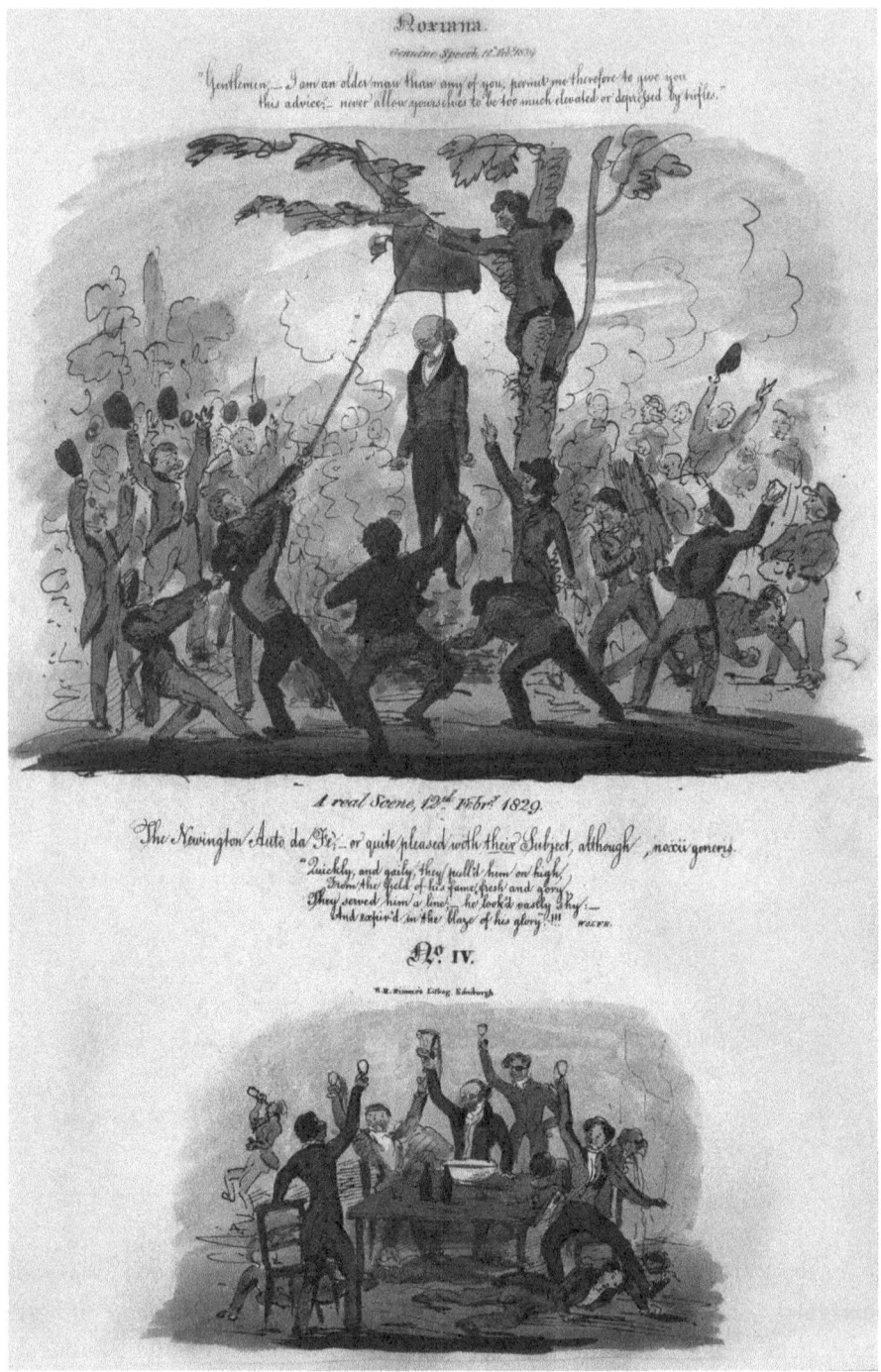

FIGURE 3.2 "The Newington Auto da Fe (top)," *Noxiana* No. IV. Courtesy of the Royal College of Physicians of Edinburgh.

AH!——can'st thou, with cold indifference, see
The hand of execration point to thee?
Can'st thou, unmov'd, hear a whole nation's cry,
To cleanse thyself from the polluted sty
Of Burke, and Hare, and all that fiendish crew,
Who, for mere gain, their fellow-mortals slew,
And sold to thee, as thou hast not denied,
Such bodies as by students were descried
Ne'er to have been interred, nay, bore, some say,
Strong marks of life, by violence reft away?
And thou didst not attempt the truth to find,
Though oft it must have flash'd across thy mind....
Art though a Scotsman——? then haste to prove
That patriot feelings can thy bosom move;
Haste to wipe out the stain thy country shares....
Art thou a son of Science? quickly, then,
Show she does not make brutes of *lect'ring* men....
Art thou a Christian?...
Assert thine innocence, REPLY, REPLY [!]
(*Trial*, "Rhymes")

Knox was known for his expertise and his oratory (Lonsdale, 130, 134). Wielding anatomy as the key to everything and never afraid to speak his mind, he nonetheless remained silent—except when he threatened legal action against the newspapers and charged conspiracy against even the colleagues who bemusedly tried to speak in his place (to Robison, March 17 and 24, 1829, Robison Correspondence).

Lonsdale commended Knox for a restraint he attributed to the doctor's elitism—which he seems to share (Lonsdale, 80–81). Whatever Knox's motivations, his silence on the matter at hand only intensified over time. On January 1, 1829 (with Burke having been condemned as recently as Christmas Day 1828), Knox asserted business as usual. On page three, the *Caledonian Mercury* continued its reporting of the West Port murders with the leader:

> Every hour some fresh tale of horror reaches us. Since our last we have been told of many things—(aye, and told, too, by Anatomists)—calculated to freeze the very blood in our veins. Murder upon system—murder almost by wholesale—has been carried on in this city for the last year and a half: and not only has it been systematically committed...it has been perpetrated upon the most refined principles of anatomical science...which must have emanated from some higher source.

But on page one, Knox held to his own practices regardless. He advertised in roaring capitals: "DR KNOX'S LECTURES on COMPARATIVE ANATOMY and PHYSIOLOGY will this year commence on the first Monday in May, at *half past twelve* o'clock." Over the years to come, moreover, Knox proved indefatigable.

On the heels of the trial, Knox dashed off three letters to Robison, including one on an amazing scrap of paper about two and a half by six inches: "I continue to investigate notwithstanding the shameful attempts of my private enemies to disturb my mind. The great anatomical fact I communicated to you.... I deem it one of the most important Anatomical enquiries & discoveries which has been made since the time of Vesalius"—perhaps this was the paper suppressed by Scott (Robison Correspondence). By 1830 the doctor was back in full form. He delivered his "Observations illustrating the Laws which regulate hermaphroditical appearances in the Mammalia" to the Royal Society of Edinburgh with characteristic persistence: it took three meetings—with Scott in the Chair for March 1 (Royal Society of Edinburgh General Minute Book January 1824–May 1843). Knox was unavoidable in print, too. *The Races of Men* (1850) stirred up the scientific community. Here, his transcendental anatomy generated theories that are (for us) paradoxically racial and radical, but that made a substantial contribution to the discussions behind Darwin's theories and to anthropological discourse (Richards). Knox wrote the gentlemanly crowd-pleaser *Fish and Fishing in the Lone Glens of Scotland*, as well (1854). He figured largely in journals, especially as a contributor (from 1846) and later editor for the *Medical Times and Gazette* (Bynum et al., 42). Historians argue that journals were essential to the dissemination of medical knowledge in the nineteenth century, but they also note their social uses. Bynum suggests that Knox used the *Medical Times* to recuperate his career; Roy Porter posits a more assertive strategy, asking whether a "publishing doctor" was "a public benefactor [or] was he a self-serving self-publicist?" (Bynum et al., 12). In his popular writings, Knox certainly fought his old causes. For instance, as the one-time Conservator of the Museum for the Royal College of Surgeons of Edinburgh, forced out after the Burke and Hare scandal, in 1846 he used the pages of the *Medical Times* to damn all such collections (even his own) and to argue for the unique value, predictably, of dissection (Knox, "Anatomical Museums").

Further, the doctor who Lonsdale claims invoked the anatomist Vesalius's sufferings under the inquisition and covertly claimed the role of martyr in front of his students rather than explain himself to Edinburgh, continued to align himself with the great, the good, and the sacrificial (Lonsdale, 111–12). In his *Great Artists and Great Anatomists* (1852), Knox weirdly argues his case under cover of Michaelangelo:

> At every court there are men of rank and influence, devoid of all taste. They are the natural enemies of men of genius—genius which they hate and abhor. They

well know that men of genius can never become courtiers, nor bend to titled mountebanks...walking backwards like apes and jugglers before one of their frail fellow-creatures; hence men of genius are hated...oppressed, crushed down, and, if possible, destroyed, or treated with sovereign contempt, neglect, or silence, which amounts precisely to the same in the grand struggle of life. (*Great Artists*, 175)

Knox the "man of genius" claimed the crown of martyrdom, yet gave no account of himself, even though the story of Burke and Hare seemed made for the anatomical and anthropological rendering in which he was so expert. Rather, he asserted his knowledge and connections, and presumed his place in Edinburgh's elite and enlightened systems. He ignored his role in the scandal that was Burke and Hare.

By 1858, Knox had been silent on the subject for thirty years. For Scots, it consequently verged to the bounds of memory, and yet remained uncomfortably unresolved. Lacking a direct reply from Doctor Knox, the vague facts of 1828 invited a discussion perhaps less and less grounded in reality, and more and more unpredictable. As dearth of information, loss of memory, and cultural anxiety pushed events beyond assimilation and toward trauma, Scots, in rising desperation, tried to take control of Doctor Knox's tale. In one respect, the task was easy: Knox continued to make enemies. When he competed for the Chair of General Pathology at the University of Edinburgh in 1837, his application stressed that the Chair's establishment was "a political job of the very worst description," and that Knox thus finds himself at odds with a "junto"—people a dispassionate observer might consider the eminent men of the university (*Letter*, 6; *Second Letter*, 1). Nor could Knox resist naming his students, with their high-class connections, or numbering them—even if he had to recall notorious events: "In the winter session of 1828–29, the number of Medical Students entered in my Books was 504, being perhaps the largest Anatomical Class ever assembled in Britain" (*Letter*, 7 n.1). Not surprisingly, the sitting professors now recommended abolishing the position Knox sought—they even volunteered to pay a pension that the retiring professor would customarily have received from his successor (qtd. *Second Letter*, 1–2). In 1847, a scandal in which a student presented bogus qualifications from many lecturers was pursued against one as fraud: Robert Knox, who had loudly accused his medical brethren of careless record keeping (Rae, 134–46). The Royal College of Surgeons of Edinburgh stopped recognizing his lectures and informed licensing boards nationwide; when Knox went to London, they tried to block him there (153–54). The Edinburgh that could not get at Knox directly used his ongoing poor judgment to punish him obliquely.

Knox found his march of intellect impeded and rerouted at every turn. In 1838, one George Johnston chortled: "I have had an odd letter from the famous or infamous Dr Knox—proposing to establish a new Scientific journal &c!! I wrote him as odd an answer" (UE MS Dk 6.20/164). And whether because of surreptitious dealings among the Edinburgh elite, or because his declining reputation undermined his finances, Doctor Knox fell out of first one and then another of Edinburgh's enlightened institutions. He had to give up his museum conservatorship in 1831 (Rae, 106–9), left Edinburgh in 1842, and was removed from the roll of the Royal Society of Edinburgh in 1848 (for reasons unspecified; Kaufman claims nonpayment of fees in "Frederick Knox"). Then by the late 1850s, and with the doctor thus beaten down, Scotland's authors were poised to tell his festering tale for him, ready or not.

Lacking data and explanations, however, those who would define Doctor Knox, Burke, and Hare found themselves relying not on philosophical systems, but on systems of narration. In 1861, Alexander Leighton insisted that he had wrought what facts there were into chronicle. In 1858–59 and again in 1864–65, David Pae attempted to explain horror according to the predictabilities of sensation fiction—reaching sales of 84,000 in the newspaper serial alone. But both authors found themselves on the downside of dialogue. Where intellect stood challenged by its march, and systematic thinking was undermined, nineteenth-century history had to invoke religion as the only way to explain the strangeness of 1828. Leighton and Pae, with their narrative strategies complicated by this moral imperative, struggled to contain Burke and Hare and Doctor Knox within the chronicle and the novel. The trio resisted containment, in turn disrupting literary form and thus the very possibility of meaning—historical, religious, or any other kind. They actually brought modes of knowing, genres, terms, and meanings into contention. In each successive moment, the attempt to tell their story thus falters into meaningless repetition. In yet another way, we cannot get to grips with it. Worse, because we cannot express the reality of Burke and Hare and Doctor Knox their difference is multiplied; this implies the impossibility of ever resolving our tale. Consequently, Scotland trends further and further toward the compulsion that signifies only national trauma in the process of cutting always deeper.

SOMETHING CATCHING? HISTORY, RELIGION, AND THE SYMPATHIES OF FICTION IN ALEXANDER LEIGHTON

Thirty years after the event, Leighton and Pae each may have imagined a straightforward task—one that should, by mere passage of time, yield at last to chronicle and story. Leighton could afford to be optimistic, for he commanded two modes of control. A Dundee-born writer with Edinburgh medical training, he was a master of the spooky and the silly as well as the annalistic and the moral. From 1836, he served as contributor and editor for *Wilson's Historical, Traditionary, and Imaginative Tales of the Borders, and of Scotland*. This popular series bore the epigraph from Walter Scott:

> Old tales I heard of wo or mirth,
> Of lovers' sleights, of ladies' charms,
> Of witches' spells, of warriors' arms;
> Of patriot battles won of old,
> By Wallace wight, and Bruce the bold.[2]

After his brush with Doctor Knox he would go on to combine the anatomical plot with his favorite themes and modes in the pleasant tale of "Mrs Corbet's Amputated Toe." Mrs. Corbet dies from a gangrenous toe belatedly amputated; medical students extort money from her husband by tricking him into buying back her supposed skeleton (known by its missing toe), though Mrs. Corbet lies peacefully in the grave. Leighton contextualized medical and historical oddities in the chronicle or the strange tale, and either way he confined them within a genre.

As we might expect, then, the title to Leighton's text, perhaps lifted from the epigraph to Buchanan's record, *The Trial*, implies a horror but also a judgment and thus a conclusion for this story that everyone was having trouble bringing to an end. *The Court of Cacus* references Virgil's *Aeneid*. Hercules ravages the den of Cacus, "foul with human gore," and

> ... grasps his prey.
> The monster, spewing fruitless flames, he found;
> He squeez'd his throat, he writh'd his neck around,
> And in a knot his crippled members bound....
> Roll'd on a heap, the breathless robber lies.
> The doors, unbarr'd, receive the rushing day....
> Next, by the feet, they drag him from his den.
> The wond'ring neighborhood, with glad surprise,
> Behold his shagged breast, his giant size,
> His mouth that flames no more.
> (Book 6, trans. John Dryden)

At last, at least by allusion, we see inside Knox's dissecting room, and the doctor, we know, will get his comeuppance—presumably with Leighton as the avenging Hercules. Advertisements confirm *The Court of Cacus* as a necessary tale—a national trauma now confined in narrative:

In this volume the reader will find, for the first time, a narrative of the deeds of Burke and Hare, which will ever be remembered as the most extraordinary in the annals of a civilised people.... The Author has disposed the lights and shadows of this strange chapter of modern history so as to retain the absorbing interest of the story, without revolting the feelings of his readers; and has endeavoured to make the book a great moral lesson.[3]

Leighton's preface then specifies:

being satisfied that what has really occurred on the stage of the world, however involving the dignity of our nature or revolting to human feelings, must and will be known in some way... nay, was intended to be known by Him through whose permission it was allowed to be, I consider it a benefaction that the knowledge which kills shall be accompanied by the knowledge which cures. (*Court*, iii–iv)

The chronicle is impelled by religion; together, this mode and purpose of telling metaphorize events as a national cure whereby, we ultimately discover, medicine and malpractice produce God's will in the form of the Anatomy Act (79). In a familiar plot of nineteenth-century evangelical politics, time lines out causes into the effect of religion's grand narrative (e.g., Gladstone in Hilton, 342–43).

Enlightened and religious thinking here coalesce, for the novel's stadial notions of progression from savage to civilized complement teleological plots. Leighton aligns himself, his "public," "society," and "human feeling" (*Court*, iii). We readers constitute an advanced stage in a combined and doubly compelling narrative; Burke and Hare figure as a story of times past, kept comfortably apart from "our" moment. Such a "grim romance, so rich in specimens of a bypast phase of society," sets off "our social ameliorations" (11). Telling this tale is the literary equivalent of geology, by which "underlying strata in the physical world... tell us of a rudeness in Nature's workings from which she progresses to more perfect organisms" (11–12). The horrors of Burke and Hare belong in other times and to a more primitive people. And it is as a symptom of other times that they are allowed to test and inform the present. Within "the ways of Providence," Burke was "permitted to be an agent, selected after due care by the devil, to push and force those passions by which a Christian country, with a name renowned throughout the world for virtue, had been scourged and scathed to a climax" (78). Burke is actually sent to realign persons and plots and serve the causes of social and religious progress.

Burke and Hare thus stand as symptom and warning, but not as threat. They are out of time, and readjust our time, only by special permission from God. That is, they fill the role of exception within system. Burke and Hare fit the logic of enlightenment and religion both: they could fit Malthusian patterns, and Hare belongs to "the scroll, whereon were marked in fire the names of the reprobates" (83).

Yet their retrogression contravenes stadial imperatives, and they enjoy no Grace—"studying them in the distance, [it] had flown past them as an impossibility" (110). They manage to be conventional outsiders within the systems of enlightenment and religion, but outside these systems, too. In either case, importantly, they are therefore not us. Although "the world, notwithstanding grave faces and simpering moralities, contains within its circumference only a trifle fewer rogues than inhabitants, the residue [are] God's own—stern beings who have fought the devil at his own weapons and conquered" (216). In a book resonant with what "we have seen," and "we know," "we" participate in that "recoil of the good which isolates the criminal from the smiles of fellowship and the help of society" (e.g., 216, iv, 122).

Leighton works very hard to delimit the story of Burke and Hare. Despite his precise categorizations, however, the transposition of Burke and Hare into the period's dominant narratives and apparently straightforward systems points back to the difficulties that necessitated such cautious rearrangements of past and present in the first place. Leighton, in fact, protests too much. On the one hand, all is God's will: "the increase of depravity is the progression of degrees, all according to that law of nature whereby God wills to act by the regular process of cause and effect, each change helping another" (66). We live in God's "Great Drama" (77). But on the other hand, it is Burke and Hare (and perhaps Doctor Knox) who disport themselves on the stage. They enact the "play of the forenoon, and the melodrama of the night" (84). What is more, Hare is "a kind of lover of the play" (235). Predestination notwithstanding, these characters upstage the director. And they upstage not only God, but his stage manager Alexander Leighton. Their actions exceed the logic of the script, manifesting, Leighton admits:

> that irregularity... in the plot which imparts to the acting the incongruity so difficult to the analyses of the time. But while it in some measure interferes with the unity so congenial to the romancist... it presents us with a picture of human nature never before witnessed out of the domain of extravagant fiction. (170)

That is, Leighton's strategies, directed through Burke and Hare, point not to plot resolution but to themselves as stories.

Fiction begets fiction. One symptom that the narratives of enlightenment and religion cannot express or contain this tale is that although Leighton obsessively emphasizes these two discourses, the story again and again requires different terms and tries out different systems. None of these work, either. Hare, "With a low animal brow...justified the phrenologist by discovering no power of ratiocination" (102). Leighton therefore claims we might "term him...a fool or semi-idiot." He declares in some relief: "We thus get quit of the heavy imputation which the doings of such a man cast upon our kind." But immediately, the author has to admit: "Burke had both thought and sense to an extent which was rather a surprise to those who conversed with him"—in fact, he stimulated a debate about the validity of phrenology. Leighton tries psychology but recognizes that "after all this information, which was so industriously gleaned, the psychologist was not satisfied" (102). He even channels early Darwinian theory: "within the moralities of our species we have gorillas far fiercer than any brother or sister of that 'splendid specimen' described by Du Chaillu" (137). And as these supplemental systems pile up yet fail to resolve the story of Burke and Hare, they reveal themselves as competing fictions participating in an ever more anxious and many voiced conversation.

Under pressure to explain the same problem and so occupy the same literary space, Leighton's burgeoning discourses clash, contaminating one another. For instance, Leighton begins with what must have seemed a fitting metaphor: in a context where enlightened medicine invokes a religious perspective, he describes the combined crimes of medicine and mammon as "diseases" requiring "the cure which God has vouchsafed to our keeping" (6). Leighton considers events "a benefaction," presuming "the knowledge which kills shall be accompanied by the knowledge which cures" (iv). No doubt the metaphor was irresistible. It allowed the medically trained moral author to diagnose, in his phrase, "the real pathology of repentance" (255). But the combined weight of medical and religious expectation fractures the metaphor. Events are too awful for expression, even in the medical system that gave rise to them. Tales of horror are heard "from the lips of an ear-witness," and (most problematically if Leighton ever wanted to practice medically, as opposed to socially) Hare is "an apparition to the retina of the ear of mankind" (57, 80). Society's wounds gape again when the doctor as author cannot suture criminality even within the codes of metaphor. Indeed, this failure points to the story of Burke and Hare and Doctor Knox as a looming sign not readable according to any system. Lacking any clear meaning, it remains an ever-present danger.

With the bonds of metaphor broken, with even such limited restraint impossible, danger comes home to the reader. Worse, we may constitute that danger in ourselves. Leighton uses one term to align religion and enlightenment: "sympathy." Through Adam Smith and David Hume and on to the sentimental Victorians, sympathy in its various modes binds together the community of the good. Leighton thus predictably foregrounds the language of community against Burke and Hare, noting that "poor people feel intensely for each other's sorrows" (149). Sympathy is the test of the human. Helpfully, in 1828, Burke and Hare were devoid of it and fell beyond its reach. *Murderers of the Close* applauded the Edinburgh mob: "If they could have sympathised with the monster...we should, indeed, be afraid that the moral sense of the nation...was altogether extinguished" (*Murderers*, 265). Mild Mrs. Hughes wrote to Walter Scott: "it may be very unfeminine to say I am rather glad at the savage display of feeling at the execution of the wretched Burke: surely it was meet that his end should not be considered with the forbearance, & in some cases the sympathy which attends that of an ordinary criminal" (Letters to Scott [1829] NLS MS3908: 65). But it was the power of sympathy that brought Burke and Hare uncomfortably close to the good people of Scotland.

If Burke and Hare represent the underside of God's plan, everyone else must somehow be set on the right side of the equation. Knox's students, however, pose a bit of a problem, so Leighton seeks to address it by his transformative term: sympathy. The students now figure as sympathetic ingenues: "generous and well-bred youths [who] never entertained a suspicion of murder"; their dubious naïveté is "honourable to their estimate of mankind"—they are just too good, too sympathetic, to suspect (*Court*, 89). Yet the students' "sympathy" also connects them to less virtuous possibilities. It does not bond them with other people, rather it connects them to the selfishness of getting ahead. "The ardour of the study of anatomy was in the youth, and it was there from sympathy; yea, for years before, the Square and the College had been under the fervour of competition" (8). Their "sympathy" links them to that other side of Smith's social theorizing, the commodity capitalism that drives the wealth of nations. The students' sympathy encourages them into the graveyard and to the trade of bodysnatching. There, they are unsympathetic in themselves and to us: "Science became the Nemesis of the dearest and most sacred affections.... The midnight enterprises...were death to those feelings of a Christian people [that are] a natural and necessary part of a social fabric" (26). In fact, driven by "sympathy" to trading in bodies, Knox's students align with Burke and Hare. And if Burke and Hare trade in bodies, they too, then, draw near us through sympathy.

Not surprisingly, as a limit term subject to such qualification on the side of the good, "sympathy" turns out to be porous for Burke and Hare. Notoriously, bodysnatching epitomized the antisocial cost of commerce. Ruth Richardson tallies it up: "Corpses were bought and sold, they were touted, priced, haggled over, negotiated for, discussed in terms of supply and demand, delivered, imported, exported, transported"—and as we have seen, they were also manufactured and taken to market (Ruth Richardson, 72). Burke and Hare's innovation was recognized from the first as one in trade (*Murderers*, 1). Through system, trade turned to "traffic" (2, 43). Hare was a "calculating villain" determined to "purchase his own safety" (39).

However, it is part of Burke's business to emulate sympathy. In *The Court of Cacus*, he relieves a police officer of one hapless drunk, destined to be a victim, "with much apparent sympathy"—the crowd even "backed the sympathiser" (Leighton *Court*, 148). As for Hare, he makes a nonsense of this system, for in him we hear "the whine of self-sympathy" (252).

All Leighton's discourses and their metaphors come to nothing in the annals of Burke and Hare. They stand revealed not as defining systems but as fictions playing through and perhaps exploited by the self. They point, then, to us. And this is where Leighton's supposed limit term, "sympathy," at once reaches its zenith and collapses in a heap. The evils of Burke and Hare, Leighton concludes, are written in "sympathetic ink" (*Court*, 150). Thus it is only by our own breath, in ourselves, that they become visible. The sympathy that should bind the community and set us apart from Burke and Hare, once let loose as metaphor, brings us horribly together.

Perhaps this is why, in *The Court of Cacus*, Leighton stands back from the story he tells. "The romance-writer will come," he says, "at present, we are content with the office of chronicler" (161). Even Leighton's cautious chronicle inadvertently exposed systems as fictions and fictions as unstable, exploitable, and dangerous. Rather than healing the wounds of 1828, this book manifests them cutting deeper, and trenching ever wider. Through the multiplications of dialogue and the infections of metaphor, the scandal of Burke and Hare figures more and more as unintegratable anxiety about the Scottish self.

RELIGIOUS IMMUNITY? EVANGELISM AND THE LIMITS OF FICTION IN DAVID PAE

David Pae held to fiction. In 1861, Leighton's strategy demonstrated the difficulty of embracing this story as fact by continuing to leave out its central detail. Though he invokes history and religion to explain Burke and Hare, Leighton never looks closely at Doctor Knox. He hints at the doctor: Knox was known as one-eyed, and Leighton characterizes him as "the monoculous"; he implies a link between "Cyclopic" crimes and the doctor through his nickname "old Cyclops" (Leighton *Court*, 86, 181; Lonsdale, 275). Knox is guilty of "winking toleration" (*Court*, 204). From his window, he turns his sights dangerously on those who would gaze upon and understand him, "threatening to shoot the officials of the law if they dared to question for the ends of justice so innocuous and ill-used a victim of public prejudice" (222). He wants to "subjugate all people to his will," using the interestingly visual strategy of "whitewashing" (228). Yet Leighton cannot get a clear view, so we are left with "suspicion" (229). In 1858, however, Pae had already placed Knox at the center of romance.

Doctor Knox occupies the middle eight chapters of the serial novel *Lucy, The Factory Girl* (1858–59).[4] This means that again, the story of Burke and Hare stands central to a religious plot. Since 1853, Pae had been famous as a millennialist. In that year, he published *The Coming Struggle*, which read current events according to prophecy and placed Britain prominently within the events of the last days—due to begin in 1866. In the context of the revolutions of 1848, "the end has come.... [In the prophets we can] trace almost accurately the regular course of events down to the beginning of the thousand years" (rpt. in Pae *Lucy*, 308). Burke and Hare and Doctor Knox fit nicely into this tale of millennial progress. Indeed, Walter Scott had initiated the discourse in 1829, when he brought together the day's most popular (and Scottish) millennialist and prophet, Edward Irving, and the horrors of the West Port: "Whether we shall at last eat each other, as of yore," he joked to Maria Edgeworth, "or whether the earth will get a flap with a comet's tail first, who but the reverend Mr Irving will venture to pronounce?" (*Letters*, 11:128). Irving's theological heir, David Pae, was ready to pronounce, and the grand narrative of millennialism, with the end in sight, should force an end to Burke and Hare and Doctor Knox.

Lucy, then, stands firmly situated in two dominant and dominating narratives, for (with its subtitle "The Secrets of the Tontine Close") the tale is also undeniably a sensation novel. The advertisement in its host newspaper, the *North Briton*, makes clear the story's position between fact and fiction, religion and sensation:

> This tale will embrace many phases of character, and contain much that is fitted to interest, to amuse, and to instruct. The plot is a very fascinating one.... It takes in most of the phases of Glasgow life, but deals principally with those of labour and crime—with honest industry and dishonest actions. It will take the reader into the homes—the humble but virtuous homes—of the city operatives... into the mansions of merchants and employers... and into the haunts of vice and crime, where in dark closes and secluded buildings are congregated those who have bid farewell to honesty, sobriety, and virtue, whose industry is exerted in the direction of fraud, robbery, and even murder. And yet, dark and romantic as the tale will appear, it will be true, awfully, solemnly true. (*Lucy*, xviii)

Of course *Lucy*, with Doctor Knox relocated to Glasgow, and an entirely fictional cast of supporting characters, cannot be "true." But it can be simultaneously millennialist and truthful, and factual yet fictive. Moreover, in a Glasgow sensation novel religion and medicine inevitably meet. Pae's city includes "lovely domestic scenes... mansions... and dark closes and secluded buildings." In an era when evangelism and medical reform together had turned to social engineering via sanitary reorganization of whole cityscapes—particularly Glasgow, and particularly through

Irving's mentor Thomas Chalmers—light, in the end, will shine into every window, illuminating and regularizing the landscape of Scotland (Brown, ch. 3; Gilbert; Day). With an appropriate place for everything, and everything healthily in its place, this novel should put Doctor Knox in *his* place.

What bonds the sensational, religious, and medical narratives is the community in which they are necessarily enacted. Pae shows us a community at risk. The place reeks of contagion that extends from the warrens of the Tontine Close with its "underground chambers, into which no light from above could come.... suggestive of crimes and deeds of darkest character" to a "handsome house in Blythswood Square" by way of a vast new cotton mill (Pae *Lucy*, 21, 234, 219). Here, human sympathy meets its test:

> Beneath the strong, whirling, bubbling, seething, foaming river of city experience there is an undercurrent continually flowing. Busy as men are, buying and selling and getting gain, they must, per force, endure the experience of their human natures. The storm of trade and commerce rushing above cannot enable them to get quit of the hopes and fears, the passions and feelings of the heart. These were meant to be ministered to by commerce... unfortunately men have reversed the order and made the heart the minister of commerce, crushing, or trying to crush, its warm and true impulses into the cold, narrow, selfish views which the mere commercial spirit engenders. (217)

In this industrial era "Newgate novel," rife with competition and commodification, children are stolen and their rights usurped, women fall, men are hurt. Villains abuse private relations and public trust. Daniel Dexter, who has stolen his six-year-old niece's inheritance and cast her on the world, all to support his business, declares: "Bah!... We must all play the game of life as skilfully as we can, and if others suffer by our moves, that is their misfortune, not our blame" (9). The narrator can only lament: "God help thee, thou little lamb [Lucy]!... human fiends... will sully thy budding nature with the pestilential breath of direct sin" (20). Commerce connects the socially sick to the spiritually pure, spreading like a disease of the soul.

Thus far, *Lucy* refracted the pervasive feeling that Burke and Hare and Doctor Knox had disrupted community. Indeed, J. G. Bertram, Pae's editor at the *North Briton*, himself published *The Story of a Stolen Heir* in the same year as *Lucy*. Here, Burke's sister-in-law receives stolen children (with all the threat of burking that implies), thereby subverting inheritances and undermining families. However Pae's book features not just Burkean villains, but also its Thomas Chalmers: the aptly named Mr. Clanworth, "a true religious philanthropist," who carries the generosity of Christianity to the city's darkest places (*Lucy*, 142). It even has its public-spirited doctor: "a smart, mild man, of middle height, with a frank, open countenance.... he was one of your free-and-easy sort, off-handed and good-natured, a careless sort of fellow, who was not accustomed to stick at trifles"—"Doctor Knox" (125). Together, they should constitute Glasgow's social ministry, working to heal mind and body.

Furthermore, the human spirit proves resilient: "it will not be so tutored and trained [toward commerce and competition]. It will assert its true instincts" (*Lucy*, 217). Usually, "between the selfishness and cruelty of Mammon and the heaven-directed desires of the heart...there is a bitter contest, in which the heart generally comes off at the worst" (217). This community, by contrast, constantly rebuilds itself under all attacks. Women fallen into commodity give a kindness they never received; new families are formed from the halt and the lame; old families get reconnected despite the gulf of sin that has intervened. And from the start, we readers form part of this unlikely community. But interestingly, we are invited to join on our ability to decide who belongs and who cannot. "You already don't like this middle-aged man, then?" the narrator asks us of Dexter. "[You] are convinced that he is not one of the best of men; nay, you are prepared to find him, on a closer acquaintance, heartless, unscrupulous, selfish, cruel...? Well, it is a thousand chances to one that you are right" (5). However in Pae's discourse of atonement and inclusion, even democracy, villains repent and atone. Dexter, forgiven, abases himself before family and God (283–85). Only one person cannot fit: Doctor Robert Knox.

Knox appears in the novel's second "lost child" plot. Here, he is invited by the community in formation to attend to a child reminiscent of "Daft Jamie." Jamie was the simple and malformed victim whose death particularly appealed to pathos and evoked outrage in 1828. Edinburgh had known Jamie well, and held him in affection. His murder provoked much sentimental and accusing poetry. For instance:

> You was simple, inoffensive,
> Loved by all where e'er you went,
> And their little bounties cheer'd you,
> And their smiles made you content....
>
> You who bought and used his body,
> Surely you was much to blame,
> In concealing thus a murder,
> For you must have known the same.
>
> If your conscience had allowed you,
> But for once the truth to tell,
> But the craft had been in danger,

Had you stopped these imps of Hell.
(Lines Supposed to Have Been Written by Mrs Wilson)

So Pae's Doctor Knox is brought front and center in a test of community that unites religion, medicine, and the West Port murders.

Alas, the doctor fails. Knox efficiently diagnoses corporeal ills, but there is something about Willie (the Jamie surrogate) that he cannot evaluate. With his "large lustrous eyes...set in a wan and pale face," Willie is "unusually striking" (*Lucy*, 103). Knox is duly struck. "'I never, in all my life—saw—such—eyes,' muttered the doctor.... 'Wonderful they are—positively inexplicable.... Such a depth, such a lustre, such a far, wondering, searching light. I *never* saw such eyes'" (127). Of course, for the doctor, the way to understanding this oddity lies through anatomy. And obligingly, the patient dies. Thereafter follow grave robbing and the threat of dissection for the commodity that is now poor Willie. But Knox has completely missed the point. He not only disturbs the community of the living here but also the hosts of heaven. For Willie's lustrous gaze is not anatomical: it comes from the soul.

Worse, Knox is given criminal connections. His anatomical obsession makes him the link between the various plots of lost wills and stolen children, bringing Willie's community into danger. When Knox needs a couple of bodysnatchers (to disinter Willie), he turns to Shuffle and Sleek—the same caricaturish lawyers who have already bilked Lucy out of her inheritance. They, in turn, connect his activities to murder, suggesting that "our friends.... would have had one or two [bodies] a month ago, but [we were] disappointed" (*Lucy*, 148). Those "one or two" would have been the freshly murdered bodies of Lucy and her protector, Sal (70). So if Knox is associated with criminals, implicated in murder, and made the conduit for vice, surely he is finally placed as unpleasant fact in fiction? As the rest of society regularizes, Knox should stand exposed. At last, we might imagine, the doctor gets what society thinks he deserves.

Yet this plot, too, fails to express Doctor Knox. Although Knox stands in the middle of the novel, he arises in a subplot. In addition, we see Knox at an undetermined date. The story concludes, after a time lapse, "very near the Glasgow of modern times"—which would be 1858 (*Lucy*, 217). Within the novel, it is twelve years, plus a few, since we met Doctor Knox. This places Knox sometime previous to 1846. But when? Knox worked briefly in Glasgow after his 1842 departure from Edinburgh, and between stints as a peripatetic lecturer and in London (Rae, 125–34). Yet no one recognizes him for previous nefarious pursuits in the sister city. Then in the middle of the book, after only a moment of community and religious upbraiding, the doctor falls from view:

Dr Knox was standing... before a large table. On the table lay an object.

The missionary [Mr. Clanworth] sprang forward and arrested the doctor's right arm. A moment later, and the ruined temple would have been spoiled. As yet it lay in all the completeness in which death had left it.

The doctor turned quickly round.

"What means this intrusion?" he demanded angrily.

"Forbear—touch it not," said the missionary....

"By what authority do you thus dictate?" asked the doctor....

"By the authority of God and nature!" was the impressive reply.

"How! What mean you?"

"This is Willie's father" [Clanworth's brother].

The doctor fell a pace or two backwards, and remained mute. He durst not utter another word in such a presence....

(174–75)

This is the last we hear of Doctor Knox. In fact, lacking Knox, Pae eventually wrapped up his serial in other terms, and rather abruptly. His publisher complained: "This is very strange.... the least thing you could have done was to have intimated your intention of closing a fortnight or three weeks ago.... you know the custom [of giving notice that a serial will conclude]" (from James Bertram, April 6, 1859, Pae papers). Knox, his plot displaced to Glasgow and unfixed in time, proves a slippery subject— perhaps a subject we are reluctant to grasp—even when constrained by the deterministic narratives of sensation and the end of times.

It is a testament to the interest and the anxiety generated by the West Port murders—and their salability—that Pae returned to them in 1864. If Leighton had found himself embroiled in dialogue between systems rather than with Knox, and Pae had so far extended only a cautious, thoroughly fictionalized grasp in the direction of the doctor, with Knox dead since 1862, surely now Scotland's authors could get a grip on him, and make him speak as national plots required. *Mary Paterson* promises that this will be the case. Bearing the subtitle "*The Fatal Error*" and the tag "A Story of the Burke and Hare Murders," this serial novel makes the 1828 scandal the heart and fiber of its tale. Mary (see figure 3.3) was the "girl of the town" murdered by Burke and Hare, recognized by Knox's assistants, pickled for months in order to demonstrate perfect musculature at the appropriate time, and meanwhile, it was said, sketched by student artists in positions disturbingly reminiscent of Venus—simultaneously classical and vaguely pornographic (*West Port Murders*, 126; Paterson, 6–9; Lonsdale, 101 and n.1; Kaufman, "Another Look").[5] Pae's narrative follows this cynosure of the medical gaze from her girlhood through her encounter with Helen McDougal to the Edinburgh of Burke and Hare. It also

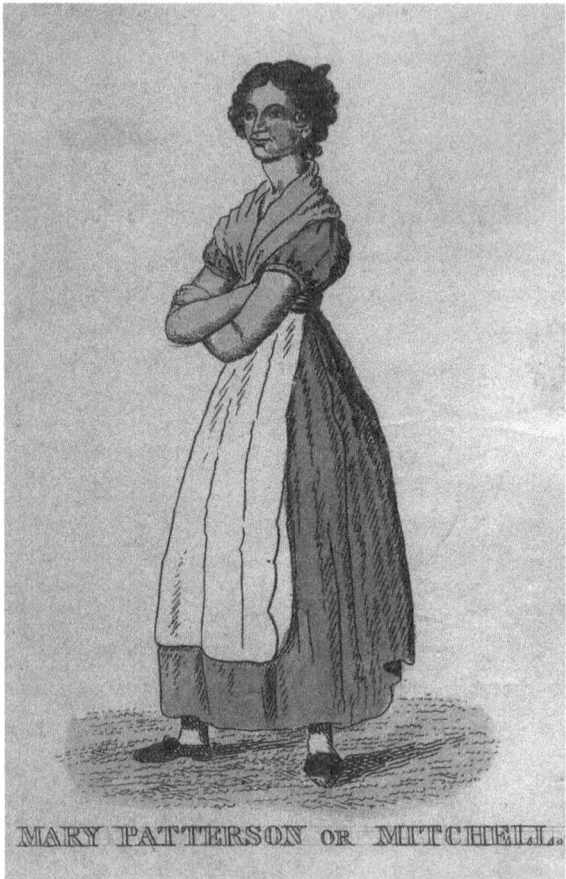

FIGURE 3.3 "Mary Paterson or Mitchell." Contemporary print, tinted. Courtesy of the Royal College of Physicians of Edinburgh.

tracks the fictional ramifications of Mary's life through her friends and descendants. The newspaper preface makes the strategy clear:

> Those who are old enough to remember the time will readily testify that a sensation equal to that which the discovery of these murders produced has never occurred since, and we doubt much if it has its parallel in any age; while at the present day, after the lapse of nearly forty years, the names of Burke and Hare are invested with horror, though the nature and details of their crimes are but partially known to this generation.
> In the following story the history of these crimes will be fully embodied.
> (*Dundee... People's Journal* [DPJ], July 9, 1864: 2)

The West Port murders are slipping from memory. At this moment when testimony is still possible, fiction will lock them within the sequences of history. Now, presumably, we will achieve the poetic justice of embodying the anatomist and his assistants on the dissecting table of prose and subjecting them to the public gaze. But even still, Pae comes no closer to the doctor.

The story is suffused with poetic justice. Not only does everyone get what they deserve, the story's success was itself a victory over Knox and his cohort. Burke and Hare notoriously preyed on their own people, the underclass of Edinburgh. *Murderers of the Close* worried that the victims' low status delayed the discovery of their murder—for who cared about them (*Murderers*, 176)? Knox increased this anxiety, for he abjured any criticism as merely the work of the mob. When Edinburgh gathered outside the lecture rooms where he continued to teach but not to explain, Knox posed his students against these "ruffians" as a "phalanxed body of gentlemen" against cowards, and in 1870, Lonsdale shows the force of that opinion by repeating it—the problem arises from "The lowest rabble of the Old Town," "surging *plebs*," a "clamorous mob" (Lonsdale, 111, 79, 81). Notably, then, Pae first serialized *Mary Paterson* in the *Dundee People's Journal*.[6] The *Journal* was a paper of and for the people, remembered on the death of its publisher, John Leng, as "a new departure in journalism... made possible by the cheapening of paper, improvements in printing, and the abolition of the stamp duty. Its appeal was made principally to the intelligent working classes" ("Memoir," *Evening Telegraph and Post* December 13, 1906). William Donaldson places it "in the forefront of advanced Liberalism" (Donaldson, 28). The paper "campaigned ceaselessly for extension of the franchise, and a whole range of social and economic reforms, particularly those affecting the working class with whose interests [it] remained identified." At the time of *Mary Paterson*, the editor was William Latto. Donaldson calls him "a typical Victorian autodidact... studying English grammar while he worked from a text book attached to his loom" (28). Under Latto, the *Journal* manifested "unique openness to its readers... [eager] to act as a platform for their opinions and experiences," and the paper not only printed working-class correspondence, it "[commissioned] and [printed]... leading articles by working men" (29). Its international reputation for liberalism was such that in 1864—the year of *Mary Paterson*—Garibaldi wanted to visit (to John Leng, June 1, 1864, DCL Leng Collection). Graham Law notes that by the time *Lucy* appeared, the *Journal* was already "issued in a number of regional editions and thus one of the most widely circulating weekly papers published outside London" (*Lucy*, viii). *Mary Paterson* helped push sales from 61,200 the week before it began, to 68,900 in the week Mary was murdered, and on to 84,000 the week it concluded (each week's sales figures appear in the next issue). The story of a fallen woman and her murder proved too much for the tender readers of one Yorkshire paper, for there the story was pulled "in consequence of the unusual sensational character of some of the incidents, and the repeated remonstrances of many of our subscribers."[7] In Scotland, however, the story sold exponentially, and built a career for David Pae, the miller's son. In 1869, he became editor of the *People's Journal* (*Lucy*, 304). At last, it would seem, the people were getting to take control of their traumatic past.

Of course, the story may have taken so well because it fitted generic expectations exactly. At a time when Scotland was deep in temperance campaigns, Mary's fall leads her to drink, and drink leads to death. Historically, Burke and Hare and their victims swam in a sea of alcohol. Now that fact meets the requirements of the moral tale. Pae himself was a noted advocate of temperance. His papers include a frustrated letter from J. G. Bertram, his editor at the *North Briton*, declining Pae's suggestion to attack intemperance head-on: "if you mixed with *all classes* of the public of Edinr as I do, and did not confine yourself to a few teetotal [friends] you would long ago have been of my opinion.... The kind of paper you would like the N. B. to become is no doubt a good kind, but my dear friend *it wouldn't pay*" (from J. G. Bertram, August 6, 1858, Pae papers). And Pae duly collected Horatius Bonar's tract on "Christian Witness-Bearing against the Sin of Intemperance" that decries censorious attacks on the drinking public as ineffective (Pae papers). Certainly, by the time he wrote *Mary Paterson*, Pae had figured out how to go about his temperance campaigning both more overtly and less directly. His Burke has "idle inclinations and drunken habits"; the first victim has "one failing—a liking for whisky" that she shares with most subsequent victims and that prepares her for slaughter (Pae *Mary Paterson*, 46, 56). The narrator imagines the response at Surgeons' Hall: "Wasn't the Scotch a whisky-drinking people, and hadn't these creatures died of *delirium tremens*?" (76). And he comments that victim Joe the Miller "was one of many thousands whom strong drink has enchained and destroyed" (81).

The characters of *Mary Paterson* also participate in the sentimental "kailyard" plot then under formation in Scotland: Mary wilfully leaves her father's house, and her departure causes his death, for "Nae suner had yer father read yer letter than he gied a deep groan and fell back in his chair. He had taen a stroke o' palsy, and ne'er spak' again. In four oors he breathed his last" (14–15, 44). Readers caught this plot, too—even responding, at Mary's death on October 1, 1864, in appropriate verse:

In grief she went to Edinburgh,
And lived a life of shame,
Until that murderers, Burke and Hare,
Extinguished her name.

All ye young maidens beware
How youth's gay moments fly;
And you should have yourselves prepared,
Ere you in dust do ly.
(*DPJ* October 8, 1864)

Furthermore, this kailyard plot echoes a religious dynamic: Mary listens to "the voice of the serpent" in the whispers of her lover, and thus "fell, 'fell by her own consent'" (*Mary Paterson*, 6, 4). "What can be said in extenuation of her folly, her crime?" the narrator ponders: "Not much. After all that could be said, it was crime and folly still" (4). Even on the brink of her falling victim to Burke, it is still Mary's sexual and religious plot that matters: "The daughter of the God-fearing Scotch elder was not ignorant that she yielded to what was sin, and what no love or sanction could cover, and the Divine law of consequence recognises no palliation in the betraying circumstances" (112). Mary thus bears the blame of Calvinism alongside the pathos of sensation. Finally, with Mary fallen from her father's house by wilfully giving over her will to another, she originates the standard plot of the lost will. The final third of the book revolves around her illegitimate son, his usurpation, and his return to his own.

Importantly, this combination of generic imperatives opens new pathways toward closure in the story of Burke and Hare. Now, the murderers can be staged as both villainous and reprobate. Burke "had confessed his crimes, but neither with regret nor remorse. Humanity, which he had crushed out of him did not return, even at this last hour of retribution" (*Mary Paterson*, 227). That aberration finally allows readers the satisfaction of a just response. At Burke's execution, "All ranks and classes were there.... the immense majority was composed of respectable and intelligent people, come there not to gloat over the spectacle of a human being put to death, but to satisfy their indignant and outraged feelings" (225). Indeed, "Humanity"—acting out Mrs. Hughes's dark side—"would not have been true to itself if it had acted towards these wretches in any other way" (253). And fiction allows Hare's wife, in her flight, to be swept from the deck of a ship to drown in the no-man's-land of the Irish Sea (262). McDougal, hounded from Edinburgh (see figure 3.4), now freezes to death in a field, and "Weeks after, when the heavy and long-continued snow-storm slowly vanished...the dead emaciated body of a woman was found lying on the ground far across the moor.... It was impossible to identify the body, for the hungry rats or other vermin had eaten away the flesh off the face" (*Mary Paterson*, 251). More positively, the Grays, who in reality discovered the body of the last victim and refused to be bribed into silence, are recast by fiction into unfortunates undermined by intemperance. In the context of religion and sensation, their story transforms into a redemptive tale of atonement with all the additional gratification of sentimental resolution.

The novel's assemblage of genres provides some closure even to the period's vexed question of the sensation novel. Dallas Liddle argues that in the 1860s, "many reviewers who were also working novelists...agreed that [sensational themes and techniques] produced not only bad and immoral art, but inferior social criticism and incorrect psychology" (Maunder ed., 98). Pae's newspaper preface declares:

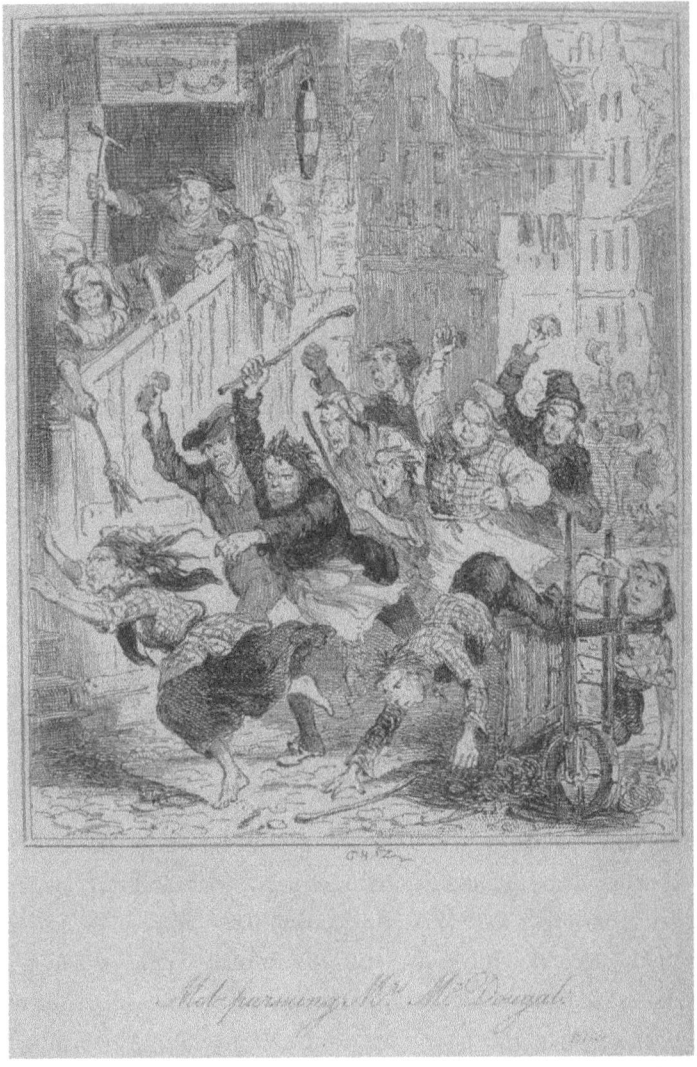

FIGURE 3.4 "Mob pursuing Mrs. McDougal." Engraving by "Phiz" (Hablot Knight Browne, illustrator for Charles Dickens), from Camden Pelham, *The Chronicles of Crime, or The Newgate Calendar* vol. 2 (London: T. Tegg, 1841), opp. p. 173. Courtesy of the General Research Division, The New York Public Library, Astor, Lenox and Tilden Foundations.

It seems fitting that at a time when sensation novels are so popular, and so vehemently denounced by certain critics as monstrous conceptions, utterly untrue to nature, that the narrative should be reproduced of deeds so utterly surpassing in atrocity anything described in nature, if for no other purpose than to show that the sensation novels of the present day do not produce such gross exaggerations of human wickedness as their decriers assert. In fact, after such atrocities as the Burke and Hare murders, it is impossible for any romance writer to depict either fabulous or exaggerated deeds of human crime; and, *provided they carry faithfully and prominently their lessons with them*, the production and popularity of stories of this character is not to be deplored. Human nature is not to be improved by "concealing its worst deformities." (*DPJ* July 9, 1864: 2)

To effect such closure, however, Pae steps away from the terms of the originating tale.

Like *Lucy*, this serial novel falls into the three-decker form. *Mary Paterson* focuses first on the heroine's fall, then on Burke and Hare, and ends by tracking the protagonists' various friends and descendants through to a displaced atonement and redemption (in rural Scotland, then Ireland). All this is made possible by emphasizing the theme of community. At the start of the book, Mary meets Helen McDougal, who acts as midwife for her illegitimate child and introduces her to Burke well before she gets to Edinburgh, thus destroying the traditional community; at the close, Mary's faithful lover James Crawford incites righteous indignation at Burke's execution, upbraids her seducer, acts as substitute parent for her child, marries the abandoned love of Joe the Miller (aptly named "Lizzie Fairbairn"), and retrieves Mary's fortune for her son. This is just a sampling of the novel's tightly woven relationships. Yet even so tight and tidy a weave cannot bind Doctor Knox. He never figures fully as himself, or in the terms of the scandal.

Pae does come close. His journalistic speculations about what the doctors know verge to conclusions:

> Here was a man, a perfect stranger to these doctors, who offered a dead body for sale, and it was bought and no questions asked—not one simple interrogation as to how the body had been procured; and not only so, but an invitation was given to bring more.... Was it possible that the idea never occurred to the doctors that the subjects which they bought so freely, and paid for with a comparatively large sum, *might* have been got in a criminal way?... We cannot think so. We are forced to believe that with them the exigencies of science were made paramount, and that they made it a point to ask no questions, lest they should be put in possession of dangerous knowledge. But the fact is, the principle of their procedure was immoral.... it was impossible that a system, illicit in every sense, should not lead to crimes of the worst description; and of these crimes we must consider the doctors *presumptively* guilty. (*Mary Paterson*, 52–53)

Moreover, Pae holds Knox specifically in mind. When Burke and Hare deliver their first, naturally dead body to Surgeons' Square, "a smart, fussy, self-consequential man, wearing spectacles, entered.... This was Doctor Knox who rapidly ran his eye over the

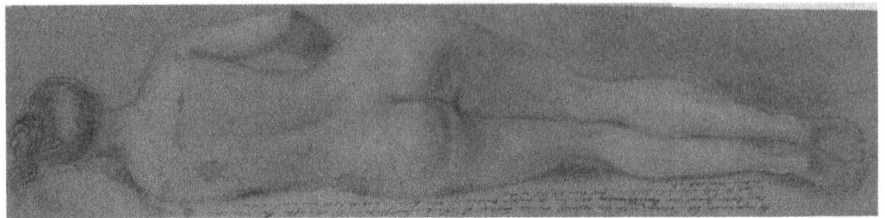

FIGURE 3.5 Sketch of "Mary Paterson," [1828?]. Courtesy of the National Library of Scotland, Ry.III.a.6 (5).

body, and simply said—'Seven pounds ten'" (52). For the first time, too, we see Knox bend over a corpse—the body of our fallen heroine, Mary Paterson (see figure 3.5):

> The corpse was cold now, but not stiff and when the murderers tossed it roughly upon a dark table, it lay there like a reclining marble statue, beautifully faultless in all its proportions, while the long tresses of hair, which had once been the pride of the wearer...lay coiled upon the snowy neck, and trailed half-way along the table....
>
> Knox...ran his eye slowly over the motionless form.
>
> "She has been a *very* pretty girl, that," he remarked after several moments of silent inspection. "Upon my word I never saw a more beautiful body."
>
> ...So pleased was Dr. Knox with the "thing" that he told his cashier to give fourteen pounds for it—the largest sum these men had yet received for the articles in which they trafficked. (*Mary Paterson*, 123–25)

We even see Knox at the moment of exposure. As the Superintendent of Police, officer Fisher, Walter Gray, and the police surgeon inspect the box containing the last victim, they are interrupted, hearing:

> a loud, authoritative "Hem" behind them, and, turning round, they beheld Dr. Knox standing in the cellar.
>
> "What's the matter, gentlemen?" he asked....
>
> "We have come about this body which was brought here last night," replied the [police surgeon]. "There is a suspicion that it has been murdered."
>
> "Murdered!" echoed Knox. "Oh, nonsense—ridiculous!"...
>
> "May I ask, doctor, if you have got any other bodies from this man?"
>
> "I decline to answer the question," was the answer, very stiffly delivered.
>
> "But the ends of justice may require an answer," observed the superindendent.
>
> "Once for all, sir, allow me to say that I decline answering all questions," said the professor, in a cold and haughty manner. (170)

Nor does the doctor ever answer—no more than he answered in 1828 or in *The Court of Cacus*. But interestingly, here, the case is not his to answer.

By the logic of the plot, the cause of Mary's demise lies not in Doctor Knox's dissecting rooms, but in her first fall and subsequent drunkenness. Mary has been marked and held personally responsible as intemperate since the beginning of her novelistic career, when her lack of sexual restraint leads to alcoholism. One drunken bout, which occurs after she has caught sight of her seducer in Edinburgh, prepares her drinking companions, Mary Haldane and her daughter, for sacrifice (*Mary Paterson*, 71–76). Another puts Mary side by side in the pub with Burke on the prowl (113). Further, although a doctor begins Mary's downward career, it is not Knox. Rather, it is Duncan Grahame: "a young man—young in years, but old in the knowledge of sin. He had been two sessions at the Edinburgh University, and there had his knowledge been acquired.... The youth was a medical student" (4). Sin and medicine are linked, but in the personal crime of sexual intemperance and seduction.

Nonetheless, doctors are brought close to responsibility. Grahame is the student who recognizes Mary on the slab (124). Picking up from the *Caledonian Mercury*'s suggestion that Burke acted with medical advice or implements, Pae has Grahame's doctor-for-hire, attending on the fallen Mary, teach Burke how to commit his crimes (*Mercury* January 5, 1829: 3; January 8: 2). Pleased at the fee for dealing with Grahame's by-blow, Burke ponders other easy ways of making money. Doctor Ford gives him ideas, gossiping:

> Were I a stronger man than you, or had another to help me, I could have you dead in a quarter of an hour, and leave nothing by which the best doctor in the country could say how you had died....
>
> All that I would have to do would be to press my hand firmly on your nose and mouth.... Then I would leap upon your chest with my knees.... In two minutes, I tell you, you would die for want of air. (*Mary Paterson*, 31)

The doctor even recommends making the victim "helplessly drunk." Lest we should miss this connection, before she freezes in a snowdrift, Helen McDougal happens upon the doctor, and makes it for us: "'You once told Burke the way to do it, and he never forgot it.'... Dr. Ford was struck dumb.... He felt that, however unintentionally, he was remotely connected with the Burke and Hare murders" (243). But even as Ford is connected, Knox is summarily set aside. Not only did he not entice Mary Paterson to her doom, not only did he not teach Burke and Hare their trade, the grand authority of Helen McDougal declares: "[Knox] didn't know they were murdered.... People may say as they like, but he didn't know it" (243). The doctors are held responsible, but not for what anybody actually did in Surgeons' Square. The chain of causes and effects yet again fails to link in Doctor Knox.

We might presume, however, that the voice of the Fourth Estate settles matters. The story opens by reminding readers of its national context:

> A more respectable or a better respected man than old Andrew Paterson did not live in or near the village of Kirkton. This little Scotch village is.... very near the centre of Scotland, and in close proximity to scenes consecrated forever to the memory of the nation's struggle for independence, many of its inhabitants were strongly tinged with the nobler Scottish characteristics—religious and national. (*Mary Paterson*, 1)

The newspaper version of the novel emphasizes steady steps toward bringing this national tale to a close at last. There, the tale ends in two chapters over two weeks— XLII: "After Twenty Years," and XLIII: "The Fate of Hare—Conclusion" (*DPJ*, April 15 and 22, 1865). In these two chapters, the plots of the lost will, legal and religious, are wrapped up together: another woman fallen and scorned, who has restored Mary's child to his inheritance, tells the end of William Hare. "We shall, in our turn, relate it to the reader in our own words," the narrator says, going on in the newspaper: "and it will be found to form a natural conclusion to the tale" (*Mary Paterson*, 408; *DPJ*, April 15: 2). Then newspaper and novel end together:

> And so, kind reader, we bring this "owre true tale" to a close. It has led us into a very dark region of human cruelty and depravity. We have had to chronicle deeds and depict scenes which must have made the flesh creep and the blood run cold. Our sympathy, our pity, our indignation have all been stirred; but have we not, even in this dark and murky sphere of human crime, obtained glimpses also of human love and goodness? and [*sic*] have we not seen, on the whole, the workings of justice and mercy?—teaching us that for wrong-doing there is punishment, and for right-doing ultimate peace and prosperity—that there is for repentance forgiveness, and for brave and patient endurance deliverance and rest. Let us learn these various lessons, and live and act under their influence, never forgetting to offer, in utmost earnestness of soul, the daily petition—"LEAD US NOT INTO TEMPTATION, BUT DELIVER US FROM EVIL." (*Mary Paterson*, 413)

Reprinted in the *Sheffield Daily Telegraph*, the novel pushes the point further again, concluding its preface: "[this story] WILL ALSO CONTAIN lessons of important instruction, and scenes of fairest beauty, to prove the more glorious truth, that man's origin is divine, and his true aspirations heavenward" (October 28, 1865). Echoing Leighton's concerns—and more than once—Pae assures us that this tale really is finished.

In fact, the story is done to death in the massed terms of chronicle, fiction, and religion. It ends in a flurry of reprobacy and retribution—what Pae calls "the very acme of poetical justice" (*Mary Paterson*, 412). Edinburgh had longed to do away with William Hare—"The Burke Mania" recounts the practice of "Hare Hunting" in 1829 (RCPEd STR-SM 5.22). Now Mary's seducer, long since cast out of Edinburgh and fled to penury in Ireland, recognizes Mr. Hare, a man on the tramp and at the end of his rope. This proves to be literally the case, for the loose-lipped Doctor Grahame, who has (fittingly) declined into alcoholic intemperance, drunkenly tells the locals, and a mob summarily hang the West Port murderer. Society's avenger, however, turns out to be the unwitting son of Hare himself. That son next kills the doctor, then flees and dies in the morass of Ireland (*Mary Paterson*, 408–12). "Poor Mary!" Pae sums up. "Her wrongs were now avenged as far as earthly retribution could go" (412). Furthermore, in a coincidence we are repeatedly told is "wonderful," Mary's son by Grahame is at hand for the denouement (407, 412). The sins of the fathers are thus both visited on and removed from the children. In an upsurge of Grace this boy, now gratefully fatherless as well as motherless, stands a restored heir to the knowledge of God and the petty cash.

These are the ways of Providence. Memory, which might fade or wander, is restored and even trumped. Fiction supplements the "strictly historical" story of the newspaper preface, allowing a resolution at once poetic and, in religious terms, the Truth. Yet this is a false memory, and not just because it depends upon fiction. Pae's story, too, undermines its terms. We are told again and again that this is a tale motivated by intemperance; Mary and a succession of victims fall through a wilfulness metaphorized as drunkenness. But the worst of criminals, William Hare, does not fit the pattern: "He was so utterly callous and hardened, so cruel and pitiless, as to be able to do his part of the deed without either a previous stimulant or a subsequent sedative. There was still a faint shadow of humanity in Burke's soul, but none in his—he seemed to be wholly a fiend" (*Mary Paterson*, 178). Through Hare, intemperance actually becomes a sign of the human, and Hare himself therefore falls outside categorization.

Similarly, although the book works and works to fold the events of 1828 into fiction, with all its impetus for cause, effect, and resolution, William Burke is a past master both at telling a tale and at making himself part of someone else's story. Time and again he claims kin with some unfortunate and thereby draws them to their death: "Och, musha! and is this yer own self?" he exclaims to one old woman, "pretending to recognize her" (*Mary Paterson*, 58). Before long, she gives him the key to her plot: "Maybe ye was ane o' the Irish child's [*sic*] that lodged next door wi' Katy

Finlayson?" "Sure, and I was," Burke lies, "I thought you would remember me" (58). Where history cannot be systematized, and is rerouted through the dialogical forms of fiction, we should be careful who we talk to in the street. Fictions can be replotted, and memories can be remade. They can even replot themselves. By this text's own logic, then, justice, is "poetic," not real, and the Truth may be merely poetry—a sensation novel, after all.

THE PREDICAMENT OF PROPHECY: TRUTH OR FICTION?

Pae himself may have known the impossibility of constraining the past within the codes of fiction. He may even have understood the past's variability within the supposedly trumping discourse of prophecy. His millennial tract, *The Coming Struggle*, stood as a response to the Enlightenment and to its methods. When it was published in 1853, the world seemed fallen into disarray. The past was confused, the future unclear. For Pae, the answers lay in prophecy. But "authorised interpreters," those who proceeded within system and code, from Pae's perspective had confused things further (*Lucy*, 308). With the end of times upon us, David Pae would set us right. Pae invoked the Truth, "throwing off a host of commentaries" (308). But his inspiration itself had a source and a method. Pae referenced the American John Thomas, who had recently been heard in Britain (1848; Thomas's followers were known as Thomasites, and later, Christadelphians). In his efforts to render prophetic text as present fact, Pae clearly credits Thomas: "Dr Thomas of America was the first to find the key" (*Lucy*, 308–9). Thomas, however, thought that Pae had plagiarized him, misquoted him, and ripped him off. He immediately rewrote Pae's pamphlet and reissued it under the same title, but added a preface that sliced up David Pae:

> [*The Coming Struggle* takes] several vulnerable positions...[and draws] unscriptural conclusions....
>
> ...I have expurgated it....I have made three hundred and twelve corrections on the thirty-two pages, which have materially altered the sense....
>
> I am not able to say who the artist is that has undertaken to work up my published ideas of things into "The Coming Struggle."...Be he whom he may, he must be greatly astonished at the success of his doings. Seventy-three thousand sterling six-pences must have afforded him a wonderful profit on the copy of Elpis Israel, out of which he fabricated his pages.[8]

The Truth, apparently, is not universal, but bears a copyright. So Pae, of all people, is reworked through the discourse of prophecy into a literary robber baron. But in

1881, Thomas himself would be accused of intellectual dishonesty for his *Anatolia*. David King, editor of the *Ecclesiastical Observer*, charged him with "unblushing plagiarism," noted that Thomas had accused others of theft, and gave what he considered damning parallel text from Thomas's *Anatolia* and Granville Penn's *The Prophecy of Ezekiel concerning Gog* that shows the traffic runs the other way.[9] By this evidence, from the 1850s forward, prophecy does not reveal present truth within past documents. It cannot establish even the logical sequences of significant time. Rather, prophecy tussles over fact and reveals itself as contingent fiction.

This contingency resides in the author. And Pae demonstrates in *Lucy* that he understands himself to be part of the problem. The story features a novelist—a Mr. Hay—in search of truth, and sure he can find and describe it:[10]

> [the Glasgow underworld is] the very place for me. It is a part of my present business in the city to visit a place like that. I have come here, sir, to study Glasgow, for I mean to describe it. I am a writer, sir—a gentleman of the press—a—a novelist; but I take care, sir, to have all my fictions full of truth. I never exaggerate, and always maintain a high tone of morality. (*Lucy*, 63)

But the novelist is a hopeless naïf—here, he is talking to the criminals of the book unawares. Then throughout the novel, the writer who should be able to connect events, decode the nefarious plot, and rescript the good, misses his cue: "Dear me—dear me," he quavers when hearing the voice of the "Captain" who kidnapped and tortured him, "I should know it—I should know it.... Very strange. Can't remember where I heard it; but I did hear it, and that lately. Very singular—very singular indeed" (189). Thus incompetent, the author stands implicated in a plot that continues because it lacks the intervention he should be able to accomplish. Moreover, by his obsession with authorship, his fascination with crime, and his ignorance, Mr. Hay becomes a hinge in that plot. As we hang on his words and wait for revelation, the Captain comes ever nearer to murdering Lucy and her protector. The author lacks authority, and in his likeness to the anxious and ineffectual reader, he brings evil into the community. Well might *Mary Paterson* conclude: "LEAD US NOT INTO TEMPTATION, BUT DELIVER US FROM EVIL" (*Mary Paterson*, 413). The author cannot help us.

There is thus no system, no discussion, no voice that can put an end to the scandal of the West Port. Back in 1829, *Blackwood's* had joked that Walter Scott declared the story too hideous for his pen. Alexander Leighton and David Pae found the tale still impossible to tell once and for all. They had such trouble coming up to the mark that Lonsdale would later mock them as the "prosy and prophetic," and dismiss them as "highly sensational" (Lonsdale, 97, 101 n.1, also 105). Evidently, Burke and Hare and

Doctor Knox, as an extension of the Enlightenment's methods, but not its principles, had stepped beyond its bounds. They could not be contained by known philosophies or stories. Indeed, the attempt to confine them within the logics of society merely provoked dialogue, for they did not fit. Dialogue revealed the difficulty of closure. Worse, channeled through Burke and Hare and Doctor Knox it threatened systems, collapsing fact and fiction, history and religion into the impossibility of meaning. The harder Leighton and Pae try to resolve the story, even after thirty years, the more it escapes containment. Efforts to control it begin to show as a repetition compulsion that keeps open Edinburgh's psychic wounds by scratching at their scabs. Perhaps Walter Scott was right, the West Port murders were better left alone—but through Leighton and Pae, the sickness could only spread.

> I had never set eyes on him before.... I was struck besides with the shocking expression of his face...with the odd, subjective disturbance caused by his neighbourhood.... I set it down to some idiosyncratic, personal distaste...but I have since had reason to believe the cause to lie much deeper in the nature of man, and to turn on some nobler hinge than the principle of hatred.
> —*Jekyll and Hyde*, 54.

4

Dissecting the Doctor

MR. JEKYLL, DR. HYDE, AND ROBERT KNOX

IN 1861, ALEXANDER LEIGHTON wondered with the Edinburgh of 1828, "Where are the doctors?" (*Court*, 237). At the end of *The Court of Cacus*, he was wondering still. Moreover, despite his best efforts, David Pae failed to help in *Lucy*. And the longer Knox refused to present himself for public dissection, the more his story festered and its infection spread. Then in 1862, Knox died—but still the story lurked untold. Mary Paterson was laid to rest, but not the tale of her anatomist.

So in the 1880s, Robert Louis Stevenson again probed the wound caused by Doctor Knox. First in "The Body Snatcher" and then in *Strange Case of Dr Jekyll and Mr Hyde*, Stevenson opens the doctor to the cleansing air of public inspection. Most important, given Walter Scott's concern about malevolent doctors and the curative powers exercised by authors, Knox "rides off on no back" of Robert Louis Stevenson (Scott *Journal*, 571). The author, as supervising anatomist, now makes the reluctant doctor lay out his own case. Robert Knox at last dissects himself.

By 1881, Robert Louis Stevenson held Scottish history much in mind. Stuck in Pitlochry with his mother and his medicines, but also a new wife, he sought gainful employment. Unexpectedly, he learned of Aeneas Mackay's retirement as Professor of History and Constitutional Law at Edinburgh. Poor student and delinquent lawyer though he was, Stevenson immediately pursued the position with unusual energy and persistence. He wrote to Mackay, hoping he was not ill, but after two lines of polite inquiry got down to business: "may I ask if you have promised your support to any successor? I have a great mind to try" (June 21 [22], 1881, Stevenson *Letters*, 3:194). With a candor that no doubt disarmed, dismayed, and dissuaded his various referees, he continued:

> The summer session would suit me; the chair would suit me.... I only wish it were a few years from now, when I hope to have something more substantial to show for myself. Up to the present time, all that I have published, even bordering on history, has been in an occasional form, and I fear this is much against me.

Indeed it was. Barry Menikoff considers Stevenson a serious candidate, but Stevenson's historical fiction was largely yet to come, and the map of Scottish academia had changed since the underqualified John Wilson ("Christopher North" in the *Blackwood's* attack on Knox) had seemed an acceptable candidate for the Chair of Moral Philosophy in 1820 (Menikoff, 22–26). Susan Manning describes a new disciplinary structure and professional tone to mid-century Edinburgh University that would have made Stevenson's 1881 venture more of a lark ("A View"). Though professors responded politely, and friends enthusiastically, it is well to note the gentle irony from Stevenson's pal Walter Simpson:

> I went down & gave your father a note of the voting today.... He seemed a little disappointed but I suppose that was paternal. I was not—did not expect you would do as well. Why did they take the patronage from the town council [?] Shopkeepers can at least appreciate learning as a worshipful thing; but these lawyers get it into their heads that a knowledge of the law is learning. So help me they do. (Beinecke MS5506, qtd. Menikoff, 25–26)

Simpson was happy to report "how unanimous people were in admitting your true position in literature"—but Stevenson was applying for a chair in law and history, not rhetoric or belles lettres.

Stevenson knew perfectly well that his candidacy was "a mad thing." (Stevenson *Letters*, 3:198). He joked to Sidney Colvin:

> Great and glorious news. Your friend sincere goes forth to war; His blood red banner blows afar; He Louis the bold unfearing chap Aims at a professorial cap, And now besieges, do and dare, The Edinburgh History chair. Three months in summer only it Will bind him to that windy bit; The other nine to range abroad Untrammel'd in the eye of God. Mark in particular one thing: He

means to work that cursed thing: And to the golden youth explain, Scotland and England, France and Spain: Their quaint beliefs, their various rites, And why they are such b——— s———.

So Stevenson understood what referees meant when they replied he was "too late" (3:198). Writing wryly to Mackay, who had responded by remembering Stevenson's absence from his classes, the author conceded, "Every one tells me that I come too late upon the field, every one being pledged, which, seeing it is yet too early for any one to come upon the field, I must regard as a polite evasion" (3:201). Nonetheless, he was enough invested to take seriously the vague suggestion that he stand anyway, as "it might serve me against the next vacancy." Therefore it is not surprising that at Pitlochry, both literally and figuratively uncertain of his own place in history, Stevenson produces "The Body Snatcher." As official Edinburgh gently undermined Stevenson's notion of his historical credentials and role, the author told a tale too ticklish for the professors to tell, showing that he was not "too late," at least in literature. In fact, he was first. Robert Louis Stevenson told Doctor Knox's secret.

The story of Burke and Hare and Doctor Knox by now had slashed its way into memory, but never been tidied away into history. Furthermore, the medical community was only too happy to seal the wound rather than heal it. When Alexander Leighton and David Pae tried to dissect Doctor Knox through chronicle and fiction in the 1860s, Henry Lonsdale, Knox's student and assistant turned biographer, immediately intervened. Lonsdale's Knox was a hero who, in Africa, "Mounted on his famous Arabian mare, that could travel ninety miles 'apparently without the slightest fatigue,' and armed with a rifle of marvellous aim…single-handed achieved wonderful things" (Lonsdale, 13). So striking were Lonsdale's biases and omissions (or so mild his irony) that William Roughead mocked in 1935:

> Seldom is the life of a great and good man written with such gusto and devotion as is the biography of Dr. Knox by his admirer and former student, Dr. Lonsdale. Dr. Knox had but one eye, and never saw more with it than suited his convenience; Dr. Lonsdale, equipped with the usual number, fails totally to see either spot or blemish in the character of his hero.… [T]he partiality of the author for his "subject" has blinded him as we find, to sundry wrinkles in the Doctor's moral make-up. (Roughead *Knave*, 320)

Lonsdale addressed the Burke and Hare scandal, but detailed no murders except that of the hapless Mrs. Docherty—which as we have seen, never fully connected with Doctor Knox (Lonsdale, 74–76).

Significantly, Lonsdale sketched a picture of Knox well within the new Victorian idea of the doctor. This Knox was an earnest pioneer of anatomy, with remarkable medical ability, humanitarian tendencies, and a genial private temperament. In time, the doctor's name

> was like a sign of freemasonry; and his Edinburgh associations often proved a bond of attachment to the veriest strangers in all parts of the world. By the camp-fires of Canada, under the Indian verandahs, in the tented field, on the heights of Balaclava, and wherever military or naval surgeons have congregated for forty years past; hours of *ennui*, anxiety, and danger have been robbed of their trials, and even made cheery, by the introduction of the famed anatomist's name. (Lonsdale, 283)

To Lonsdale: "Everybody was made happy at Knox's fireside. The intellectual and the humorous could not fail to be pleased with mine host's talk and joke that always set the table in a roar. Knox at home was Knox triumphant; his cheery words and affable manner were as exhilarating as draughts of champagne" (223). The doctor of 1828 was sealed within and sheltered by the Victorian emphasis on medical community—though that community, ironically, increasingly depended upon the regulation Knox had lacked.

As medicine regulated itself, in fact, Knox's story became even less tellable. The new medical ethics focused on professional etiquette rather than on public service; knowledge was privileged and practice was secret—not something to be shared with the common man. Ivan Waddington notes that from 1803, when Thomas Percival's *Medical Ethics* began the discussion, through 1853, when the British Medical Association set up a "medico-ethical committee," doctors focused on their relations not with their public or even their patients, but with their colleagues (Waddington, 36–37). Such regulation was particularly needed in Knox's time—specifically "as a result of the cutthroat competition of the 1820s and 1830s" that brought Knox to grief (Searle, 126). Records of the Royal College of Surgeons of Edinburgh are rife with complaints from one doctor against another. In 1822, a letter from Liston to the authorities at the Royal Infirmary is returned, for it "seemed to contain Reflexions injurious to the character moral and professional of some of the most respectable Members of the Royal College" (May 15, 1822, RCSEd Records 1822–28). In 1826, Doctor Hunter, an "examinator," received anonymous letters blaming his high demands for a student suicide. Hunter complained that he had been hissed by students in the course of his daily rounds (ibid. March 4 and 24, 1826). Even Knox's abhorred Doctor Monro had to defend himself against charges that he did not teach enough (November 11 and 25, 1823). As late as 1845, a correspondent to the *Lancet* pleaded for a change: "must we continue to live on, hoping for better feelings and deportment in those who have hardly a fair word to use for their brother?" (qtd. Waddington, 41). And *Lloyd's Weekly Newspaper* of 1856 demonstrated that such attitudes could track and widen current divisions, for tellingly, it decried individuals who squeezed in to the profession "by some little back door Scotch university" (qtd. Bynum et al., 113). In this context, Knox's complex tale might reduce into one of failing to get on with his colleagues in Scotland and now England, who in turn did not much support him.

Moreover, Knox might appropriately keep his own counsel. Jeanne Peterson describes a "new division between consultant and general practitioner" that arose just as surgeons, apothecaries, and physicians were aligned in a more regulated discipline (Peterson, 28). With this renewed class division of medical responsibility, the doctor's distance from the rabble became more important: his dark knowledge was recast as the occulted expertise of an elite. Silence became a symptom of the decorum appropriate to rank (91). In addition, Petersen notes: "Medical men claimed—and the lay world began to accept—their right to power based on their special knowledge. The *Times* in 1880 acknowledged the basis of medical authority in 'skill and knowledge'" (187). Under this kind of regulation, Knox might never have had a charge to answer—he had done what was necessary for his craft. He also would not have been required to tell his tale.

In the developing field of medicine, Knox's case looked more and more like a stitch-up. A history that had never been fully told might no longer be recognized as needing to be told. Worse (or better, depending on your point of view), in 1865, medical historians say, everything changed, because doctors actually started to cure people. With the advent of anesthesia and antiseptics, doctors gained some grounding for their godlike elevation. Digby summarizes that when Lister's 1865 use of antiseptics combined with the 1840s discovery of anesthesia: "major internal surgery was possible.... There was a striking difference between the earlier operating theatre, grimed from long years of use and with surgeon dressed in frock coat, and that by the end of the century where hands, instruments, and patients' skins were awash with carbolic" (Digby, 95). Attention shifted from the suspect experiment—that could kill—to the successful treatment—that should cure. So by 1881, when Stevenson turned his attention to the story of Doctor Knox, that story stood on the cusp between unacceptable experiment and positive (therefore exculpatory) effect. It was liable to fall out of memory, and all the more in need of being told. Not surprisingly, then, the Stevenson who could not make himself an authority on Scottish history rips into history and medicine. Wielding a medical metaphor once more at the cutting edge, he retells the story of Burke and Hare—and especially of Doctor Knox.

CUTTING INTO THE PAST: "THE BODY SNATCHER" AND THE GOTHIC TALE

"The Body Snatcher," written in 1881 but not published until 1884, figured as a dark tale in the midwinter tradition—like Dickens's *A Christmas Carol*. That is how it was pushed by the *Pall Mall Gazette* for its Christmas Extra. In a succession of ads, the gazette hyped the story, bringing it progressively to center stage until it featured not in one or two but in three special sixpenny editions—with an appropriately lurid cover.[1] The magazine gushed:

> Mr. ROBERT LOUIS STEVENSON, one of the most powerful imaginative writers of the day, whose vivid picture of the 'Suicide Club' has frozen the heart's blood, whose 'Treasure Island,' written for boys, has fascinated a Prime Minister, and become a classic, has consented to write for us a vivid GHOST STORY, and when ghosts are walking Mr. Stevenson is at his weirdest. (ad. "Christmas Extra," *PMG* December 5, 1884: 16)

Graham Balfour, Stevenson's cousin, remarks on the "gruesome and unauthorized methods of advertisement"—Sidney Colvin remembered "sandwich-men carrying posters so horrific that they were suppressed, if I remember aright by the police" (Balfour 2:6; Stevenson *Letters*, 5:35 n.1). Ernest Mehew reports "a procession of corpses with coffin lids" (Mehew attributes this to "Markheim," dropped from *PMG* and replaced by "The Body Snatcher," but it more sensibly applies to Stevenson's resurrection tale [5:35 n.1]). Clearly, Stevenson was providing the gazette with what it wanted.

Stevenson himself thought the story "horrid"—awful enough for the genre, no doubt—and gave it a modernist twist with its lack of concern for ultimate morality, its focus on the shock, and its pleasure in style (Stevenson *Letters*, 3:204–5).[2] But the tale nonetheless expressed Scotland's complex realities. Its composition in 1881 coincided not just with Stevenson's pursuit of the Chair in History and Constitutional Law, but also with the setting up of a Royal Commission to regularize access to medical training; its publication in 1884 coincided with new requirements for standardized exams—"similar arrangements were made in Scotland" (Parry, 129; 130, also Stacey, ch. 3). In 1881, the story's role as counter narrative to Scotland's official history (with its newly recuperated tale of Scottish medicine) was evident in its planned location within *The Black Man*. This collection was supposed to feature similarly dark and alternate tales, such as "Thrawn Janet" and "The Devil on Cramond Sands" (Stevenson *Letters*, 3:188–89). Perhaps this lurking context explains why "The Body Snatcher" was too "horrid" to complete at a sitting, short though it is.

Stevenson wrote to W. E. Henley that he had taken "a scunner" at the tale and chose to break from writing it (Stevenson *Letters*, 3:200). And well he might, for here, Stevenson anatomizes Doctor Knox and his assistants in gory detail and with slow deliberation. We read backwards toward catastrophe from the moment a great London doctor is called to attend a case at a rural English pub. Macfarlane, this scion of Edinburgh's medical patriarchy, encounters the "parlour sot," who turns out to be his old acquaintance, the decayed doctor Fettes ("The Body Snatcher," *PMG* "Christmas Extra": 4). Mysteriously horrified to meet Fettes, Macfarlane flees into the night, leaving Fettes to terrify the locals with a tale of his student days. It is a tale of Doctor K___, and of murdering to dissect. But however titillating this story may be for an English audience, it cuts through one protective layer of Knox's story after another to open the festering sore beneath.

As a student under K___, Fettes receives bodies for dissection. One evening, he recognizes a subject as a prostitute recently alive, but Macfarlane, his senior and "clever, dissipated, and unscrupulous to the last degree," persuades him to keep quiet ("The Body Snatcher," 7). Macfarlane is pretty glib about it. He says: "practically speaking, all our subjects have been murdered" (7). Before long, Macfarlane himself presents Fettes with a recognizable corpse, that of the senior student's familiar demon, Mr. Gray. Introduced by Macfarlane, Fettes has joked to this man: "When we dislike a dear friend of ours, we dissect him" (8). Now, Fettes is complicit in such a case. Shortly thereafter, Fettes and Macfarlane take a bodysnatching trip. In the dark of night the corpse, sitting in the gig between them,

> fell now upon the one and now upon the other.... Still their unnatural burden bumped from side to side, and now the head would be laid, as if in confidence, upon their shoulders, and now the drenching sackcloth would flap icily about their faces.... [T]he bundle...seemed somehow larger than at first.... [S]ome nameless change had befallen the dead body...it was in fear of their unholy burthen that the dogs were howling. (12)

And of course, since this is a sixpenny shocker:

> The light fell very clear upon the dark, well-moulded features and smooth-shaven cheeks of a too familiar countenance, often beheld in dreams by both of these young men. A wild yell rang up into the night; each leaped from his own side into the roadway; the lamp fell, broke, and was extinguished; and the horse, terrified by this unusual commotion, bounded and went off towards Edinburgh at the gallop, bearing along with it, sole occupant of the gig, the body of the long dead and long dissected Gray. (12; see figure 4.1)

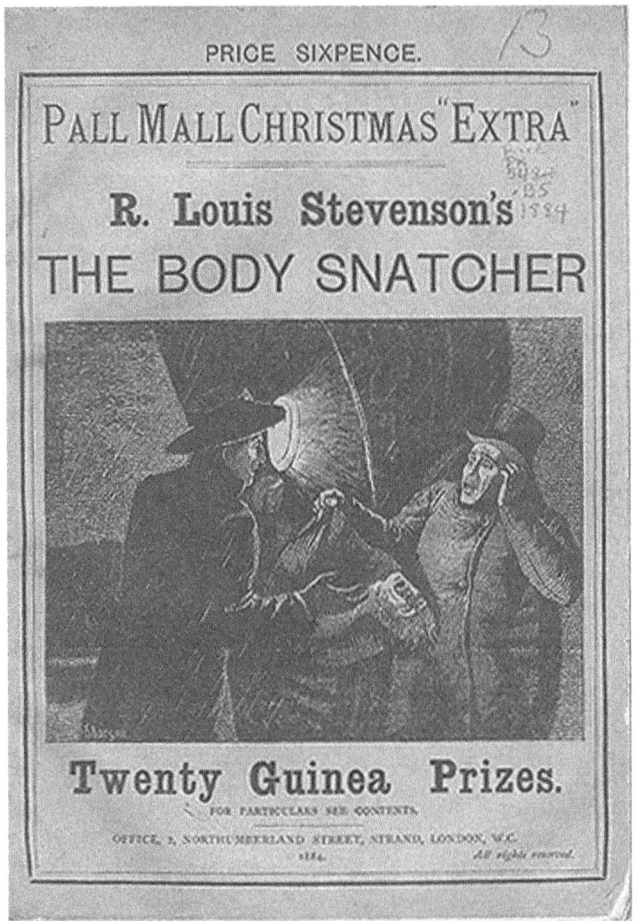

FIGURE 4.1 "The Body Snatcher," *The Pall Mall Gazette*, 1884. Courtesy of the Irvin Department of Rare books and Special Collections, University of South Carolina Libraries.

The transposition that matters here is not that of Gray into corpse and dissected cadaver into Gray, or even of Gray, the hero who exposed the Burke and Hare murders, into a villain within this plot. What matters is how Stevenson connects Macfarlane and Fettes back to William Fergusson, Knox's assistant, and binds Macfarlane to Knox himself.

Layer by layer, Stevenson cuts through the obstructions to Knox's tale. Fettes, as the student who recognized a prostitute on the slab, and Macfarlane, as the assistant who has become a London phenomenon, recall Fergusson. Although today historians debate about which student recognized Mary Paterson—or if any of them actually knew her in the way of "business"—nineteenth-century rumor settled on Knox's primary assistant.[3] Also, Fergusson was named as the one to make away with Daft Jamie's recognizable feet (Edwards *Burke and Hare*, 129). But Fergusson became Knox's star pupil, and he went from the Burke and Hare scandal to attend on the rich, famous, and royal. In 1840 he was appointed Professor of Surgery at King's College London. He became Surgeon in Ordinary to Prince Albert in 1849, Surgeon Extraordinary to Queen Victoria in 1855, then in 1867 her Sergeant-Surgeon. By the time Lonsdale wrote, Fergusson was a baronet (since 1866). This stratospherically successful student in recent years had been invoked as a belated guarantor of Knox's respectability. Lonsdale touted him as "William Fergusson, who owed nearly all to Knox, and now occupies so proud a surgical position in the metropolis" (Lonsdale, 281). And Lonsdale unctuously recounts that Fergusson, "on joining the Royal College of Surgeons, naturally offered homage to his master" (275).

Wolfe/"Toddy" Macfarlane directly references Doctor Knox, too. This student dresses like his flamboyant teacher, wearing: "the finest of broadcloth and the whitest of linen, with a great gold watch chain and studs and spectacles of the same precious material…a broad folded tie, white and speckled with lilac" ("The Body Snatcher," 4). As Lonsdale remembered:

> Dr. Knox was wonderfully got up in the way of costume, and perhaps the only lecturer who ever appeared before an anatomical class in full dress.… Knox, in the highest style of fashion, with spotless linen, frill, and lace, and jewellery redolent of a duchess's boudoir, standing in a class-room amid osseous forms, *cadavera*, and decaying mortalities, was a sight to behold, and one assuredly never to be forgotten. (Lonsdale, 125–26)

He was thus to be remembered through Wolfe Macfarlane.

And the evasive Knox is anatomized down to his last secret when Fettes recognizes the prostitute. Macfarlane challenges Fettes, "why did [K___] choose us two for his assistants? And I answer, because he didn't want old wives" ("The Body Snatcher," 7). K___ has told his assistants, "Ask no questions…for conscience' sake" (6). So Macfarlane recalls Doctor Knox when he declares: "'The next best thing for me is not to recognize [this corpse]' he added coolly, 'I don't'" (7). Through these resections of the past, Knox is culpable: "the lightness of his speech upon so grave a matter was…a temptation to the men with whom he dealt"—not just Burke and Hare, but Macfarlane and Fettes (6). As Stevenson presents him through the elegant Macfarlane, Knox knows what is going on and himself is fully implicated in murder.

In the Edinburgh of 1828, Knox refused the public gaze. According to legend, and perhaps in fact, when the police came to investigate him, he stood at the window "threatening to shoot [them] if they dared to question for the ends of justice so innocuous and ill-used a victim of public prejudice" (Leighton *Court*, 222). MacGregor quotes from a contemporary newspaper: "he swore at them...and threatened to blow their brains out" (MacGregor, 157). And Lonsdale imagines a Knox resplendent in "military cloak...sword, pistols, and Highland dirk" who claimed that he "would have measured a score of the brutes [the rioting crowd]" (Lonsdale, 110). But now the "ruffians" get a good, satisfying look at Knox in the person of Toddy Macfarlane on the run. He is caught between the curious eyes of his cab driver, and the wondering locals.

> White as he was, there was a dangerous glitter in his spectacles; but while he still paused uncertain he became aware that the driver of his fly was peering in from the street at this unusual scene, and caught a glimpse at the same time of our little body from the parlour, huddled by the corner of the bar. The presence of so many witnesses decided him at once to flee.... But his tribulation was not yet entirely at an end; for even as he was passing Fettes clutched him by the arm, and these words came in a whisper, and yet painfully distinct, "Have you seen it again?"
>
> The great, rich London doctor cried out aloud with a sharp, throttling cry...and, with his hands over his head, fled out of the door like a detected thief.... Next day the servant found [his] fine gold spectacles crushed and broken on the threshold. ("The Body Snatcher, 5)

As in all thorough autopsies, the gazer has become the gazed upon. Caught within the public eye, Macfarlane cum Knox not only gives up his authoritative perspective, with his "throttling cry," he suffers the ultimate humiliation. Joining sixteen victims before him he is, at last, "burked."

Finally, an author had exposed the doctor's secret. But more, Stevenson laid out a web of connecting fibers that tied fiction back to fact. Honoring his predecessors and establishing his own community of authorship against that of the doctors, Stevenson in his little shocker referenced a history of once failed and now bonded attempts to connect Doctor Knox to his 1828 dissections. The horror of the animate corpse haunted gothicized tales during the era of the resurrection men. In 1821, John Galt told of "The Buried Alive," who revives on the dissecting slab under galvanic experiment. After the Anatomy Act of 1832, the story maintained its vigor. An 1838 story in the *Buchan Clown*, "The Lost Will," features an apparent rise from the grave, and then a corpse that, when galvanized, achieves a temporary animation to sort out an inheritance plot. "A Night in a Dissecting Room," published in 1878/79, presents a cadaver that rises as an effect of an unsteady support beneath it (Ranking). And these stories had taken a Knoxian tone. The fictions and histories that critiqued and supported Knox foregrounded such tales in their run-through of the doctor's context in resurrection times. David Pae's 1858 novel, *Lucy*, connects Knox with grave robbing, criminality, and the accusing cadaver: the bodysnatchers have exhumed poor Willie, and the one carrying the boy feels something

> move up and down upon his cheek, and, when he felt it, he became absolutely frozen with horror. The head of the corpse lay on his shoulder, and it seemed as if it had lifted one of its cold hands and was passing a finger to and fro on his face.... Then the wind, which had been gently blowing for some moments, came in a gust and lifted the white covering from the face of the corpse. Ben felt as if compelled by an invisible power to turn his head, and there he saw two large glassy eyes staring fixedly at him. (Pae *Lucy*, 160)

Leighton, in his attack on Knox's "court of Cacus," gives the story's provenance in the (perhaps apocryphal) exploits of a bodysnatching Edinburgh student:

> just as F—y got to the road...the grasp he had of the shroud began to give way.... [T]he feet of the corpse, coming always to the ground, resiled again with something like elasticity, so that it appeared to him as if it trotted or leaped behind him. Fear is the mother of suspicion, and the idea took hold of him that the body was alive. He uttered a roar,—threw his burden off, and crying out to his friend, "By G—, she's alive!" jumped into the gig. His friend was taken by the same terror, and away they galloped. (Leighton *Court*, 40–41)

Stevenson's story of animation fulfilled two generations of literary striving. For the community of authors, it finally pinned Doctor Knox to his own dissecting slab.

Of course, the story was a shocker. The *Pall Mall Gazette* had wanted gothic horror. When Stevenson decided he could not "put a skeleton" into "Markheim," he turned to "The Body Snatcher" as "blood-curdling enough" (Stevenson *Letters*, 5:35 and 41). And that is the level at which England received the story. But although this was a terrible tale, "The Body Snatcher" did not cut close to the English bone, indeed the *Gazette* found it needed to insert "A Key to Mr. Stevenson's 'Body-Snatcher'" in a subsequent issue (*PMG* February 3, 1885: 6). A gory follow-up note about cadaver teeth and dentistry appeared in "Occasional Notes" for the gazette of February 4 (3). This public was titillated, but not deeply affected.

Scots, however, felt the knife, and knew its portent. Joseph Goodsir, brother to one of Knox's foremost students, expostulated about the story in its "bilious coloured wrapper with coarse & hideous wood cuts, the whole having a decidedly 'penny dreadful' appearance" (NLS MS170: 48–67, see 2).[4] Goodsir heaped opprobrium on the tale and its teller, calling "The Body Snatcher" a "gruesome—and...craven sketch"; uncharacteristic of the "genial and pleasant author of 'Travels with a Donkey' and the 'New Arabian Nights'"; "juvenile" (3–4). After this rant against artistic and adolescent awfulness, he gets to the point:

> That [the story] should have been given to the public at all is a matter of very questionable taste.
>
> The fact of Mr Stevenson being himself an Edinburgh man would have presupposed his better acquaintance with the facts upon which he founds his story, and above all have made him think twice before reviving the memories of one of the darkest series of crimes that have stained the annals of his native city....
>
> It will be said, of course, that the "Body Snatcher" is only a piece of Fiction. A pleasant piece of Fiction certainly—to attach the stigma of cold blooded deliberate murder to the names and memories of men who have relatives, and friends, and admirers amongst the few still living of his many thousands of pupils.
>
> Was it out of delicate consideration for their feelings that Mr Stevenson made use of the K___ when he well knew that he might just as well have written KNOX.[5]

Goodsir stressed the Irish origin of the crimes, asserted that authoritative Edinburgh vindicated Knox from the "vulgar *fama clamosa*," and excused each of Knox's demonstrators by name (6, 9, 14–17). He held the line of cultural, class, and medical community, but he well knew that for Scots, Stevenson's gothic tale had cut to the heart of the case of Doctor Knox.

The story was not reprinted in Stevenson's lifetime, or in Colvin's edition of the author's works (Stevenson *Letters*, 5:41 n.2). Was it too horrific for England, and too specific for Scotland? Whatever the case, Stevenson went on to slice his subject even finer. Goodsir had challenged the author:

> Should these lines meet Mr R. L. Stevensons eyes we would ask him to take the trouble to read Dr Henry Lonsdales 'Life of Robert Knox.'... Should he do so, we venture to predict that his own love of fair-play, of truth, and of justice, will lead him to regret the penning and still more the publishing of the Body Snatcher. (Goodsir, 12–13)

Stevenson may now have cast an eye over Lonsdale's biography, but he may equally have read George MacGregor's *The History of Burke and Hare*, which came out in 1884. MacGregor, a Fellow of the Society of Antiquaries of Scotland, was no apologist for the doctor. In a book that claims to supplement the burgeoning "fugitive literature" by giving "due prominence to the medical and legal aspects of the whole subject," he works up to a crescendo of celebration for the Anatomy Act, and questions for Doctor Knox (MacGregor, v, vi). In his closing chapters, MacGregor reminds his readers that "In the eyes of many, [Knox] seemed a greater criminal than even Burke and Hare" (234). While this is "much too harsh a judgement," Knox nonetheless echoes Leighton's Burke as:

> A despair to the physiognomist... [and] not less a difficulty to the psychologist. There seemed to be no principle whereby you could think of binding him down to a line of duty, and a universal sneer, not limited to mundane powers, formed that contrast to an imputed self-perfection, not without the evidence of very great scientific accomplishments. (235–36)

In 1828, Doctor Knox was hard to pin down. Figuratively and literally, MacGregor reminds us, he had bolted out the back door to "Portobello, where, it [was] supposed, the Doctor burrow[ed] at night" (239, qtd. from *Edinburgh Weekly Chronicle*). So despite his intent to trump the "fugitive literature," MacGregor concludes with an appendix of sad, unfocused, and frustrated ballads and poems that still await the explanation and analysis of Robert Knox.

Perhaps this is why, instead of regretting his work, Stevenson took another, deeper detour through England and anatomy, this time entering by the doctor's back door— in the neighborhood of Henry Jekyll. MacGregor had stressed the lack of closure to Knox's case. The committee that ultimately investigated Knox, MacGregor insists, intended "to clear Dr. Knox from the aspersions cast upon him; and this was a result far from satisfactory to a very large section of the community.... However, the matter was allowed to rest there" (MacGregor, 244). Knox, MacGregor hinted, still had not spoken. Now, under the pen of Robert Louis Stevenson, Doctor Knox would at last dissect himself in the persons of Doctor Jekyll and that other, often forgotten doctor, Mr. Hyde.

CHEMICAL DISSECTION: DOCTOR JEKYLL MEETS DOCTOR KNOX

What can *Strange Case of Dr Jekyll and Mr Hyde* have to do with Robert Knox? The novel appeals far beyond Scotland through its London doctor and its double life assisted by chemistry. A long tradition of criticism places *Jekyll and Hyde* as a psychological tale, a tale of the professions, a story of "queer street," a deeply misogynistic work, and a standard story of the Scottish double or proto-modernist other.[6]

In the Scottish context, critical talk connects Stevenson's doctor with that other Edinburgh criminal of note, the city worthy and housebreaker Deacon Brodie. After all, the Stevensons owned a wardrobe built by this craftsman (now at the Writers' Museum, Edinburgh); the Deacon lived a double life; Stevenson had already coscripted the play *Deacon Brodie; or The Double Life* with his friend W. E. Henley. All of these have merit—though we might dwell less on the Deacon, for it is a sketchy, scene-chewing piece that reductively themes duality and is most notable for Stevenson's dislike of it (a dislike manifested in his use of the language of body-snatching and burking not to give Brodie's tale thematic resonance but to degrade it).[7] However, Stevenson himself characterized *Jekyll and Hyde* as "a gothic gnome…[from] a deep mine, where [it] guards the fountain of tears" (Stevenson *Letters*, 5:163). That mine ran deep. Shortly after the novel's publication, Stevenson suggested that his "old Scotch Presbyterian preoccupation…itself morbid.…[t]he Scotch side came out plain in *Dr Jekyll*" (5:212–13). This was a mine full of Scottish memory, as indicated by the text's oddly sentimental dedication:

> It's ill to loose the bands that God decreed to bind;
> Still will we be the children of the heather and the wind.
> Far away from home, O it's still for you and me
> That the broom is blowing bonnie in the north countrie. (*Jekyll and Hyde*, 4)

In *Strange Case of Dr Jekyll and Mr Hyde*, Stevenson binds the phrenological and psychological conundrum that was MacGregor's Doctor Knox to its factual past using the creative memory that is fiction. Through Stevenson's reconstruction, the doctor at last feels the knife and begins to stir.

Of course, Jekyll is an experimental chemist, whereas Knox was an anatomist. Jekyll is a polite London professional complete with cane—which Roy Strong calls "medicine's most distinctive prop, symbolizing the public presence of the Georgian physician"; Knox is distinctly a Scot, elegant only in attire (Strong, 149). But Robert Louis Stevenson knew his medicine and its transpositions and transformations inside out. In 1856 George Allarton defined gradations of doctor. He catalogued:

> the SCIENTIFIC DOCTOR, much respected but seldom wealthy, and the FASHIONABLE DOCTOR, always seen at the opera, and 'a *darling* doctor' with 'the gentler sex'. Next was the LITERARY DOCTOR, eccentrically dressed and with little practice…and, finally, the PHILOSOPHICAL DOCTOR, renowned and eminent through 'giving his affection to those collateral subjects which the man engaged in practice cannot give.' (Loudon, 205)

Jekyll and Knox are both recognizable as the "Philosophical Doctor," interested in systems and speculation, but not much to be seen on the wards.

Stevenson understood all about doctors and the stories they represented. The year before he penned "The Body Snatcher," he was in Davos under the care of Doctor Ruedi, "a boss human being.... He is going to attack me in every tender spot and make my life a burthen to me—said so, straight out.... The doctor is to put me on hours for every mortal thing.... To blow the gaff on the cigarettes...!" (Stevenson *Letters*, 3:113). Ruedi was Stevenson's idea of a doctor—"Dr Ruedi, whom we all adore," and "my oracle" (3:118, 121). Moreover, the author's supposed lung disease and nervous prostration made his doctors central players in his relationship with his parents. When he fled Edinburgh in 1873, Stevenson turned to the doctors. The obliging Dr. Clark composed a masterpiece of vague diagnosis that allowed Stevenson to put the English channel between himself and his parents: Mrs. Stevenson reported, "[Clark] tells us that Lou's nervous system has quite broken down, that his lungs are delicate and just in the state when disease might very easily set in. When I ask if I ought to go [abroad] with him, [Clark] said: 'No, he wants a complete change of everything'" (1:350).[8] In Davos, when the parents wanted Stevenson to come home, the author replied, "Ruedi allowed me to go home, on condition I stopped neither in London nor in Edinburgh, but went, via Glasgow, to some one spot in the highlands," and so, he explained to his mother, "on the whole...I should stay here" (3:154). A few days later, he suggested his father come to nearby Ragatz for treatment, but kept his own distance through the doctor: "Ruedi does not wish me to go so low. You must judge what is to be done by Ruedi's letter" (3:156). Clearly, Stevenson understood medicine as a story that could be used to shift realities.

In "A Chapter on Dreams" Stevenson hints toward a deep, troubled, specifically medical and Scottish source for *Jekyll and Hyde*. He dreamed first of the scene at the window; he dreamed next of a transformation scene. But before that, apparently, he suffered a persistent nightmare about surgery, set against the curative powers of chemistry:

> he studied...at Edinburgh College.... in his dream-life, he passed a long day in the surgical theatre, his heart in his mouth, his teeth on edge, seeing monstrous malformations and the abhorred dexterity of surgeons.... All night long...he climbed the stairs [of an Edinburgh tenement]...and at every second flight a flaring lamp with a reflector. All night long, he brushed by single persons passing downward—beggarly women of the street, great, weary, muddy labourers, poor scarecrows of men, pale parodies of women.... [He dreamed persistently] enough to leave a great black blot upon his memory, long enough to send him, trembling for his reason, to the doors of a certain doctor; whereupon

with a simple draught he was restored to the common lot of man. (Stevenson "Chapter," 129–30)

"He" was Stevenson himself. And in this little passage, the author placed the Edinburgh and activities of Doctor Knox (complete with dexterous medical villains and downward sliding victims from the slums) alongside the transformative powers of modern chemistry. From this very deep mine of memory and medicine, he would get at the mystery that was Robert Knox.

Mystery, indeed, is the primary medical phenomenon that binds doctors Jekyll and Knox. Jekyll hoards his chemical secrets like an up-and-coming professional in the knowledge market. Moreover, he is secretive with everybody. Jekyll will not listen to the most gentle concern. He tells Utterson: "I do not care to hear more," when the lawyer seeks to understand his relationship with Mr. Hyde; "This is a matter I thought we had agreed to drop" (*Jekyll and Hyde*, 22). Nor will he speak: "You do not understand my position," he insists, only offering misleadingly, "it isn't what you fancy." And he stresses, "this is a private matter." Jekyll is thus aligned not just with medical professionalism, but with Knox, the arch secret-keeper who, MacGregor had recently reminded, refused to speak and declared that those who spoke against him would be subject to law for defamation.

Knox and Jekyll also meet through ideas about the mind as an organ characterized by the secrets it keeps. MacGregor had reintroduced consideration of Knox's physiognomy and psychology, but the threat of disjunctive behavior that binds the doctors runs through the history of medicine itself. Anne Stiles and Julia Reid have recently located *Jekyll and Hyde* within the period's shifting theories of the double brain. The standard reading of the novel as an early psychological text now gains scientific heft. Certainly, the double brain as tracked by Anne Harrington operates through *Jekyll and Hyde*. Harrington notes in the 1860s and 70s an upsurge in: consideration of the gaps in memory (Harrington, 71); arguments that different brain hemispheres have different functions (40–41 and 82–83); theories that set a civilized hemisphere (65) against a lurking animal brain (40); and interest in the asymmetrical brain (62–63). Jekyll, with his imprecise memory and smooth face yet sly expression, and Hyde with his undeveloped personality and brutal tendencies, fit many aspects of this developing model—as might Doctor Knox.

Yet scholars have connected Jekyll and his double to a different doctor, invoking the work of Ernst Haeckel, with its focus on ontogenesis (see Mighall, 151; Naugrette). Certainly, in Pitlochry in 1881, still writing "The Body Snatcher," Stevenson ran down a "comic Bunctionary" that included himself and "Haeckel—the Man with a Tail" (Stevenson *Letters*, 3:208–10). Haeckel theorized that an organism's biological development reprises the species' evolutionary development—that is, over time each being runs through the stages of its species. Children, in this context, are "primitive." Such a notion might explain the younger, animalistic Mr. Hyde. But in the history of science, we do not have to reach so far to find a map for him.

Robert Knox's later career turned toward anthropology, for anatomy allowed systemic deductions about species development. In his well-known lectures about *The Races of Men* (1850), Knox argues that since different species display the same anatomical phenomena in their young, but diverge in maturity, the history of the genus is embedded in every species. From this perspective, all aspects of the species are present at once in every organism. As Evelleen Richards summarizes:

> the successive appearance of new forms or species is "no new creation, but merely the development of forms already existing in every natural family.... To institute a species all that is required is to omit or cause to disappear, or cease to grow some parts of the organ or apparatus already existing in the generic being." Humanity was, of course, subject to the same laws. (Richards, 398)

Mr. Hyde seems to be subject to these specifically Knoxian laws. In fact, with his role as a throwback that Jekyll tries to throw out, but his potential to show many aspects of the doctor, he fits the theories of Darwin or of Haeckel only in part. He is a much better match for Robert Knox's theories, and thus the story points, once more, to the Scottish doctor himself.

Notably, too, the later Knox focused on "moral" anatomy. Richards observes that "Knox differed from the majority of his ethnological contemporaries in placing far more emphasis on the 'moral' than on the physical differences between the races."[9] In so doing, Knox came close to another area of medical indeterminacy: did illness result from a failure of the will? With causes still vague and treatments uncertain in their logic, never mind unreliable in their effect, a substantial division of Victorian medicine focused on medication by moral fiber. An 1878 guide to *Davos-Platz: A New Alpine Resort for Sick and Sound* stressed that:

> common sense and a strong will are the great means of recovery. Many people die because they have not the energy to live.... [T]he duty of spontaneous self-management cannot be too strongly impressed upon all who suffer from the chronic disorders which here find alleviation and cure.... No one can help [the patient] as they can help themselves; their very existence is often, as it were, given into their own hands, to retain or cast away as they choose.[10]

No wonder Davos made Stevenson feel mentally plugged up. And again, in his need for a good dosing of moral fiber, Hyde reveals his doctor to be of a Knoxian type.

Still, Knox was not a chemist, and chemistry is the operational science in *Jekyll and Hyde*. However, if anatomy was the foremost medical science in 1828, in the 1880s chemistry stood at the cutting edge. In the Edinburgh of 1847, James Young Simpson brought chloroform into medical use; in 1865, in Glasgow and then in Edinburgh, Joseph Lister pioneered antiseptics; through the 1870s and 80s, discoveries in organic chemistry came fast and furious from the laboratory of Louis Pasteur.[11] This shift in medicine was recognized by the founding of the specialized journal *Annals of Chemical Medicine* in 1880 (Bynum et al., 78). It is this combination of achievements that makes 1865, for some medical historians, "the moment when real progress first began in medical therapy" (Wootton, 4). This was chemistry's Knoxian moment of triumph.

Stevenson and his friends benefited from and fully appreciated these advances. In 1875, Stevenson first met W. E. Henley, at the time under Lister's care in Edinburgh for tuberculosis of the bone (Stevenson *Letters*, 2:117 n.3). Henley describes his treatments vividly:

> There was a long cut across the foot, from ankle to ankle, dividing vessels, tendons & everything, & laying open the affected bone, which in its turn was scooped out (gouge and pliers), so that a large triangular cavity was the result, the apex of which pointed to the toes. This cavity was filled with strips of lint in carbolic oil.... I have seen my foot since then, & I can assure you... that the aspect of it is not calculated to put me in spirits. (December 18, 1873, Henley *Letters*, 14–15)

Small wonder that he also wrote a poem in honor of chloroform:

> Behold me waiting—waiting for the knife.
>   A little while, and at a leap I storm
> The thick, sweet mystery of chloroform,
> The drunken dark, the little death-in-life.
>   (Henley *In Hospital*, 6)

As for Stevenson, in 1880 he had all his remaining teeth dug out and replaced with dentures (Stevenson *Letters*, 3:79). Bob Stevenson, the dental historian, points out that to survive such a major set of extractions, the frail author must surely have undergone anesthesia and, one might add, antiseptic treatment (Bob Stevenson, "Stevenson's Dentist").

Yet as with anatomy, this moment of triumph for chemical medicine also tested the discipline. For all its advances, medical chemistry stood at the margin of quackery and of trade. Anne Digby notes that the fact and language of quackery persisted well into the nineteenth century (Digby and also Bynum and Porter, *Medical Fringe*). The word "empiricism," crucial to the new sciences, bound chemistry to quackery, for quacks were "empirics," in that they randomly used what worked (Cowan, 4–5, 39). Quacks thus compromised the careful processes of experimental chemistry. Furthermore, as tradesmen selling their goods, quacks broke down the bounds between the public and the elite profession of medicine. The doctors' anxiety about being misrecognized as quacks produced a whole range of protective commercial and social behaviors. First, doctors should not sell drugs. Digby observes that "Self-promotion through advertising or the selling of medicine came to be seen as the attribute of the quack or those lower in status, such as the chemist" (Digby, 61). Certainly, one doctor anguished:

> are we a profession or a trade, are we gentlemen or are we not.... [M]edical practitioners, the members of a learned and liberal profession, should be gentlemen.... [Those counted as gentlemen regard] our profession as a profession strictly and not as a compound of a profession and a trade.... [A] gentleman must not engage in *retail trade*. (Parry, 131–32)

Rather than selling drugs, doctors should charge for services. The Manchester Medico-Ethical Association insisted in 1879 that "medical men *should, in all cases, base their title to remuneration upon the value of their time and skill*"—and specifically not on sales (Parry, 150). A doctor's office should not be his home or (notably), home and office should have two different doors that would distinguish business from social life and help maintain his status. As the century progressed, aspiring practices boasted: "a corner or double-fronted house together with a separate surgery entrance" (Digby, 38). Thus in 1879, Walter Rivington classed doctors according to how evident were the tools of their trade:

> I. The *Dispensing order*... may be again sub-divided into two chief groups of sub-orders—(a) *The surgeon-chemist*, or the red-bottle and blue-bottle practitioners, who combine the work of medical men with the retail business of a chemist. An open shop is kept, with glass-cases containing tooth brushes, nail brushes.... (b) *The surgeon-apothecary*, with an open surgery and a red lamp. No retail trade is done but advice and a bottle of physic is given for a moderate sum.... As the scale is ascended the surgery retires more and more into the background, until it reaches the interior of the dwelling, where it is no longer exposed to the vulgar gaze. At last it disappears entirely, and the second sub-order is attained, or—II *The non-dispensing or consultant order.* (Rivington, 55)

Digby observes, too, that "[quacks] were always other people, and the term appears to have been frequently used as a non-specific kind of abuse" (Digby, 27). Not surprisingly, Robert Knox had embraced the discourse as he emphasized his status as a medical man. He loudly declared any doctor who lacked training in pathological anatomy a "quack" ("Anatomical Museums," 308–9). Anatomy was the only safeguard against "that flood of quackery which, like an ocean tide, continually threatens the embankments of a highly cultivated country." Without it, "Homeopathy, hydropathy, and numerous other quackeries, would speedily overspread the fair field of medical science." Knox maintained the distinctions of medicine, and anticipated the nineteenth century's obsession with separate space, with his rooms in Surgeons' Square, his house in Newington Place, and his bolt-hole at Portobello. But as an anatomist with a backdoor trade in bodies Knox, too, had collided with commerce and quackery—and opened his door to that rash chemist, Doctor Jekyll.

It is important to note, as well, that pharmacy was itself an experimental science with uncertain substances, processes, and results. Robert Louis Stevenson, enthusiastic customer of spas from Dunblane to Pitlochry and Davos to Saranac Lake, was also an incorrigible self-medicator. Stevenson happily ingested authorized substances that would make a modern doctor quail. At the harmless end of the scale, he treated his supposed tuberculosis with doses of fresh air (see Bradley); in December 1884, however, we find him in bed treating "Bloody Jack" or hemorrhage with an "injection of ergotine"—which by 1913 was recharacterized as "A powerful astringent alkaloid… used to produce contraction of the uterus."[12] Later, he takes to doses of "Gregory's powder," a preparation of rhubarb, to which we might ascribe his occasional bouts of (colorfully described) diarrhea (Stevenson *Letters*, 5:190–91). Meanwhile, his wife Fanny was dosing herself with lemons—and arsenic (3:121). And the same pages that touted Stevenson's "Body Snatcher" declaimed the virtues of Beecham's Pills, a strangely universal modern specific that meets the prime criteria for quackery. In twenty-eight stacked short ads, Beecham's—at the time largely a laxative—claims to treat "Bilious and Nervous Disorders…Indigestion in all its forms…Sick Headaches…Giddiness…Costiveness and Scurvy," and of course, "Female Complaints" (gsk.com/about/history.htm; *PMG* February 2, 1885: 5). It is "Worth a Guinea a Box," "Adapted for Old and Young," "Recommended by Medical Men," has "Saved the Lives of thousands"—and so on. As Charles Cowan wrote in his 1839 treatise on *The Danger, Irrationality, and Evils of Medical Quackery*, "No statement [on behalf of a drug] is too extravagant for belief," especially the ludicrous claim to "[*Cure*] *all or many diseases by one remedy*" (Cowan, 9, 15). By 1895 Beecham's was selling a million pills a day, including Sundays, for an annual turnover of £360,000 (Terence D. Turner, 162). Beecham's made grand claims; people like Stevenson believed them; and chemical medicine thus stood perilously close to

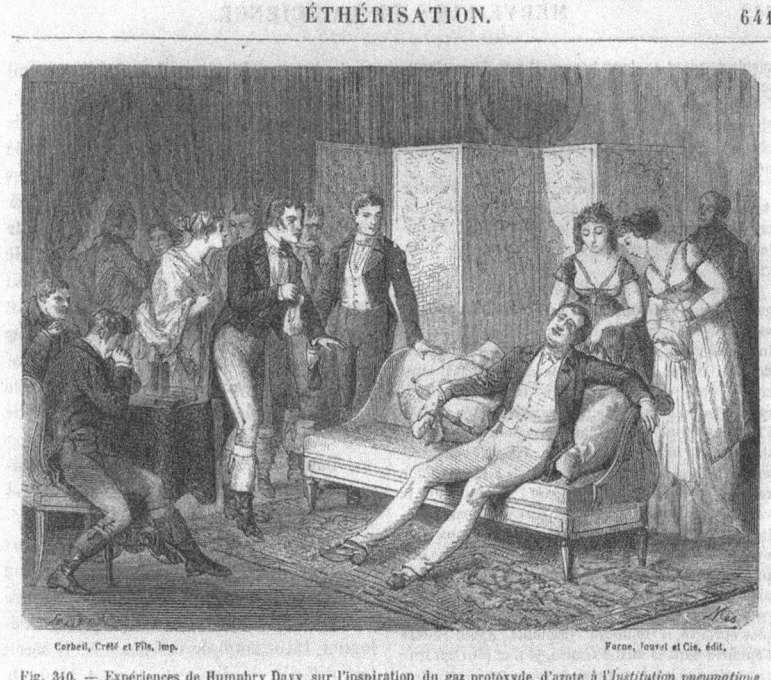

FIGURE 4.2 "Expériences de Humphry Davy sur l'inspiration du gaz protoxyde d'azote a l'*Institution pneumatique* de Clifton," Louis Figuier, *Les Merveilles de la Science*, vol. 1 (Paris: Fourne, Jouvet, 1891), 641.

Beecham's pills. In these circumstances, it is not surprising that Louis Pasteur's discovery of a treatment against rabies—featured in the *Pall Mall Gazette* just after Stevenson's tale—was energetically refuted eight days later.[13] How could enquiring minds know the difference between quackery and organic chemistry? Louis Pasteur could as easily be Doctor Jekyll—or even an incautious anatomist like Doctor Knox.

Nor should we forget that chemical medicine could upset the boundary of body and brain that so confused Edinburgh in the case of Doctor Knox, became a wonder in Doctor Jekyll, and was the conundrum for Pasteur in his investigations of rabies. Anesthesia, in particular, canceled memory and mind, leaving only the inanimate—or disturbingly animate—body. Although Humphry Davy declared himself "absolutely intoxicated," by his 1799 experiments with nitrous oxide, he later felt he risked "sinking into annihilation" (Paris, 56, 67; see figure 4.2). Stevenson's best friend was Walter Simpson—they lived across from one another in Heriot Row and Queen Street. The writer probably heard about after-dinner experiments by his friend's father: Professor Simpson's guests would try a succession of substances for the good of science—and slip slowly under the table (Neuberger, 2). He may equally have heard from the Simpsons the cautionary tale of Doctor Horace Wells (Swearingen, 101). Wells was a pioneer of anesthesia, but he lost his medical reputation after a public experiment failed to send the patient beyond pain. He subsequently became addicted to chloroform. Then in January 1848, after a weeklong self-experiment, Wells assaulted two prostitutes with sulphuric acid. In a fit of remorse, he committed suicide, taking chloroform, then slitting an artery.[14] Alongside this, we might consider that the nineteenth century had recently experienced medical poisoners by the handful—such as William Palmer (who did away with his five children, his wife, his brother- and mother-in-law, and a friend before being caught in 1856) and the emigrant Scot Thomas Neill Cream (who up to 1881 murdered several lovers plus the husband of one—though he claimed it was their epilepsy and may have been his nostrum for the affliction that did them in). Apparently, chemistry brought the inside out, revealing the monster within the doctor. Experiences coming from Stevenson's nearest neighbors, friends, and his medical treatments made clear that mind and body ran separately amok when doctors became the center of their own experimental worlds. This chemistry opened the way to Mr. Hyde—and it also remembered Doctor Knox, strangely split between science and selfishness.

Importantly, however, the anesthesia that separated brain from body and divided the mind could make you expose yourself. Doctor Knox refused to talk, and Doctor Jekyll proves equally reluctant. He insists that his relationship with Hyde is "one of those affairs that cannot be mended by talking" (22). But narcotics could bring on the talking cure. Davy described how under the influence of nitrous oxide:

> My bosom burns with no unhallow'd fire,
> Yet is my cheek with rosy blushes warm;
> Yet are my eyes with sparkling lustre fill'd;
> Yet is my mouth replete with murmuring sound;
> Yet are my limbs with inward transport fill'd;
> And clad with new-born mightiness around. (Fullmer, 215–16)

Anesthesia produced an afflux of bodily power, and also of talkativeness (see figure 4.3). So much so that advertisements for the entertainment potential of narcotics stressed the liberating effect of nitrous oxide, but equally that things would be kept within the bounds of respectability. The American medical student turned showman, Gardner Quincy Colton, advertised "A Grand Exhibition" in 1844:

> The effect of the Gas is to make those who inhale it either Laugh, Sing, Dance, Speak or Fight... according to the leading trait of their character. They seem to

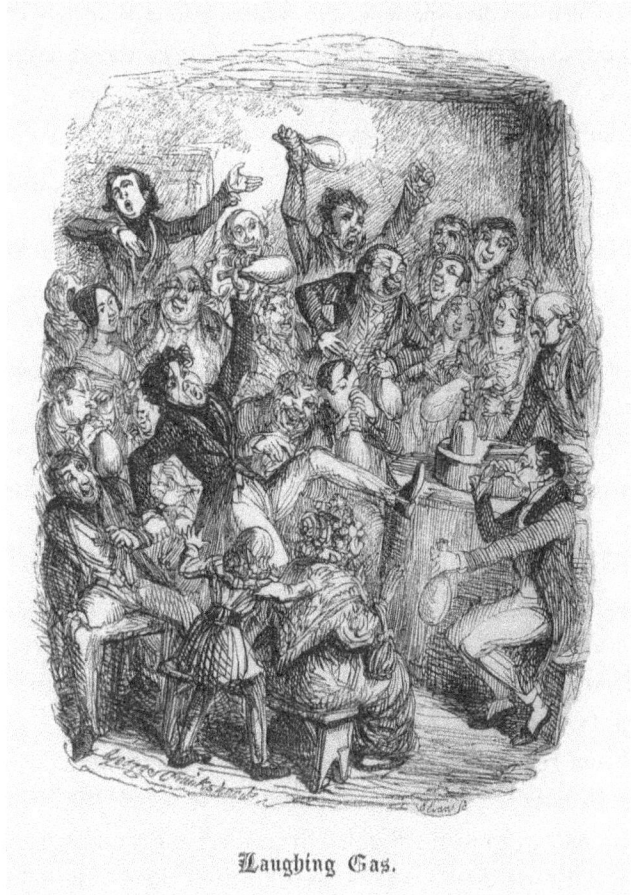

Laughing Gas.

FIGURE 4.3 "Laughing Gas." Line drawing by George Cruikshank, from John Scoffern, *Chemistry No Mystery* (London: Harvey and Darton, 1839), frontspiece. Courtesy of the Wellcome Library, London.

retain consciousness enough not to say or do that which they would have occasion to regret.[15]

No one, the posters emphasized, would act too strangely or talk too much. But speak, as body and as mind, is exactly what Hyde and Jekyll do.

In 1829, R. K. Greville joined *Blackwood's* to complain: "Knox...[says] he kept silence in compliance with the advice of his Counsel—*I* thought [this] had an ugly sound about it" (to Sir William Jardine, February 12, 1829, UE MS Gen 422D). Knox was just a bit too "philosophic." But in *Jekyll and Hyde*, the undiagnosable Mr. Hyde demands explanation. Of course, society cannot explain him, and produced by chemistry at the cost of memory, gesturing from the pit toward man's worrisome multiplicity, Hyde does not and perhaps cannot explain himself. As the site of an "unknown disgust, loathing and fear" for all who meet him, Hyde might recall the revulsion conventionally experienced in earlier fictions by upright citizens in the presence of bodysnatchers (*Jekyll and Hyde*, 18). "On the Pleasures of Body-Snatching" (1827), for instance, worries that "I do not know how it is, but there is something peculiar about P—'s eyes—something that one looks at a second time…because he cannot help it; it produces a disagreeable feeling—a kind of chill" ("Pleasures," 364). Hyde might even point to the "secret sin" of Burke and Hare that for Alexander Leighton produced "that recoil of the good which isolates the criminal from the smiles of fellowship and the help of society" (Leighton *Court*, 122).

Still, we need not wonder unduly, for Hyde's body speaks for itself. When Hyde takes his watery green medicine, his transformation is one that a trained doctor like Lanyon can read. Lanyon's word choice reveals the reality embodied in Mr. Hyde: "he reeled, staggered…staring with injected eyes…he seemed to swell—his face became suddenly black and the features seemed to melt and alter" (56–57). In the process of dissection, veins and arteries might be injected with colored wax so that they could be distended and displayed independently of the body. So Hyde reveals himself as a medical preparation. His transformations run back through the changes of death—the melting and altering—and connect him to the decaying, dissected, injected, and preternaturally vivid body in an anatomist's laboratory. Chemistry points through Hyde toward Doctor Knox.

But is *Jekyll and Hyde* convincingly a response to the long-dead doctor? The text quietly yet persistently claims Knox as the problem to which Jekyll will now speak out the answer. MacGregor had reminded the readers of 1884 that the incisive Knox "was not sufficiently gratified by the pouring forth of the toffana-spirit of his sarcasm. He behoved to hold the phial with refined fingers, and rub the liquid into the 'raw' with the soft touch of love" (MacGregor, 236). Toffana was a compound of arsenic, lead, and belladonna, held responsible for numerous deaths. So for MacGregor the anatomist verges to quack and self-absorbed chemist—the type of Doctor Jekyll. More, MacGregor reactivates a long trail of association between Knox and chemistry through the Doctor's supposedly poisonous personality: MacGregor quotes Leighton (Leighton *Court*, 20)—who may draw on Sharpe's preface to the *Trial* (*Trial*, v). As for Jekyll, his emphasis on chemistry places him in a direct line of descent from Doctor Knox and experimental medicine. Utterson comes in by Jekyll's front door, passing through the old surgical theater to the chemical cabinet, and implying a medical progress from ancient to modern. But Hyde has entered first, through the back door. The anatomical past and the chemical present are in important respects one and the same. Julia Reid reminds us, too, that Stevenson's Printer's Copy "contains a couple of deleted passages in which Utterson speculates that Hyde may be Jekyll's illegitimate son" (Reid, 99). Again, Mr. Hyde directs our awareness from the modern era to its origins. Indeed, in a time when dissection and vivisection were not much separated, and only at the point of pain, Hyde's vague proclivities gain meaning from his tendency to "torture," and "[lust] to inflict pain"—though Knox was against vivisection, the exploits of Burke and Hare irrevocably linked him to its horrors (*Jekyll and Hyde*, 63, 70).[16] It is only a misdirection, then, not a mistake, that Utterson and Poole first look for the missing Doctor Jekyll in the disused theater, which occupies the "far greater proportion of the building," "filled almost the whole ground story and was lighted…by the [chemical] cabinet" (48). Jekyll and Hyde, separated by a door, then locked together by a broken key, at last align in the same space when Utterson breaks down an inside door and exposes a secret— there they both are as one. Early in the text, a little girl going for the doctor is trampled by the juggernaut Hyde (9). Little does she know she has found her doctor.[17] In fact, we all have found this dark inner doctor—and he is an anatomist by descent.

Oscar Wilde complained that "the transformation of Dr. Jekyll reads dangerously like an experiment out of the *Lancet*" (Wilde, 973). For Stevenson, however, medicine serves as a narrative strategy. The author deploys modern medicine not so much to get at facts, but to get at truths long deferred. The transformations of chemistry that produce Mr. Hyde are simultaneously transpositions in literature that access Doctor Knox. And Stevenson shows us early on in the book how they might work. Mr. Hyde and Doctor Jekyll divide medicine by time and place, according to their titles. Through the nineteenth century, governing bodies trying to regulate medicine quarreled over who had the right to which terminology: "Doctor" was a term of high art accorded to those with a Scottish degree, to the chagrin of medical men to the south (Sir Robert Christison to [Dr. Greig], June 10, 1860, UE MS Gen 784/9/1; Loudon, 203). So Mr. Hyde also points through Doctor Jekyll back to Scotland. The Edinburgh doctor who attends the little girl may realize as much, for he recognizes Hyde/Jekyll instantaneously: "emotional as a bagpipe," he turns "sick and white with the desire to kill him" (*Jekyll and Hyde*, 9). And if we consider that, according to MacGregor, at least, police had to force the door to Knox's lecture room, then as Mr. Utterson breaks down Jekyll's door, in the fictive terms wherein this story lives, present finally gains access to and accomplishes retribution against the past (MacGregor, 157). So by running forward the history of medicine from anatomy to chemistry, Stevenson gets at the tools to diagnose the peculiar pathology that was Doctor Knox.

THE DOCTOR DISSECTS HIMSELF

The pathology of the past is laid open, for now, in the context of Mr. Hyde and thus equally under the influence of the strange green potion, Dr. Jekyll speaks. Indeed, talking through his "Full Statement of the Case," he dissects himself. In "The Body Snatcher," Fettes terms the dissection of Gray a "dreadful process of disguise," and rues that he "made no deductions" ("Body Snatcher," 10, 4). However in Knox's period, dissection was supposed to serve the purpose of deduction and detection. Southwood Smith's 1824 argument on the *Use of the Dead to the Living* presumes that dissection is a stage toward detection: "error is inevitable, without a knowledge of anatomy... in all these cases error is fatal: in all these cases anatomy alone can prevent the error—anatomy alone can correct it. Experience [in itself cannot lead to] detection" (Southwood Smith, 6). And Lonsdale credited Knox with a "keen eye, equalling that of a French detective"—in some cases, anyway (Lonsdale, 98). Now that obscure subject, Doctor Jekyll, investigates his own medical and legal case. Under Stevenson's chemical knife, he undergoes a moral dissection, peeling back the layers of his own secretive self.

Lonsdale says that in 1862, just before Knox died, the doctor who had been a great orator but nonetheless maintained a "noli me tangere" relationship to the murders of Burke and Hare, "spoke of writing his life, and gave as a reason that he could explain the terrible events of 1828 better than any other person living, and further, that he would be able to prove his entire innocence" (Lonsdale, 273, 102, 393–94). Knox had waited thirty-four years too long. For Stevenson in 1886 this was exactly the problem with Jekyll qua Knox: he is dishonest with himself and with us. Jekyll insists that "Though so profound a double-dealer, I was in no sense a hypocrite" (*Jekyll and Hyde*, 58). Stevenson disagreed, stating bluntly, "The Hypocrite let out the beast Hyde... who is the essence of cruelty and malice, and selfishness and cowardice" (Stevenson *Letters*, 6:56–57). So when Stevenson's doctor begins to spell out the legal and medical case, he does not give exculpatory facts. Rather he undertakes a dissection of hypocrisy, and makes a turn toward apology.

Early in his story, Jekyll says how much he has suffered—just like Knox, who offered no sympathy for the victims of Burke and Hare, but loudly declaimed "Scarcely any individual has ever been the object of more systematic or atrocious attacks than I have been" (*Mercury* March 21, 1829: 4). Jekyll characterizes himself as "the chief of sinners," but cancels out this realization when he claims also to be "the chief of sufferers" (*Jekyll and Hyde*, 36). He hides behind community, like Knox behind his committee, writing to Doctor Lanyon as "one of my oldest friends" (51). Then he betrays fellowship when, as Hyde, he dares Lanyon to share in a community of dreadful knowledge: "a new province of knowledge and new avenues to fame and power shall be laid open to you," he tempts, "under the seal of our profession" (56). Not surprisingly, then, by the time we get Jekyll's full statement, the community that supports a profession and that in reality recuperated Doctor Knox is in disarray. Lanyon is dead, and Utterson perplexed. But now the doctor, for a wonder, explains, protects community, and apologizes—a gesture so difficult for any doctor, never mind Knox and Jekyll, that books have been written on it and today hospitals design policies to support it.[18] In his own hand, this doctor details events, even though he cannot fully explain them; he judiciously decides to keep his one medical secret, the formula—though in part, he keeps this secret because it does not work; he comes close to apology, at least as Henry Jekyll who stood "aghast before the acts of Edward Hyde"; and he even may be said to atone with his—or their—death (49, 63).

And crucially, Jekyll peels away the layers of cause and effect, linking himself to the past and to present horrors:

> The veil of self-indulgence was rent from head to foot, I saw my life as a whole: I followed it up from the days of childhood... and through the self-denying toils of my professional life, to arrive again and again... at the damned horrors of the evening. I could have screamed aloud. (*Jekyll and Hyde*, 68)

In fact, Jekyll now detects his life as a slow dissection of the self. He began in his laboratory where "Certain agents I found to have the power to shake and to pluck back that fleshly vestment" (59). He ends, that dissection complete, "severed... from my own face and nature," the inside man turned out like an anatomical preparation (73).

For years, Edinburgh had wondered how to come to grips with Doctor Knox. Now, emulating the mob that in 1828 sought to lay hands on the anatomist, Utterson breaks down the door. And for Edinburgh, the lawyer at last takes a good long look at the doctor. Then he takes up Doctor Jekyll's last will. Finally, the doctor speaks for himself. Doctor Knox is laid out in Doctor Jekyll's prose. Stevenson, that Scot and suffering medical subject, has performed a poetic revenge on the doctors: in *Strange Case of Dr Jekyll and Mr Hyde*, Stevenson's doctors dissect themselves.

READING THE ENTRAILS AND PRESCRIBING THE FUTURE

The contemporary audience set a trend for later readers by recognizing that this short tale carried unusual freight. *Punch* knew the story bore an excessive emphasis—to be revealed by the last chapter—but could not quite tell what it was:

> "Let us never refer to the subject again," said Mr. STUTTERSON.
>   "With all my heart," replied the entire human race, escaping from his button-holding propensities....

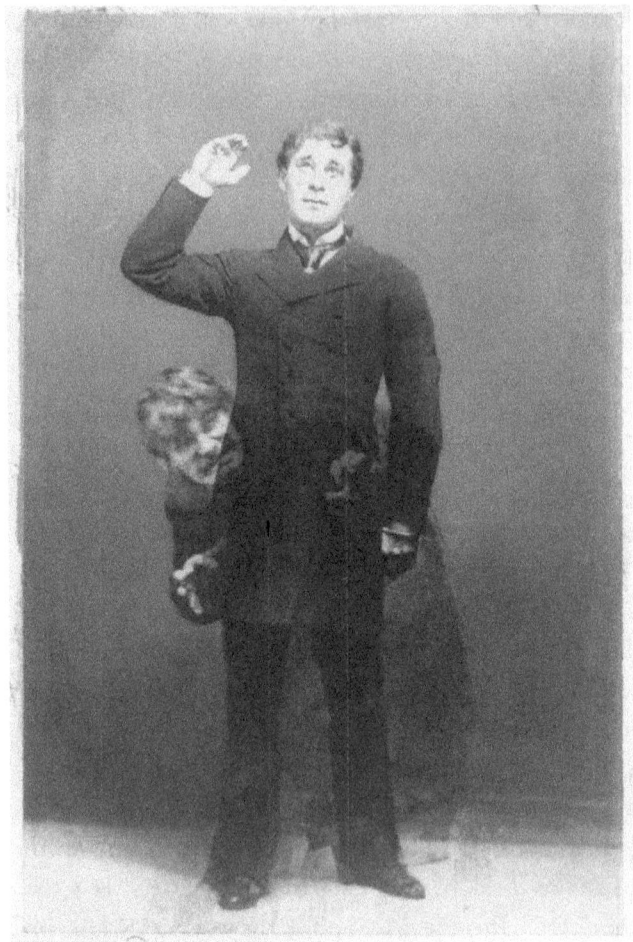

FIGURE 4.4 Richard Mansfield as Jekyll and Hyde. Courtesy of the Library of Congress.

..."Don't speak to me about TREKYL—[says Dr. ONION]—he is a fool, an ass, a dolt, a humbug, and my oldest friend."...

...[STUTTERSON] went to visit Mr. HIDANSEEK. He found that individual, and asked to see his face.

"Why not?" answered the little old creature.... "Don't you recognise me?"

"Mr. R. L. STEVENSON says I mustn't," was the wary response: "for, if I did, I should spoil the last chapter."

...Then Dr. ONION went mad with terror....

"Was it the whiskey?" asked STUTTERSON.

"Wait until the end!"...

CHAPTER THE LAST.—*The Wind-up.*

> ...I, TREKYL....had no fixed idea how it would end when I began, and I trust you will see your way clearer through the mystery than I do, when you have come to the imprint. (February 1886, in Maixner, 208–9)

However, like the Edinburgh doctor, the general public got it—even the London readers made the right connections, although *Jekyll and Hyde* was not, strictly speaking, their tale.

To a degree, Stevenson's story was trumped by recent events: before the author could receive much in the way of reviews, Jack the Ripper began to terrorize the capital (1888). But the popular response is informative. As "autopsies examined what looked like earlier autopsies," journalists connected the Ripper's exploits to those of Burke and Hare. Harkening back to Camden Pelham's *New Newgate Calendar* of 1841, which celebrated police and their supposed powers of detection in the Edinburgh crimes, the populace complained that (in contrast to the present moment) Burke and Hare's case had been investigated and resolved by an alert people and an active government (Warwick, 114; Curtis, 149; Warwick, 30). Rumor burgeoned that the Ripper led a double life between criminality and respectability. Specifically, writers were convinced (prompted by *Jekyll and Hyde*?) that the murderer—who did have a penchant for dissection—must be a doctor (Curtis, 224–29). One even "condemned the steep rise in the price of corpses since the heyday of Burke and Hare" (225). Most tellingly, Richard Mansfield, the actor playing Jekyll/Hyde in a new stage production (see figure 4.4), was accused of being the Ripper (Danahay *Strange Case*, 16, and *J&H Dramatized*, 35–39). The play had to close!

Embracing the market for horror, and diagnosing the trauma that was Doctor Knox, Robert Louis Stevenson had bonded his London and Edinburgh doctors. The two now stood for medicine, criminal malpractice, and murderous dualism for a wider public. Together they were poised to take on a whole new career in film and genre fiction—outside Scotland.

There is nothing very uncommon about you,
—Dr. Knox, *The Anatomist*

5

Anatomizing the Audience

JAMES BRIDIE, MELODRAMA, AND THE MOVIES

DR JEKYLL AND MR HYDE went some way to explicate and so to assuage the anxieties Knox provoked. Stevenson apparently thought as much, for when he next gave an outing to the uncanny body in *The Wrong Box* (1889), with his stepson Lloyd Osbourne, the story took a comic turn. Uncle Joseph, supposedly dead in a railway accident, blithely wanders around England even as the body misrecognized for him is crammed into a barrel, then a piano case, and passed like a parcel between horrified recipients. This carnivalesque tale transposes the body in the box into a pending joke in a folk narrative when the last unwitting recipient, having stolen the cart with "Uncle Joseph," hurtles off into the night. The events of 1828 have been evacuated of threat. They are incipient in society only as a good story.

A "good story" it was, as evidenced by its new career in colorful, cheap editions. The publisher Hugh Jamieson of Edinburgh enthusiastically plagiarized Leighton. Jamieson's stripped-down text appeared between pink soft covers emblazoned with the famous line drawing of Daft Jamie. The inside cover of this *Life and Times of Burke and Hare* (c.1900) indicates the story's audience niche: it advertises *The Best Song Book*, *The Champion Song Book*, *The Famous Song Book*, and *The Holiday Song Book*. History has become urban legend and has aligned with parlor ballad. In c.1910, publisher D. R. Burnside of Glasgow produced a more fictive version, complete with couthy and comic neighbor Sandy M'Nab: *Burke and Hare: The Body Snatchers* (inside subtitle: *Their True Lives*). It too bore a soft cover—this time displaying both Daft Jamie and his hideous (and lively) murder. Advertised on its inside cover, we find the companion texts *Willy Reilly: A Story of the Penal Days in Ireland*; *Sappho: A True Story of Life in Paris*; and—from which we might derive much context for this series featuring Burke and Hare—*Fanny Hill: A Fascinating Story of London Life*. (John Cleland's *Fanny Hill* was a notoriously pornographic "country girl comes to big city" eighteenth-century novel.) The back indicates a financial niche, too. It tempts with "Courting Cards" which promise "Roars of Laughter, useful for those in love, and those who would like to be very good for Pic-Nic Parties going on a Holiday"—four packets for six stamps, "all different," and importantly, "sent in Sealed Envelope."

In the larger market, the story took a turn toward genre fiction. Published in London, Hargrave L. Adam's 1913 *Burke and Hare, The Story of a Terrible Partnership*, begins in Gothic tones: "The story I am about to lay before my readers is one of an exceedingly sordid character.... [we shall] see how these human ghouls, vampires and stoats lived" (Adam, 5). It, too, makes one in a series for sales. The Pearson edition lists it with *The Sale of a Soul*, "an ideal [book] for holiday or train reading"; *The Terror By Night*; "and other Notable Sixpenny Books." Adam's edition did double duty. Republished by the Mellifont Press [1936] it began a career as "true crime," featuring alongside *The Penge Mystery* and *Pritchard the Poisoner* (both by Adam), and *Crimes That Thrilled the World*. The tale shifted along with its writer, who emphasized "true crime" as his career developed, but it easily adapted in any case: *Burke and Hare* made up one of the *Secrets of Scotland Yard* on British radio (1949); by 1952, America's CBS Crime Classics picked it up (*If a Body Needs a Body, Just Call Burke and Hare*).

What is interesting here, however, is work the tale does *not* do in Scotland. Nineteenth-century Edinburgh police procedurals, both factual and fictive, already embraced the horrors of medicine and murder, though surprisingly not of Doctor Knox. Consider James McLevy's "The Dead Child's Leg," or William Crawford Honeyman's "The Mysterious Human Leg."[1] Of course, the story may inflect pieces by that Edinburgh doctor and crime writer Arthur Conan Doyle, who lived hard by the West Port, might have seen Burke's skeleton at the university, and had his own copy of the *West Port Murders* (Edwards *Quest*, 195). Doyle's detective may have drawn his name from Oliver Wendell Holmes (Senior)—who spent some weeks in Edinburgh in 1834, meeting Knox, and later became Professor of Anatomy at Harvard (205; Holmes, 9–10). The professor had told his personal story of auto-experimentation with ether in 1870, contributing to Jekyll as well as Sherlock Holmes, perhaps.[2] For Edwards, Knox lends both coldness and bonhomie to the detective; the victimized Mrs. Docherty shows up in a claim that "One of the most dangerous classes in the world...is the drifting and friendless woman"; and Sherlock Holmes draws his proclivity for pummeling bodies from Christison's experiments on corpses to determine postmortem effects post–Burke and Hare (*Quest*, 197, 202, 196, 194). Christison, too, contributes to Holmes's self-experimentation (194). The line of descent seems clear from Burke and Hare to Baker Street. Still, Scotland's most noted crime writer makes little of this particular past.

Such an omission implies a larger point: the national investment of those who, like Scott, Pae, and Stevenson, so far make much of Burke and Hare and Doctor Knox. For others, it seems—even some Scots—by the late nineteenth/early twentieth century, their story no longer challenged beyond the conventions of genre fiction. As proof, consider the next two major documentary versions of resurrectionist times: these both arise outside Scotland and are directed to English interests. Tellingly, neither recounts the tale of Doctor Knox. The moment that had set going generations of Scottish literary and historical attempts to come to terms with the doctor simply disappears. In 1896, James Blake Bailey, librarian of the Royal College of Surgeons of England, published *The Diary of a Resurrectionist 1811–1812*.[3] The diary stands out for its firsthand account of grave robbing, its uncanny echo of Burkean days (the writer frequently admits to being "intoxsicated" [*sic*] in a way that would have delighted Christopher North), and its disconnection from northern scandal. Bailey makes a feature of not discussing the Edinburgh context for his book. "The great crimes of Burke and Hare drew especial attention to body-snatching in Edinburgh," his introduction states (James Blake Bailey, v–vi). "For this reason, Edinburgh has been omitted from the present work." Cecil Howard Turner's *The Inhumanists* (1932) leaves out Knox for an interestingly different reason:

> For a hundred years, English surgeons have remained complacent at the obloquy exclusively heaped on the head of the unfortunate Dr. Knox.... I shall have done no bad thing if in trying to tell the truth of the alliance formed between culture and crime and reveal the frightful horrors that were perpetrated by the most iniquitous set of villains that ever lived to satisfy the requirements of surgical science I help to restore the balance of criminality. (Cecil Howard Turner, vii–viii)

Turner celebrates the centenary of the Anatomy Act by detailing the bodysnatching and burking proclivities of other doctors and different places, homing in on London.

Does this double shift—to generic writing and away from Scotland—indicate that authors and historians have taken a step in resolving the trauma of 1828? Burke had suffered the pains of the law (see figure 5.1). Perhaps Knox's story now has been told, the horror viewed and integrated, allowing Scots, like their untroubled English counterparts, to escape its old, obsessive terms. Or maybe the past now seems a problem best located somewhere else—preferably in Henry Jekyll's London.

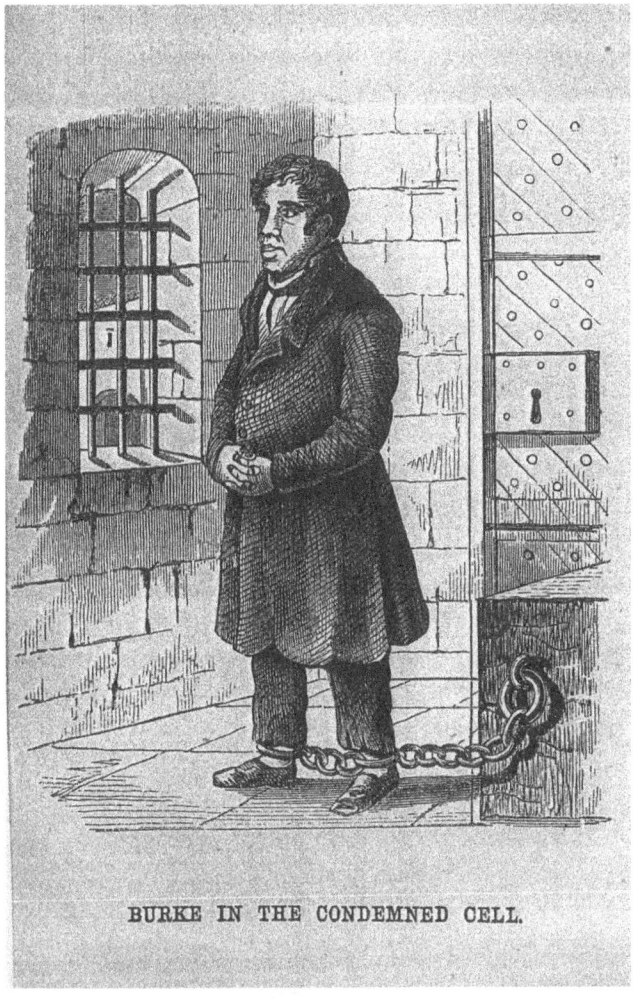

BURKE IN THE CONDEMNED CELL.

FIGURE 5.1 "Burke in the Condemned Cell." From David Pae, *Mary Paterson* (London: Fred Farrah, 1866). Courtesy of the British Library.

In fact, the general turn away from Doctor Knox and Edinburgh exposes a related but broader concern. As Dominick LaCapra has pointed out, trauma resonates not merely through victims but also, if problematically, through perpetrators—think Knox/Jekyll (LaCapra *History*, 41). We can carry this analysis further: when Scots hasten to draw the line of responsibility between themselves and Doctor Knox (as in Stevenson), or when they hand responsibility for their story over to other tellers in other places (as with these medical histories), they characterize themselves as victims now healed. But in so doing they imply anxiety about their own liability for events. So long as Knox remained silent, for Scotland he functioned as the trauma that needed to be expressed and integrated. Stevenson, by making "Knox" talk in the person of Henry Jekyll, and ironically Bailey and Turner, too, by removing him from consideration, expose the scandal's wider context. Stevenson, despite the humor of *The Wrong Box*, winds in Uncle Joseph's family and implicates strangers related only in the most tenuous way; Bailey and Turner, assertively not invested in Scotland, consequently extend the story's historical and geographical reach. Together these three imply that the box of "Uncle Joseph" can turn up on anybody's doorstep and reveal each and all of us as culpable for its criminal circulation.

DOCTORS AND LAWYERS

Though few Scots had known about Burke and Hare until they were caught, all had benefited from Knox's research—and had done so through succeeding generations. Doctors and lawyers stood particularly vulnerable by their relation to the scandals of 1828. Respectable professional identity teetered on whether any doctor was different from Knox, and whether any lawyer had played his part in policing events. Did doctors whose expertise derived from the bodysnatching industry share de facto responsibility for Knox's actions? Did lawyers share de jure responsibility for the machinations that had removed Knox from trial and made him a site for cultural anxiety? Not surprisingly, lawyers and doctors had long struggled to deal with the scandal of 1828. Leighton and Lonsdale were only the most prominent Scottish-trained medical men who so far had tried to negotiate their relation to the anatomist through prose; William Roughead is only the best-known lawyer. Leighton was a medical student who apparently did not take a degree but made much of his experience in his writing; Lonsdale studied under Knox and briefly partnered him (Rae, 125); Roughead was a Writer to the Signet (Scottish solicitor) and author of numerous criminal histories. Other doctors who wrote post-Knoxian tales and tracts on bodysnatching include Christison, who detailed his firsthand experience as the medical examiner for Mrs. Docherty in his *Life* (Christison, 1:305–11). Lawyers number Henry Cockburn, who recounted the trial in his *Memorials* (Cockburn, 456–58), and the Edinburgh-trained doctor and lawyer Samuel Warren, notable for his *Passages from the Diary of a Late Physician* in *Blackwood's* (1832–37). Over the years, professional sympathy has continued to produce writings by non-Scots with a medical or legal investment (for instance the American James Moores Ball, M.D. LL.D, author of *The Sack-'Em-Up Men*). Typically, however, the earlier medical and legal writers follow the established pattern for Knoxian narrative. They focus on Knox to celebrate or damn him—when they can bring him into view at all—and in either case they look away from the implications of their professional similarity to the doctor.

Even that lawyer Robert Louis Stevenson, in a story made up of doctors and lawyers, does not seriously impugn these professional men. Mr. Utterson the lawyer feels like a criminal, but he is not to blame for Jekyll's behavior; rather, Jekyll's activities produce Utterson as the nemesis in the shadows. Lanyon understands Jekyll's science, but the two have parted over the philosophy that drives Jekyll's criminal acts some time past. Nonetheless, through Utterson's uneasiness and Lanyon's outright decline in the context of Mr. Hyde, Stevenson hints toward the connectedness of doctors and lawyers—as individuals and in the aggregate—in a society inherently problematic. In their professional roles and as respected representatives of the wider society, doctors and lawyers needed to recognize their duplicitous part in the scandal of Doctor Knox. It was now time for all Scots to acknowledge their role in the realities of Burke and Hare.

JAMES BRIDIE: THE DOCTOR IS IN

Doctor Osborne Henry Mavor, better known by his pen name "James Bridie," was up to the task—and not just on behalf of his medical community. We might remember Michael S. Roth's concern that history writing symptomizes a problem in memory—it becomes possible because a culture is in process of forgetting its past (Roth, 10). Doctor Knox had now been carefully placed through the strategic deployment of narrative memory—his tale had been told as fiction (by anxious Scots) and laid to rest within British history (by Bailey and Turner). Having blamed him, Scots were ready to forget him at last. But as a general practitioner whose training ranged from anatomy through Freudian psychology, Bridie knew the necessity of a full diagnosis; and as a national dramatist he knew how to bring all the makers of memory themselves into painful play.

Who was James Bridie? The Glasgow doctor's writing first came to the commercial stage in 1928. When Bridie's Knoxian play *The Anatomist* was staged in 1930, the *Glasgow Bulletin* considered it "one of the very best of Scots plays," and when it went to London in 1931 Shaw Desmond described it as the work of "that extraordinary playwright, James Bridie" (*GBulletin* July 5, 1930; *LP* November 11, 1931). By 1934, Ivor Browne considered Bridie "Shavian," and Bridie's competing author, Eric Linklater, thought him a second Ibsen (*NSN* May 5, 1934; Linklater in MacDiarmid *Raucle*, 3:96). Browne stressed: "We know, when we go to a play of his, that we shall escape... the usual much ado about the couplings of nobodies," and he singled out *The Anatomist* for being "as tidily made as it is brilliantly written." On the basis of Bridie's plays, he joked, "I wish he were my doctor."

Publicly, Bridie demurred at such praise. His sardonic autobiography *One Way of Living* (1939) carries his attitude in three epigraphs. The first two situate the writer as a local and lost opportunity—the motto from Glasgow City Arms reads:

This is the bell that never rang,
This is the fish that never swam,
This is the tree that never grew,
This is the bird that never flew.

Bridie follows his compounded negatives with the double bathos of a dictionary definition: "Inertia is the property of matter by which it retains its state of rest or of uniform rectilinear motion so long as no foreign cause occurs to change that state." But next we read from Robert Browning's *The Ring and the Book*:

Well, British Public, ye who like me not,
(God love you!) And will have your proper laugh
At the dark question, laugh it! I laugh first.

Bridie laughed last, too. Despite taking ten years to graduate as a doctor ("I do not, myself, understand Anatomy at all" [*One Way*, 14]), he served well in the Royal Army Medical Corps during the First World War, then ran his own practice from 1919 to 1923. In 1923 he became assistant physician at Victoria Infirmary, and subsequently a professor at the Anderson College of Medicine. Beginning as an amateur dramatist, Bridie turned full-time and wrote over forty plays, many of them successful (*NSN* May 5, 1934; chron. and bib. in Luyben). The crucial conjunction of doctor and dramatist came when Bridie crossed paths with "John Brandane" in the 1920s. Brandane, too, was a doctor (John MacIntyre) and playwright, with a distinct commitment to "a thing very grandly called The Scottish National Theatre Society" (*One Way*, 260). Under Brandane's influence, Bridie helped to establish the Glasgow Citizens Theatre, the Edinburgh International Festival, and the College of Drama of the Royal Scottish Academy of Music. He did become his country's Ibsen or Shaw, having "put Scotland on the dramatic map of the world" (Linklater in MacDiarmid *Raucle*, 3:96).

Did the Doctor Have a Dilemma? *The Anatomist*

The Anatomist marked the turning point between Bridie's medical and dramatic careers, and the fulcrum for the doctor's "Shavian" success was his national concern. Bridie tracked Robert Knox through medical and legal histories. He claimed to have deduced his fellow doctor "from Lonsdale's Life, some Edinburgh College of Surgeons papers, some of his own writings & Roughead.... A friend of mine... was the son of a friend of Knox & the last act is based partly on an incident he described to me" (letter September 30, 1931, RCSEd). But whereas Lonsdale celebrated a heroic doctor, and Roughead chastised a Knox who anticipated "the privileges of the superman," Bridie attempted a more complete assessment of the case (Roughead *Burke*, 80). With a theater for, by, and about the people in mind, he figured his anatomist as symptomatic of a generalized complaint. For Doctor Bridie, there was plenty of contagion to track and responsibility to go around. The case of Robert Knox manifested a systemic reality—a disease already spread through doctors and patients.

How does Bridie bring Knox's human context into focus in a play dominated by its protagonist? Doctor Knox, after all, usurps a parlor drama, bringing his early ego and later problems with Burke and Hare into the Miss Disharts' home, and complicating the love relationships between proper young ladies and eager medical students. One answer lies in the play's noted discomforts: it promised "no moral.... no lesson" (*Anatomist* Westminster Theatre Program, 1931). Audiences, in fact, registered and picked at the play's apparent problems. The *Scotsman* pondered "a lamentable obscurity of purpose" in the last act arising from confusion within the supporting characters: despite nefarious events, the ingenue Mary Belle "informs [Knox] that they will never believe the stories that are going about," so "Her heart does her more credit than her intelligence or consistency" (*Scotsman* July 4, 1930). With this critique, the reviewer is drawn into the play's dynamic and provides an index to its success: the stress Bridie lays on Knox, together with the diagnosis of the doctor that he fails to provide, provokes a reflex action in those beyond the footlights. We engage not with Robert Knox so much as with his stage audience, and their responses to the Knoxian crisis at hand. In so doing, we participate in the weave of relationships that makes an implicated community. This play is all about us.

Bridie understood such relationships. As O. H. Mavor but also "James Bridie" (and "Mary Henderson"), and as doctor, playwright, and thoughtful Scot, he made up a community in himself. Indeed he enacted a play of personalities, each implicated in the others. For instance, he was an anatomist, but a reluctant one. The first time (of many) that he took the Anatomy viva, the professor "roared and howled and chuckled for a full minute. Then he said, 'Well, Mr. Mavor, I suppose it is no secret to you that you know nothing at all about Anatomy'" (*One Way*, 125). At the same time, Bridie appreciated his Glaswegian inheritance from the famous anatomist John Hunter, and his scholarly descent from Robert Knox: "Johnny Cleland had been taught by Goodsir, who had been taught by Knox, who was the patron of Burke and Hare" (16, 101). And Anatomy class cultivated Bridie's dramatic sensibilities: Professor Cleland "had a large mop of sheep's wool on his head. It was said that this was kept in position with the fat of human corpses, for, while he was demonstrating, he would frequently run his fingers through his hair" (97–98); in the anatomy lab, "The corpses were naked and bronze coloured. The general effect was rather gay. My head swam a little and I had an impulse of flight. [Another student]…smacked a corpse on the abdomen with a cheery greeting and passed on" (105). The doctor and the dramatist informed one another, standing, as both did, at the crux of medical and literary pasts and futures. Thus, Mavor finally connected with his work as a doctor when he realized the narrative drive of diagnostics and its humane application: Dr. Middleton "asked [a patient] three or four questions that seemed to have little bearing on the subject, and listened carefully to his answers. [he then diagnosed privately and]…. said we would [check] in the post-mortem room in a fortnight's time"—and they did (183); Doctor Renton "was by far the most humane [teacher]. I could not have chosen a more pleasing introduction to my kindly trade" (131–32). Bridie shone as a practitioner informed by his humanity, and a dramatist supported by his diagnostic insight. Thus he produced Doctor Knox as the enlarged and inadequate heart of a failing body politic. For Mavor/Bridie, "Robert Knox" set the pulse for relationships with broad implications for doctors, Scots, and "community" in general.

At first, Bridie's Knox seems the focus of the text. The play places the doctor in the drawing room, where he mediates between lovers Mary Belle and Walter Anderson; it moves on to show the love-crossed medical student (Walter) be charmed by Mary Paterson, then recognize her on the slab; and it concludes back in the domestic sphere, when murder has been revealed and the streets are filled with the mob against a blustering yet still lecturing Doctor Knox. This structure implies a persistent doctor, and perhaps a recuperated one. We hear echoes of Lonsdale's heroic Knox as well as Roughead's boneheaded doctor, and even Stevenson's marginally self-doubting experimental scientist. Bridie's play, it seems, like *The Court of Cacus*, *Mary Paterson*, and *Strange Case*, aims at Doctor Knox—with an overture of romance in the persons of Walter and Mary Belle, an interlude of sentiment provided by Mary Paterson, and incidental grosserie performed by Messrs. Burke and Hare.

But Bridie's few statements on Knox confuse the anatomist's role. After dismissing Lonsdale's doctor as the work of "a frank Knoxophile," Bridie indicates a possible medical moral for his story: "the shifts to which men of science are driven when they are ahead of their times. The 'mob' should be very careful in its choice of objects for persecution; for stoning the prophets is not so good for their moral [sic]" (*Anatomist*, xi, xiv).[4] However, to Alfred Wareing the theater entrepreneur, Bridie wrote that the play's first performers had "no notion that it was a parable *against* modern scientific thought" (my emphasis); to Knox's descendant, he declared that "For the purposes of the play I've definitely assumed [Knox] to be in the wrong"; and ultimately, he termed the doctor "the Scientist as Dictator" (October 26, 1830, NLS MS8181/12; December 1, 1931, RCSEd; *One Way*, 278). The anatomist provides only a contradictory center to a play that points somewhere else—perhaps back along the imprecisions of Bridie's reference to "the 'mob'" and "their moral."

Bridie's Knox manages to be multifaceted without being deep. The author stresses in his "Author's Note," "[Knox] did not usually wear a patch on his blind eye, but he definitely should in this play" (*Anatomist*, xii). The morally winking Knox is now simply half blind. Insistent on "facts" as pointing to the sum "Truth" when he presides over a trivial lovers' quarrel, he cannot—indeed, will not—recognize the truth when the fact of Mary Paterson is literally staring him in the face (22, 46–48). This Knox, who mocks the lovers and rejects Walter's concerns about Mary Paterson because "it is past the hour for sentiment," is given to posturing on his own behalf (20, 46). Courting Amelia Dishart, the married doctor falls into the clichés of romance, declaring himself a "little pink shivering boy" (63). Worse, the doctor is apt to dramatize his professional role: "I have my pistols and I will fight if necessary," he declaims, and he ludicrously exhorts his students: "I shall lead you to Surgeons' Square" (69, 71). We should be mindful, perhaps, of Bridie's later comment on sentimentality: it is "a form of voluptuous cruelty" (*One Way*, 244). Knox is contradictory rather than complex. He lacks the nuance that can inform even the least sympathetic protagonist.

So it is no surprise that this Knox claims a noble difference from other less able doctors, but for all the wrong, self-indulgent reasons. When he declares "Bob Liston is no friend of mine. I abhor his methods," the ingenue Mary Belle promptly asks, "Where do *you* get your bodies from?" Registering no irony, Knox retorts: "How should I know?" (*Anatomist*, 22–23). Even when this Knox admits blame, he does so only within the parentheses of religious and dramatic convention:

> Do you think because I strut and rant and put on a bold face that my soul isn't sick within me at the horror of what I have done?... But I tell you this, that the cause is between Robert Knox and Almighty God. I shall answer to no one else.... I shall play out the play till the final curtain. (65–66)

Some critics find here a note of contrition and hence, greatness of character. The *Evening News* congratulated actor Henry Ainley for revealing "the diffident soul of the scientist within the ogre's body" (*EN* October 8, 1931). However, any sincerity in Knox's assertion is borne down by the continued strutting and ranting. Bridie's Knox cannot help but strut and rant, whatever position he adopts. This is evident in his crucial test, when he can either feel someone else's pain and accept responsibility, or pass it on because it does not fit his reality. Walter, devastated by finding his companion of the evening in a box, accuses Knox of paying blood money for Mary Paterson. Knox does not address the issue. Rather, he turns to the lowest form of argument with the riposte, "You paid the money, Mr. Anderson, I think" (*Anatomist*, 47). This doctor has lots of form, and no substance.

Bridie's Knox finds his being not so much in medicine or its truths as through the posturings of dispute with weaker individuals—whether with sentimental Mary Belle, or conscience-stricken Walter. He thrives on opposition. "Only a fool is sure of himself until the mob denies him," Knox declares, with a witty delight in contradiction (*Anatomist*, 12). His bon mot loses its joy for us, however, when an actual mob with a legitimate grievance hounds him through the streets. "The mob are cowards to a man," this poor student of human nature declares; and though Amelia offers a corrective: "Their hatred is a dreadful thing," the doctor refuses any relationship between himself and the mob beyond mere opposition: "Dreadful? It is the only compliment they can pay me" (64). If earlier texts worked hard to integrate for Scotland the trauma constituted by Doctor Knox, Bridie's doctor has no intention of being integrated. This poses the mob sitting just beyond the footlights a bit of a problem.

Bridie makes no effort to help the audience. He seems not to want to integrate Knox. Amelia tells the doctor, "You will talk yourself out of Edinburgh," and the dramatist lets him run on and on (*Anatomist*, 65). Indeed, Bridie primes us for this excessive yet impenetrable doctor. In his note, the playwright indicates the theatrical intensity but limited dramatic potential of Doctor Knox by his massed efforts to describe him:

> He was a dandy. He wore a dark puce or black coat and a fancy waistcoat; a high cravat passed through a diamond ring.... He gestured when he lectured.
> He had a bitter heart: he had served at Waterloo and in South Africa; he was eloquent and full of bull-dog pluck.... He had a well-stocked mind and kept the largest possible proportion of his stock in the shop window. He really did contribute to Science. He was the most popular lecturer in Britain. (xii)

The declarative statements pile up, multiplying facets of Doctor Knox but not focusing through to any complex heart. Evidently, Knox sets plots agoing, but their interest does not lie with him.

Knox may be a Shavian superman, and the character offers a plum, scenery-chewing role sought by major actors from Ainley (who made a comeback in the part) to Seymour Hicks (who could have placed the Doctor alongside his Scrooge) to Alastair Sim (who built a career through the anatomist over decades).[5] But Bridie's doctor constitutes an absence in the play. Early reviewers loved the part, yet noted how Knox manages to be at once central and a gap. *The Curtain* pondered: "a character which is constantly theatrical cannot be dramatic," and the *Sunday Times* complained, "Yes, you say at the end of the first act, that's a first-class bit of painting. Now let us see the monster in action.... But we were not so to see him" (*Curtain* January 1932; *STimes* October 11, 1931). Knox is a constructed absence. Though he stands at the middle of the play, he is too dense to have the heart necessary to center it. Rather, the doctor is the rhino on which, with unconscious irony, he bases his closing lecture. Knox turns from murder and mayhem to:

> a weightier matter... "The Heart of the Rhinoceros." This mighty organ, gentlemen, weighs full twenty-five pounds, a fitting fountain-head for the tumultuous stream that surges through the arteries of that prodigious monster.... [The] rhinoceros buffets his way through the tangled verdure engirdling his tropical habitat. Such dreadful vigour, gentlemen, such ineluctable energy requires to be sustained by no ordinary forces of nutrition. (*Anatomist*, 72–73; ellipsis in original)

The supposed genius Robert Knox can only describe, not recognize himself. Evidently, it takes a rhino not to know one.

In fact, there is not much in Knox for the audience to know. Bridie's note acknowledges the difficulty and perhaps the irrelevance of trying to judge the man with the sensibility of a rhinoceros: "No solution to the mystery of Knox's attitude in 1828 is suggested. Perhaps Mary's (in Act III) is nearest the truth, though she only says it to hurt him" (*Anatomist*, xiii). Mary Belle's opinion, "I think you are a vain, hysterical, talented, stupid man. I think that you are wickedly blind and careless when your mind is fixed on something," really reaches no deeper than that we can derive for ourselves (66–67).

The Audience Anatomized

The dramatic complexity of *The Anatomist* arises obliquely, through Knox's troubled context. Knox is the rhino in a china shop, for the first and last acts of the play take place in the Miss Disharts' drawing room. In the opening act Knox comes to perform on the flute, preside over a lover's tiff, and make sheep's eyes at Miss Amelia. In the closing act, the Miss Disharts return from abroad to find shrouded furniture (that for one reviewer recalls Knox's dissecting room), riot in the streets, and a Knox at once blustering and bathetic (*STimes* October 11, 1931). This domestic background throws Knox into relief, but it also evokes the complexity in minor characters through their shifting relationships to the doctor. In anxious boys and silly girls, their easy opinions, conscience-stricken concerns, and sad compromises, the implications of Knox's ventures reach beyond the anatomy lab. Bridie, that is, tracks the dynamics of groupthink. Whether Knox is a bully or hero, a sentimentalist or himself unsympathetic, fascinating or ridiculous in his relations to women, a realist or a parlor performer, what matters, as the *News of the World* captured in cartoon, is how individuals realign as they relate to him (see figure 5.2). The doctor, with his unpredictable positions, serves as a test of character to those around him. Yet he reveals them not simply as lesser intellects or softer hearts. Rather, as they react, critique, and adjust, these serious young men and thoughtful women show themselves to be involved and implicated in the human perplexity that is Doctor Knox.

Of course beside Knox, most characters look small. David Paterson the doorkeeper verges between religious cant and petty graft as he reads the "awfu' curse" against disobeying the commandments yet haggles over the price for Mary's corpse (*Anatomist*, 39, 33, 43). To Jessie Ann, the maid, Knox's scandal offers an occasion for proud gossip about "*Our* Dr. Knox"—her response lends some credibility to the doctor's derision of the mob (52). Still, the human context for Doctor Knox gets complicated early in the play and through the least likely character. Bridie denigrates Mr. Raby as "fictitious…intended to symbolise the dog-like loyalty of Knox's students" (xiii). Raby is a comic butt. Yet he calls into question Knox's supposed great-

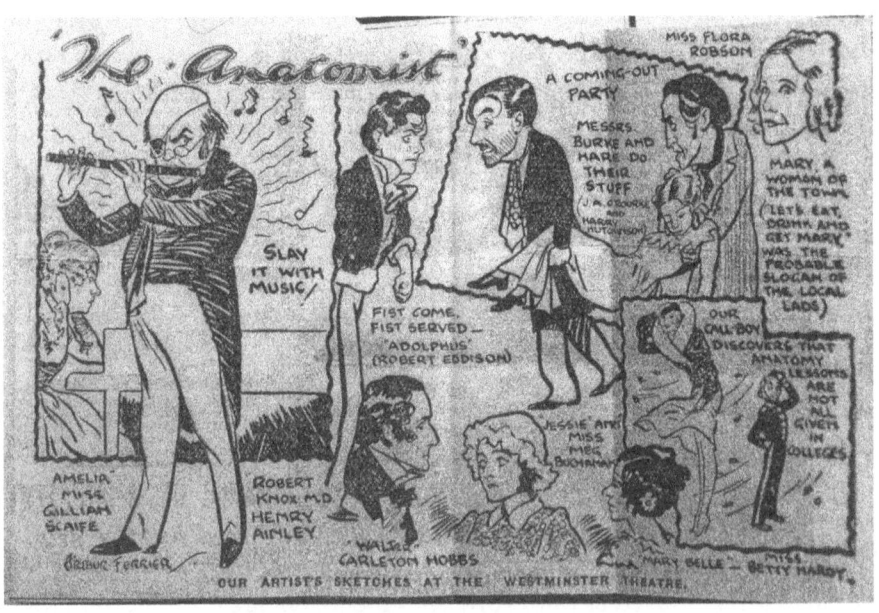

FIGURE 5.2 "The Anatomist." Cartoon from the *News of the World*, November 15, 1931. Courtesy of the University of Glasgow Library, Department of Special Collections.

ness (however wrongheaded) of character. Walter considers Raby "a dull fellow, sir, but conscientious and anxious to learn"; Knox parrots and parodies: "[Raby] is also most conscientious and anxious to learn. He ceased this evening, at my urgent request, to pursue his studies at Surgeons' Square" (8, 13). The dull Raby possesses a nobility unavailable to his hero, and undermines Knox's vaunted commitment as a teacher. Moreover, the dark questions refused by Knox swirl around this incompetent student. Walter has given Raby a head to work on and Knox bursts out: "Do you think that dissecting-room subjects are so easily come by that I can afford to have them mangled by that imbecile?" (8). Raby is the crux for the economics of anatomy that produce Burke and Hare—the more implicated, indeed, because he is so unwitting.

The noble lover Walter, righteous critic Mary Belle, and thoughtful Amelia, too, fall to complicity. Walter is embroiled in events through his naïveté. Helen MacDonald notes how the students of the past distanced themselves, citing David Paterson as receiver of bodies (Helen MacDonald, 30). As demonstrator, Walter tells Knox that arranging churchyard raids "is no part of my duty.... I disapprove of them very strongly" (*Anatomist*, 9). At the same time, he gives a zealot's clichéd endorsement to anatomy: "It isn't disgusting. It's beautiful. Lovely intricate human bodies. It teaches me to see God" (6). Apparently he has no notion of meeting God through the act of premature resurrection in the cemetery. Where, then, does he think the bodies come from, and who does he think gets them? Ignorance and enthusiasm together bring us close to culpability.

That goes for Mary Belle, too. Her counter to Walter's idealistic commitment to medicine is an equally thoughtless romanticism. She challenges Knox: "If you had the least sensibility you would feel—as Walter *knows*—that if he had been a poet or a musician or—or inspired in any way, I would have followed him barefoot through the world" (*Anatomist*, 20). Here we can only agree with Knox's riposte: "That would have been very foolish of you." And we must doubt if Mary Belle is so far removed from blame as she imagines.

No one is without some sort of guilt. Amelia idealizes the doctor: "Poor soul, he is lonely!...And he has married, we are told, so unhappily" (*Anatomist*, 2–3). So although she is generally the most mature person in the room, able to recognize contradiction and sense the anguish that may underlie it in Walter, Mary Belle, and even the doctor, Amelia, too, fails the test posed in Robert Knox. She states, with full complexity, "Doctor, it is terrible that you should be put in this position. I think of you galloping on a crusade with your eyes to the front, fixed on your goal. How could you know that your horses' hoofs were trampling poor crushed human bodies? You don't realise it yet," but ultimately she, along with all the others, aligns with Doctor Knox (65). Walter and Raby put their own safety at risk, fighting their way through the streets to protect him; Amelia asserts, "My sister and I have just heard of the monstrous things that are being said against you. We are so sorry," and Mary Belle follows up with "please believe that I and my sister will listen to nothing that anybody says" (59–60). So much for facts.

In the speech that Bridie suggests comes closest to understanding for the play, Mary Belle snaps: "Posterity will have to be very clever to judge you justly, Dr. Knox" (*Anatomist*, 67). Nor does she let Knox off the hook when he responds, "At least it will have the facts before it." She retorts: "But the excuses will be hard to find." Well said, but not just for Doctor Knox. The doctor is incorrigible, so whose reputation stands at issue here? Bridie pointed to the play's complexity when he vaguely claimed: "The 'mob' should be very careful... for stoning the prophets is not so good for their moral" (xiv). Whose moral—or "morale," if this be a misprint? The play's structure allows no one any excuses. Winnifred Bannister applauded Bridie for frying up no "Knox steaks to be consumed by the mob" (Bannister, 87). At the end, in lieu of "Knox steaks," we have Knox lecturing again. But amid shrouded furniture reminiscent of the dissecting lab, and despite the central fact of Mary Paterson, everyone is here; everyone is listening. For better or for worse, we are the mob, and our own moral/e is at issue.

In 1861 Alexander Leighton had carefully avoided implicating Knox's students. In 1921, William Roughead hinted broadly in their direction (Roughead *Burke*, 80, 87–8). Now, characters revolve around Knox, casting light on the doctor, but themselves becoming illuminated as they twist and turn. Consequently, as Bridie's play moves from a first act where characters argue over principles to a second full of hard fact and on to a final act stumbling into compromised practice, everyone is anatomized. Walter presumed that he could learn anatomy without dirtying his hands in the graveyard; fallen from romance, he imagines he can wash himself clean in the broad waters of the Forth (*Anatomist*, 40). But there are no innocents, nor any second baptism. And with Mary Paterson, the actual victim, kept in parenthesis in Act II, there is nothing to choose between doctors and ladies and even the naïve Mary Belle and thoughtful Amelia. All of Edinburgh is responsible.

Does Bridie's analysis reach beyond the Miss Disharts and their Edinburgh coterie? *The Anatomist*'s final moments disturbed and asked something of the critics. With the play newly on the boards in Edinburgh, the *Glasgow Herald* expressed disappointment: "One would have liked it better had Knox been either a villain or a martyr. In this respect the play ends lamely"—"with none of the expectations of the audience fulfilled" (*GH* July 5, 1930). The *Scotsman* understood more fully. Although lamenting the final act's "obscurity of purpose," the review turns toward the site of this lack (*Scotsman* July 4, 1930). While "The doctor storms about," he "has suddenly become a hero to his former accusers." This is where Mary Belle comes in, with her heart that "does her more credit than her intelligence or consistency." The review concludes: "[This] act is a strangely incoherent medley, most un-Scottish in its illogicality." Here lies the point. We are looking at Scots not as they suppose themselves to be, but as they are—as individuals and by the handful—in complicated circumstances. Knox provides the occasion for us to question the flawed Mary Belle and the malleable students. Thus, disputing Bridie's competence, the critic actually offers an index to the author's effectiveness, for this reviewer finds himself entangled in the illogicalities of the last act, and embroiled in a defense of Scottishness. Bridie's supposedly inadequate ending has implicated the critic.

That ending was no accident; rather, it seems part of a rigorous strategy founded in a philosophy of drama as it intersects with the theatricalities of life. Roughead had referred to "The Resurrectionist drama, of which Scotland in general and her capital in particular were the theatre" (Roughead *Burke*, 3). Bridie thematized the metaphor, even as he translated Doctor Knox into the realities of the playhouse. Knox, he claimed, "was so theatrical in his life and habit that it is possible to transfer him almost bodily to the stage" (*Anatomist*, xi). Bridie's Knox lives within the discourse of the theater. He is a "barn-storming tenor" prone to "gesturing" and can easily be interpreted as "farce" (63, 69, 5). Nor is he wrong in diagnosing those around him as indulging in "theatricals" (7). However, Bridie goes further than this. The play resonates not just with metaphors of performance, but with the consonant necessity for audience involvement and interpretation. Knox arrives in the drama to play his flute which, we are told—ironically and significantly—he does very badly (3). The ladies, however, are supposed to support him in his avocation. As for his concluding lecture, it is not unusual for the man who "would go into the lecture-hall and gesture and rant to naebody but the auld skeleton in the cauld o' the morning" (41). Lecturing is a habit of being for the doctor; his note is performance. Performance always beseeches an audience—whether a tatty skeleton, or a drawing-room assembly (41, 71). Bridie's play is thematized as a constant manifestation of performance and thus as posing the problem of what can be "real" or "true," both for and in the viewer.

That is, by dwelling on performance and resisting the drive toward critique and closure, the play turns our focus where we do not expect—toward each of us. Bridie described the play as a "fable" (*Anatomist* xi). Fables carry messages and meanings, but those meanings reside in us and are evident only through us. When the dull Mr. Raby arranges a scene, wanting "to see daybreak in the Chamber of Horrors," the view is more than he bargained for (41). It redounds upon himself as Mary Paterson tumbles from her tea chest and into his own tale. When Doctor Knox poses for Mary Belle as "Your only jig-maker," Bridie deploys the anatomist's performance as the hub for the minor characters' actions (8). What matters, and what Bridie seeks for the story of Burke and Hare, is our uneasy response in turn.

Bannister considers this Bridie's great achievement as a dramatist. "A Bridie comedy," she argues, invites the audience to "look at itself in the Hall of Mirrors"—and in *The Anatomist* Bridie offers less of an invitation than a compulsion (Bannister, 6). So who recognized themselves as mirrored in *The Anatomist*? Clearly, this was not an easy play; it posed questions about the shape of drama as well as about its meaning, never mind what it implied about the locations of meaning. Indeed, the Masque theater company in Edinburgh, which premiered the work, had no idea how to take it. Bridie complained that during rehearsal, "on numerous essential questions I put about The Anatomist they are silent" (to Alfred Wareing, June 15, 1930, NLS MS8181/7). It turned out that in trying to make head or tail of the play, the Masque was actually in the process of ripping it into shreds. When Bridie arrived for a preview, the performance bore no relation to his script:

> The circumstances were...a lot of idiotic cuts.... As they destroyed the thread of the play altogether they all had to be put back with the consequence that the leading man, a bad study, forgot 80% at least of his words & simply yammered.... the story was quite unintelligible. (to Alfred Wareing, 30 July 1930, NLS MS8181/8)

As Bridie remembered once the heat of the occasion was past, this Knox "forgot altogether the two sets of words he had learned, but carried through the part with great verve by dint of shouting 'God Almighty!' 'Damn!' 'Rot their souls!' and 'Barbara Celarent!' at suitable intervals" (*One Way*, 271). "Barbara" and "Celarent" are the first terms in a mnemonic detailing forms of syllogism—they thus provide an ironic filler for the actor trying to vamp in the part of Robert Knox. In this context, the play's unlikely "great success" indicates that Knox, though the dominant figure, was not essential to its meaning, and that the audience did get Bridie's meaning despite and perhaps because of the challenge the performance made to their understanding (271).

The play was an immediate hit with doctors. The *Edinburgh Dispatch* noted their support even on the opening night; the *Evening Standard* found in the 1931 audience "large numbers of doctors and Scotsmen, and particularly those who are both"; and Bannister considered the medical profession well represented and still appreciative in the audience for the 1952 production (*EdEDis* July 4, 1930; *ES* November 12, 1931; Bannister, 70). Doctors typified the general audience reaction in Scotland. The *Glasgow Herald* admitted that despite the failings of the last act, "there was no doubt that the audience enjoyed 'The Anatomist'" (*GH* July 5, 1930). The columnist for the *Times* stressed that the Edinburgh premiere "was warmly received," and the *Dispatch* was sure "there will always be crowds to see 'The Anatomist'" (*Times* July 3,

1930; *EdEDis* July 4, 1930). They were right. Looking back from 1955, Bannister (67) stressed that "I have not yet come away from a performance of *The Anatomist* without sharing the satisfaction of the audience in the play's ending" (though she herself rather misses the irony of that ending).

Importantly, too, all critics recognized this as distinctly a Scottish play. The *Glasgow Bulletin* touted a "Scots Dramatist's Gripping Play," and considered *The Anatomist* "one of the very best of Scots plays" (*GBulletin* July 5, 1930). The *Times* registered that the audience "showed much interest in the recounting of a famous incident in their local history" (*Times* July 4, 1930). *Time and Tide* urged "Let none assume that this is another of those too, too sweet Scottish comedies in which most of the characters are half-wits.... there is the true granite ring about the dialogue" (*T&T* October 17, 1931). That is, a hundred years after Burke and Hare, doctors and citizens stood forth, were recognized, and recognized themselves as implicated Scots in the refracting mirror of Bridie's play.

There is no doubt that Bridie viewed his project as simultaneously medical, theatrical, and Scottish. He wrote *The Anatomist* in a moment of self-consciously national dramatic endeavor with a distinct agenda for bringing theater home to Scots and Scottish theater to a wider audience. *The Switchback*, its recent predecessor, was developed under the guidance of Brandane, of whom Bridie said, "If anything comes of the Scottish Drama, John Brandane is its begetter" (*One Way*, 268). Brandane "was for the pure milk of the Gospel. He considered that the [Scottish National Theatre] Society should produce a Scottish drama by Scottish authors and, as there was no existing Scottish drama by Scottish authors, that the Society's sole function was to evoke one" (260–61). Bridie is just beginning to be recognized, too, for formal innovations that derive from his mixed agendas. The *Scotsman* caught a hint of Bridie's deconstructivist dynamic when it recognized the "clever anti-climax" that ends *The Anatomist* (*Scotsman* April 30, 1931). The *Evening News* understood that Bridie's play, although it appeared to have "no great meaning or message," was "about twice as well written, produced, and acted as the average West End success," and thereby stood as a Scottish challenge to the English theater's conventional forms (*EN* October 8, 1931). Today, Bridie stands out as the Scottish philosopher and disputant who resists the sense of an ending and, in modernist mode, directs his drama out though the hall of mirrors that is his audience (Bannister, Carruthers).

Hugh MacDiarmid and the Anatomy of Scotland

Bridie's play was not universally recognized as a work for Scotland in either its themes or its innovations. Many Scots acknowledged seeing themselves and their ancestors in Bridie's portrait of Knox's Edinburgh—the records of the Royal College of Surgeons of Edinburgh hold admiring letters to Bridie by Knox descendants, heirs to doctors, and record keepers.[6] Some arbiters of Scottish letters, however, did not recognize the Scottishness of Bridie's plays: after *The Sunlight Sonata* was performed in Glasgow (1928), Bridie notes, "The o'ercome of the song of most of the other young men of genius was that the first great Scottish play had yet to be written. In the meantime it was necessary for them to be very firm" (*One Way*, 267). *The Anatomist*, too, stumbled over its national affect: "The performance was a great success and the dramatic critics of Edinburgh said that the first great Scots play had yet to be written" (271). Consider Bridie's phrasing: "The performance was a great success *and* the dramatic critics...." Hugh MacDiarmid was one of those who did not recognize the Scottishness of Bridie's writing—and he disliked Bridie's plays in part for their very success.

MacDiarmid's attitude poses a major question for Burke and Hare as national tale—what makes a Scottish tale, and when is a story too successful to be Scottish? Given that MacDiarmid presented himself as the manifestation of things Scottish and as fearless leader for Scottish literature, we might expect him to appreciate and recognize Doctor Knox—the moreso that MacDiarmid argued for the specificity of Scottishness and its eccentricity. We might think that MacDiarmid and Knox could match on all counts. We might further imagine that MacDiarmid would appreciate Bridie's distinctly Scottish location, retrieval of Scottish history, and the play's appropriate use of Scots dialect in a vehicle for Scottish actors that boosted Scottish dramatic writing, the theater, and theater attendance. But no. And it is worth considering MacDiarmid's reasons for disliking Bridie's plays.

MacDiarmid found no Scottish drama in Bridie—or anyone else. The poet had established his opinion in 1922, when he sweepingly declared: "There has never been a Scottish drama" (MacDiarmid *Selected Prose*, 14). Indeed, he swept aside Bridie's cohort-to-be:

> I do not attach the slightest importance to the present Scottish Players' movement.... writing plays superficially Scottish—or at any rate superficially subscribing to the stock-conception of what is Scottish... [T]hese plays are in every respect inferior to English or Irish plays in their respective *genres*, and are entirely destitute of literary distinction or significance... they are not only not Scottish but anti-Scottish. (13)

In 1934, after Bridie's massive success in Scotland and England with *The Anatomist*, and the successful production of at least half a dozen other plays, MacDiarmid had nothing to say in mitigation of his earlier remarks. Rather, he added Bridie to his list of problem Scots: "Scottish arts remain almost wholly derivative," he declares.

"Certainly nothing is to be gained by hailing all our geese as swans" ("Scotland and the Arts"). MacDiarmid's criticism homes in on the fact that "Young Scottish artists of all kinds are drawn to London and become almost entirely subdued to the general art modes and material of the South." He singles out Bridie for particular chastisement: "James Bridie is not a dramatist comparable to Synge or O'Casey, and (perhaps this is the reason) he is proportionately less national."[7] That is, for a Scottish author to be recognizable outside Scotland makes him not Scots and also inferior—in equal measure. The unfortunate correlative might be that a dramatist can be considered Scottish only if unrecognizable in a larger context. From this perspective, and through his first successful London production that moved to radio, served as early TV drama, and motivated two generations of British and American movies, Bridie poses a problem.

What does it mean to succeed with a Scottish story, or as a Scot, outside Scotland? Does success demonstrate that the art and the story are powerful enough to penetrate a larger world, or have they lost their cultural specificity and been absorbed? MacDiarmid feared the latter: in 1922 he claimed that "most of these debased 'Scottish' brands of letters and drama are made in England, or by Scots enslaved by the ubiquitous and incessant suggestioning of the Sassenach" (MacDiarmid *Selected Prose*, 14). Bridie thought differently. A deep philosophical difference lay between the two authors, and it arose from their conceptions of where worth and value lie in any culture. Responding to MacDiarmid's attacks, Bridie caught MacDiarmid precisely where he prided himself—on the Scottishness of character:

> the Scottish theatre [has] taken over the delineation of character.... [I]t is possible to see, in many towns and villages in Scotland, what Scottish dramatists have found in the vein that seemed to be exhausted. Mr Joe Corrie is bringing life out of the miner's row, Mr T. M. Watson has found it in the mean streets. Mr Donald MacLaren has found West of Scotland villages full of it. (*The Scottish Character*, 20)

Bridie sees Scottishness not so much in the unique, the grand, or the distinctive, but in the ordinary—the common.[8] His philosophy motivates Mary Belle's most cutting remark to Doctor Knox, who thinks himself so special: "There is nothing very uncommon about you" (*The Anatomist*, 67). What matters to Bridie is less the difference of nations than the similarity of individuals—as we can see in the plot of *The Anatomist*.

Bridie, then, offers a competing diagnosis of Scottishness—one that many Scots, willing to see themselves as Scots, not exceptions, clearly recognized. And it was on the basis of similarity, in ironic juxtaposition to Knox's eccentricity, that Bridie's

Scottish play appropriately penetrated English culture and even gained American reference.

The Scottish author's achievement, his translation of the story of Doctor Knox into a tale not uncommon and that weaves in a larger world, was not immediately evident. At first the play was read as too different to understand. English critics, falling into MacDiarmid's stereotypes, presumptuously offered plot solutions to suit this provincial drama to the London stage. The *Sunday Times* complained that "when we return for the third act in expectation of the evening's grisly but nevertheless *bonne bouche*, we find, alas, that all is over except that those things which we know already have to be explained to ladies returning from Dieppe!" (*STimes* October 11, 1931). The play needed to be rendered into an English plot and form:

> Must not the ideal drama have concerned itself with the conflict between the man of science determined to admit no bar...and the man of normal conscience?...[T]here *was* a third act to this play [Knox's London biography], which Dr. Bridie could have found if he had bethought him of that old question of dramatic conflict.

MacDiarmid might have felt justified. A Scottish play would have to become "English" to succeed. But did success indicate such a change?

Bridie's drama actually foregrounded its difference through aggressively Scottish performance. Recurrently, critics have noted the impenetrability of *The Anatomist*'s language for foreign audiences: an American visitor to the Edinburgh production said that he "had once sat through an entire Chinese play. 'I understand as little of this one'" (*GBulletin* July 5, 1930). When the play moved to New York, it was criticized for being "Delivered by so-so actors in a haze of Scotch dialect" (*New York World Telegraph* October 25, 1932). But even a better actor, Alastair Sim, eighteen years later in London had trouble bringing the audience beyond the bar of language—or didn't try to. The *Stage* commented that "He delivers his lines with fluent ease, but often too rapidly and inaudible, a fault which all the cast might have borne in mind, considering the difficulty which the ear has in receiving Scots and Irish brogues" (*Stage* November 4, 1948). Yet Sim, speaking Bridie's (English) prose, held the audience. These foreigners may have been perplexed by the play's Scots enunciation, but they were not alienated from its ideas. Struggling with linguistic difficulty, they grasped that there was something challenging, and therefore worthwhile, in the play itself.

London critics, striving to tease it out, obsessed over the possibility that the piece was carried by its performances. The *Lady* gave a section of its review to "Fine Acting," as did the *Sunday Times* (*Lady* October 15, 1931; *STimes* October 11, 1931). The *Era* commented: "Here is Acting at its Ablest" (*Era* October 14, 1931). Critics particularly admired Flora Robson, who rose to stardom through her nuanced rendering of Mary Paterson (*Sphere* October 17, 1931; *EN* October 17, 1931). There was something "extraordinary" here, as was recognized by the Irish novelist Shaw Desmond—oddly yet significantly giving advice about national writing to the Welsh in the *Liverpool Post* (*LP* November 11, 1931). What was it?

The Anatomist, despite and perhaps because of its overt Scottishness, was able to cross national bounds. The critic for the *Evening Standard* attended the play three times to figure out how that worked (*ES* November 12, 1891). His review gives a hint: the English actor Henry Ainley has started to collect Knox memorabilia; Londoners are claiming to remember Knox and Hare in London. Just like the Scots before them, Bridie's wider audience was wound into *The Anatomist*. The Scottish story deployed national difference to tell a story of disturbing similarity. Critics might want to retell the tale according to English conventions, but the play itself, with its tortured relationships between protagonist and supporting characters, and characters and the punters in the stalls, reconstructed all audiences as potential Scots. All audiences for better, but mostly for worse, could recognize themselves in Bridie's story.

THE ANATOMY OF MELODRAMA

We can track the degree to which this play, though with "no great meaning or message," redirected the stories and practices of drama across the generations of movies that followed it, by testing Bridie's Scottish effects against those of productions that were already in circulation (*EN* October 8, 1931).

The Anatomist did not enter an empty field either as art or as drama. Bridie subtitled the play a "Lamentable Comedy," and ever since the Edinburgh immigrant de Quincey's second paper on "Murder Considered as One of the Fine Arts" (1839), authors had appreciated the blackly humorous aspect of the Burke and Hare murders. Stevenson, with his opposed characters of "Jekyll and Hyde," then Joseph Forster, the author of the lusciously titled *Studies in Black and Red* (London, 1896), contributed further to the rendering of Burke and Hare as criminal and literary high style. Marcel Schwob, picking up Stevenson's drift, had translated the two murderers into French and also into Burke "the mighty genius" who "evolved toward a kind of romanticism" recreating "the nocturnal ritual in the fog," and Hare who shared his "dilettante style of life" (Schwob, 89). Together the two achieve "the classical period of their existence," and "a beautiful, artistic effect" (89, 90). The problem of form as meaning by which Bridie challenged his audience had already been posed in short fiction.

More important, Burke and Hare had long since fallen into a competing form: melodrama. French authors Jules Lacroix and Frédéric Mercy had made them bit-players in novellas as early as the 1840s. The *Edinburgh Evening Dispatch* held *The Anatomist* against a heritage of stock productions and portable theater or "penny geggy" performances that seem to have emanated from Scotland but traveled further afield:

> Mr A. W. B. Kingston produced [Burke and Hare] successfully in the Pavilion Theatre, Grove Street [Edinburgh], many years ago. The crowds... were so great that police supervision had to be called in....
>
> To give the drama an air of respectability it was usually billed as "Bonnie Mary Paterson," although Mr Kingston [christened] it "Old Edinburgh," when he toured it with much success all over Scotland....
>
> That prince of portable theatre owners, Mr J. D. Mackenzie [was] amongst the first to produce "Bonnie Mary Paterson," either at Fisherrow, Musselburgh or Penicuik....
>
> ...Mr George Campbell...was also a power in the west.
>
> ...George Duckenfield...wrote an excellent version for Messrs Pierce and Bolton, who held premier place in the portable world for many a day [they established the New Gaiety, Ayr, in 1902]. (*EdEDis* July 14, 1930)

Industry ads that imply such plays were well known, and passing reminiscences of portable theater productions that "always packed the building," together with the lack of scripts for Burke and Hare melodramas, indicate that the plot was one so frequently presented it was easily vamped by an experienced company.[9] Entertainment notes mention "Bulwer," who "intends to strike at villany [*sic*] of a deeper dye, and [as early as 1839] is under an engagement to do what he can for Burke and Hare"; ads circulate for "'Burke and Hare.'—The Greatest Card out. Manuscripts of this Startling Drama—Terrific Situations"; actors tout their experience in Burke and Hare productions—"Johnny Matthewson, Clown, Disengaged," looks to "join any good Ballet *Troupe*" and has "a First-Class Fit-up to Lend" as well as "MSS. of 'Burke and Hare'" to sell; and "Clark's Portable Ghost Illusion, of Stewarton, Scotland," advertises for "Scotch Actor, accustomed to Daft Jemmy in 'Burke and Hare'" (*Era* December 13, 1839; February 24, 1867; March 22, 1874; September 24, 1892).[10] The play, in fact, appears to have evolved from Scotland as shorthand for a set of melodramatic types.

It seems to have met all the requirements of melodrama. The *Dispatch* recalled that "The story dealt with the love of Mary Paterson and a medical student, named John Haldene" (*EdEDis* July 14, 1930). "Daft Jamie" was a celebrated role. The paper described a famous performance that evoked Jamie's sentimental potential: J. D. Mackenzie "played the part with the traditional stoop and in his bare feet, besides carrying his snuff box throughout.... [He] could reduce his audience to tears in his final death appeal to the murderers with, 'Dinna hurt puir Jamie! Tak' a

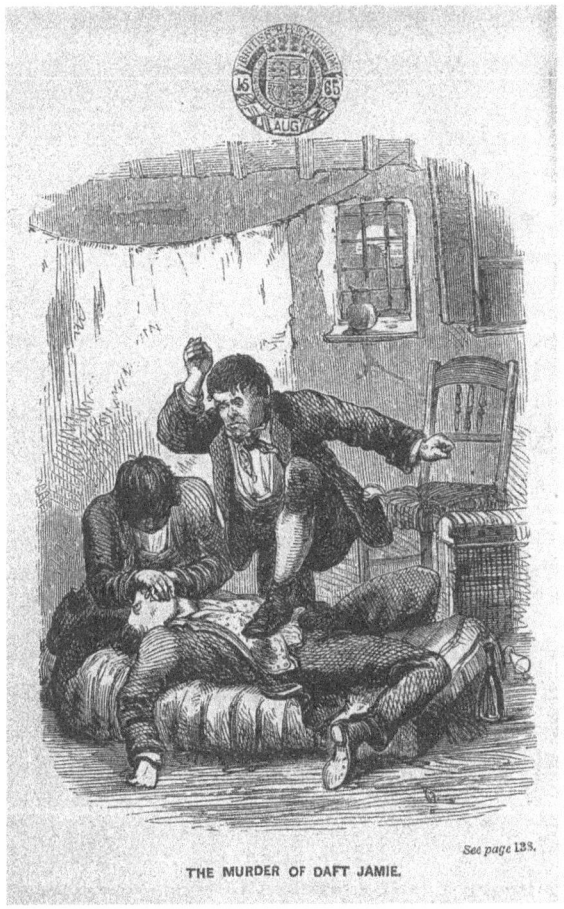

FIGURE 5.3 "The Murder of Daft Jamie." From David Pae, *Mary Paterson* (London: Fred Farrah, 1866). Courtesy of the British Library.

sneeshin!'" "Jamie" was known, too, as a comic turn, famous for lines like "Dae ye ken why my head is like frae Saturday [*sic*] tae Monday?... Because it is the weak end!" Such humor frequently turned to pantomimic anachronism: in a rendition by John Fyffe, actor/manager of a penny geggy, Jamie asks: " 'Dae ye ken why Gladstone wears blue braces and Disraeli wears red ones?... To keep their trousers up!' "[11] Even better, Jamie died in a splurge of violence and gore (see figure 5.3 for an 1866 rendition of the moment). The *Dispatch* insisted that unlike in *The Anatomist*:

> All the murders were done before the audience, who believed in realism and blood in those days. When it came to the killing of Jamie, it took three struggles before he was finally disposed of. The death of "Daft Jamie" was highly realistic, and called for strength and endurance from all three actors taking part.

A generation later, the memory had not faded, north or south of the border. In 1962 Dick Milton described "a terrific scene":

> Jamie…while being suffocated with a pillow, becomes tenacious of life and, springing from the bed, he endeavours to escape.… The stage is strewn with broken furniture, smashed ornaments, and splashed blood (red paint)…until, at last, poor Jamie, maimed and bleeding, is overpowered, and killed by a blow on the head with a hammer. A real blood-freezer!

In 1965, Jack House recalled a post-Bridie melodrama staged by the Charles Denville Company in Glasgow: "Glasgow audiences had…never seen anything like *The Horrible Crimes of Burke and Hare*" (House, 112–13). With Jamie dead, Burke says, "Who would have thought that the boy had so much blood in him" (echoing Lady Macbeth). "Now"—in the way of melodrama's easy oppositions and shocking juxtapositions—"it is time for them to go off to church." In the empty room:

> A green spotlight shines on the cupboard door and gradually the audience notice that a rivulet of some sort is coming from under [it]. It spreads slowly down the stage and they draw in their breath with terror as they realise it is BLOOD!… The Metropole was packed every night, and a large part of the audience was medical students from Glasgow University. They had already loaned a quantity of skulls and bones for the production. Every time…[Knox] appeared he had a special horrid spotlight on him and the medicals booed and hissed. (112–13)

Furthermore, in 1931 a direct heir of melodrama had taken to the boards in London, in opposition to Bridie's play.

On October 17, the *Aberdeen Press and Journal* recorded that "'The Anatomist,' is not to be the only [play] presenting Burke and Hare to London, for on Monday week a drama called 'The Wolves of Tanner's Close,' or 'The Crimes of Burke and Hare,' will be produced at the Brixton theatre." The paper added to its concern at English competition surprise that the play was "the work of a woman, Gladys Hastings Walton." Walton knew her context, writing that "'ye villains' are household words in the North—& they revel in them.… All our best murders…seem to come from the North!" (October 5, 1935, BTC EJE/001473). She sought to add the villainous duo to her repertoire of "'Frankenstein' and 'Sweeney' [Todd]." Not surprisingly, Walton's play stood out for its similarity to past melodramas. The *Manchester Guardian* noted its staging on the low-rent "south side of the Thames" by a repertory company known for "weekly entertainments of the '*Maria Martin*' and '*Sweeney*

Todd' brand" (*MG* October 28, 1931). Tod Slaughter's production (that *was* his name) even begged such comparisons. Reviewers noted that the first act introduces "the old firm of Burke and Hare. 'You want the best corpses; we supply them'" (*Daily Telegraph* December 3, 1931). They caught broader echoes, too. The *Star* celebrated the "noble sentiments uttered by the bluff sailor hero"; that "vice was shown up, and that gory deeds were accomplished with stirring realism" (*Star* October 22, 1931). This was "an admirably ghoulish entertainment, complete with orchestral tremolos, green limelight, and grand heroics in the good old style," and it seems to have been much like its predecessors in crucial details. The *Star* critic "was lost in admiration over the Scottish daftness of Bryan Bishop" (presumably, "Daft Jamie"), while the *Guardian* described familiar death scenes:

> Having seen the girl murdered—melodrama insists on that, and yet, as a tribute to gentility, the killing was exceedingly well bred, the stranglers roaring like Bottom's lion—we were privileged to see still another victim die before justice overtook the villains. And a fine fight the victim made of it before he succumbed. The house rose at the death of Jamie, the daft loon. [Geoff Carlile] quite brilliantly suggested the bird-witted intelligence of the daft ragamuffin while blending a proper amount of low comedy to fit the part of the play. (*MG* December 18, 1931)

The Wolves of Tanner's Close, aka *The Crimes of Burke and Hare*, testifies to the degree that audience expectation now drove the representation of 1828. Walton, though an astute author of melodrama, had tried to make this play into something different. Her story of Burke and Hare is sandwiched between the two parts of a (lengthy) condemned cell scene—that features none of our usual three suspects. Hare's descendant has murdered his wife, fearing that his child-to-be will perpetuate the family curse. Knox adopted him to track the descent of criminality, and he has already attacked Knox. Now, fulfilling Knox's theories and, as the *Saturday Review* points out, giving an oblique argument for preventative abortion, he awaits his death and tells a tale of the past (*SR* January 9, 1932). But the play lodged with the Lord Chamberlain and the promptbook and partbook in the Bristol Theatre Collection show the depredations of the censor and the dramatic costs of the audience's limited attention span. Walton's play appears to have been cut severely—back to the parameters of melodrama. Moreover, whatever version they saw, reviewers respond to no nuanced text, but describe all the attributes of theatrical convention—right down to that stage villain, "the small and mean and cringing Dr. Knox" (*SR* January 9, 1932).

The 1948 film *Horror Maniacs*, also known as *The Greed of William Hart*, echoes this production—as well it might, since it stars Tod Slaughter in the role of Hare/

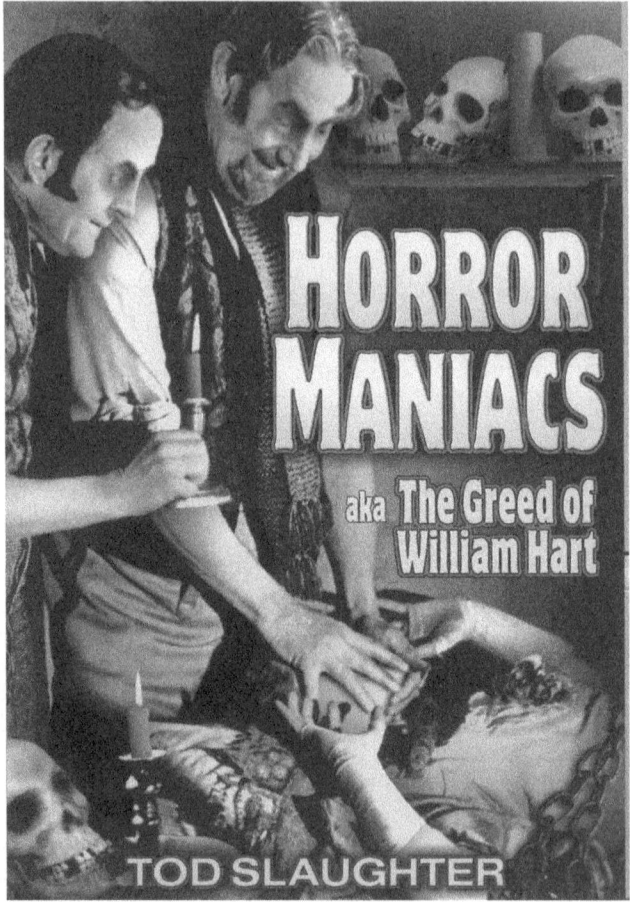

FIGURE 5.4 *Horror Maniacs*.

Hart (see figure 5.4). There are some changes: Burke and Hare and Knox become Hart, Moore, and Cox. Rumor declares that Burkean relatives threatened to sue, and the change is to protect the guilty (see *Greed* at Classic Horror website). But given that the change abandons the innocuous title *The Crimes of Burke and Hare* and adopts *Horror Maniacs* (or even *The Greed of William Hart*) for a story that everyone knew anyway, it seems likely that any such demand merely served the needs of melodrama in the market place. Name changes and legal threats hype interest in the manner of Bela Lugosi's 1931 *Dracula*, with its nurses waiting in the wings.[12] Certainly, the script is remarkably similar to Walton's, and also to N. Hastings's *Burke and Hare*, registered with the Lord Chamberlain in 1947—lines and even speeches are repeated. That similarity points up both the incestuous climate of melodrama, and the debt of all to stock scenes. The movie, too (again like the Walton and N. Hastings plays), features a sailor hero. Its Jamie descends from the character of melodrama, accomplishing sentiment, humor, and a gory death. What is more, this Jamie's comic routines come close to those now part of the character's melodramatic repertoire, and reprised in Walton (*EdEDis* July 14, 1930). The *Dispatch* remembered Jamie's crony, and Jamie's risible commentary: "'Dinna mind him, he's daft. He's a daft soul, Bobbie Aw.'" Now Jamie recounts that "Bobbie's no canny like me." And as in Walton, together they buy two glasses of beer, but Bobby drinks both: "wasnae that a daft trick?" Of course, Jamie dies in traditional lively style. Hart and Moore, meanwhile, sound like they have stepped straight from the music-hall stage: "I understand your honour perfectly, don't I Mr Moore?" "I think you do, Mr Hart."

The Slaughter play and film reveal their descent in one further, significant contrast with Bridie's *The Anatomist*. They too pose a test for the audience, but one quite different from Bridie's production. A. E. Wilson was gratified that the play revealed "the heart of Brixton beats true and sound" (*Star* October 22, 1931). Importantly, "The audience played its part as well as the actors. Tod Slaughter's Hare will often be recalled with a shudder by many a local playgoer, and so will... Burke and [the] sinister Dr. Knox. I gloated with the best of them." Slaughter's work sets a test we can pass—the audience is invited to condemn the villains and to identify with pathos. Bridie, however, tests us in a way that reworks our understanding of ourselves. Slaughter's audience can celebrate its commonality; Bridie's audience must admit and lament it. To be not "uncommon" is to be like even Doctor Knox, and thus denied the luxury of seeing yourself on the side of the good (*Anatomist*, 67).

The outward melodrama and the inward dramatic conflict competed to direct the plotting of Doctor Knox's story through the films of the twentieth century. Bridie was not afraid of competition; in fact, he considered it a necessary component of national literature. In 1949—just after the much delayed Slaughter film came out—Bridie declared: "All that I can find in the English Domination story is that the English, at one time, inundated us with their plays. If there is anything in the 'Nemo me impune lacessit' legend, we should have answered them in kind" (Bridie *Dramaturgy*, 3). Bridie himself took the battle to the enemy, and his concept of individual and community responsibility carried the day.

THE FOREIGN BODY OF FILM

We can see Bridie's effectiveness beginning with a story distinctly not his own. In 1945, Boris Karloff starred in *The Body Snatcher*, which claimed direct descent from Stevenson's tale—with Bela Lugosi as the sneaking porter in the dissecting room (see figure 5.5). This RKO film echoes major plot elements from its source: the bodysnatcher combines the roles of resurrectionist and Burke and Hare, turning

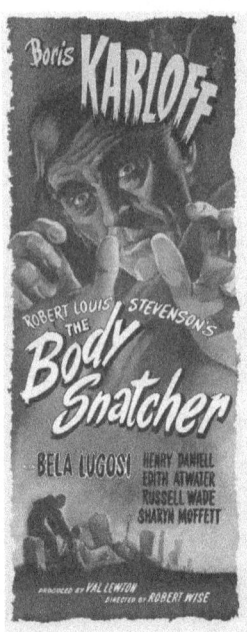

FIGURE 5.5 *The Body Snatcher*.

from snatching to murder; he also folds in the role of Stevenson's Mr. Gray, who threatens Toddy Mcfarlane (here, MacFarlane) and ends up dead. MacFarlane has moved on a generation. Now he, as successful doctor, entangles a student, and together they exhume an old lady who morphs into Gray. There are some cinematic additions, notably a pathetic, sick child who both occasions and is constantly threatened with death and premature resurrection. For our purposes, however, the movie's interest lies in the dynamic between two generations of students. MacFarlane is Knox's medical heir; he escaped justice when the snatcher took the rap for him. Having come too close already to the problem of life and death as it is complicated by Knox's bodies, MacFarlane today fears even to practice medicine. Fettes is MacFarlane's junior student, who is beloved by the sick child. Out of concern for the child—so that MacFarlane may develop the necessary procedure—Fettes solicits a fresh corpse.

The murder of a street singer (by Gray) and of Gray (by MacFarlane), as well as the death of MacFarlane (the runaway gig carries him over a precipice), all ensue. These sins of the fathers are visited back on them. But this plot takes a major turn toward complicity beyond that evident in Stevenson's original tale. Stevenson's Fettes has lived a life in decline as a result of a complicity that lacked any redeeming features; this new Fettes gets implicated in the plot not through his baser motives, but through his good intentions. He in turn re-implicates the doctor. Furthermore, MacFarlane repeats the anatomist's line to Walter back to his student: "You ordered the subject... and paid for it." Naïve Walter Anderson and the compromised Miss Disharts resonate through Fettes's role.

We might think that a 1944–48 script by Welsh author Dylan Thomas and produced at the behest of English director Donald Taylor (known for wartime information films) would escape the influence of either Slaughter or Bridie (Dylan Thomas, 135–38; Ferris, 196 and n., 220–21). Here, however, Bridie's theme of complicity takes over. Doctor Murray and Jennie Bailey repeat Walter Anderson's fascination with Mary Paterson. Early in Thomas's script Murray questions Knox/Rock's assertion that "'The end justifies *any* means'?...That is—to say the least of it—unscrupulous" (Thomas, 11). When Rock responds, "Then do not say 'the least of it.' Say 'the most': that it is *honest*," Murray, with heavy symbolism, washes his hands alongside his mentor. Murray, then, is half implicated when Jennie Bailey turns up on the slab. Rock, again like Bridie's Knox, manifests his own guilt by implicating his junior doctor fully. Murray accuses: "She was murdered by two paid thugs of yours: Fallon and Broom," and Rock bristles like Bridie's Knox before him (70):

> Thugs of *mine*, Mr. Murray? Do you remember that you yourself paid them for the last *three* subjects?... We are anatomists, not policemen; we are scientists, not moralists. Do *I, I,* care if every lewd and sottish woman of the streets has her throat slit from ear to ear?... Let her serve her purpose in death. (70)

But both men, the unsympathetic and the sympathetic, are only part of a more visibly fallen community.

Taking a line from Lonsdale that Knox, with "a world of promise...before him...put shackles to his social progress by marrying a person of inferior rank," Thomas introduces Knox/Rock's wife (who appeared in the Karloff movie), and also his religious sister (Lonsdale, 36). The one represents domesticity, the other social judgment. When Murray brings his concerns to them as supposed angels of Doctor Rock's house, they line up behind their doctor. Wife Elizabeth immediately temporizes, "Can't people die a 'natural death' in twelve hours?" (Dylan Thomas, 74). She then twists the knife in Murray: "everyone will call you murderer, too.... I thought Thomas told me that it was one of *your* duties to buy the bodies." (76). Then in the movie version (1985)—though Jennie (Twiggy) is kept alive for the romantic plot and a rip-roaring resistance to Fallon—the theme is further developed through sister Annabella. With Jennie's friend and Daft Jamie/Billie's sister serving as the victim, the religious Annabella sides against Murray with the wife who is otherwise her rival. Women, too, can be both sentimental and vicious, religious and wrong. Even enemies are alike in their complicity.

The McGregor Affair, produced for *The Alfred Hitchcock Hour* in 1964 from a 1953 story in *Ellery Queen's Mystery Magazine*, shows how far the discourse surrounding Doctor Knox had shifted to the issue of the complicit community and folded in the gazing audience. In Sidney Rowland's source tale, McGregor the porter decides to do away with his good-for-nothing wife, realizes that Burke and Hare are trading in murder victims, and places the drunken Aggie in their way. He subsequently delivers her, too, to the museum, but celebrating in the pub he himself falls victim to his employers. The Hitchcock production makes a subtle change to this American tale. It winds invented persons into this time and place so that innocents actually mimic the murderous role of Burke and Hare. A student questions the provenance of a body. Knox responds obliquely, "Young sir, what are you after?" and insists that "since the supply of bodies is not provided for by the government, we must find our own source." The student is cowed, and his companion says "Agree." These two students fold in both attributes of Walter Anderson: his concern and his complicity—the second young man is notable, in this respect, for always saying "Agree." But the main interest lies with McGregor, who provides the audience for doctors and murderers alike. This McGregor, always watching, always at the window, and eventually prying open packing cases, figures out his new marital strategy. He has thought of killing Aggie before. Extended comic sequences show him trying to hang her from a tree, but dangling himself, or attempting to drown a preternaturally buoyant Elsa Lanchester—"You'll never do it that way, McGregor," he laments: "she's a floater." He is both an innocent and a rather dark dreamer. At last, however, he is fully involved: although he does not himself murder Aggie, he "brings the beef."

The Horrors of Burke and Hare (1971) appears like *The McGregor Affair* in its humor, and unlike *The Anatomist* for its broad turn toward cockney comedy. The credits play rowdy doggerel over vivid woodcuts:

> In the land of bonny Scotland,
> It's not very bonny today....
> Watch out! Don't let 'em catch you,
> Or you'll end up on a slab! ...
> Burke an"are, beware of 'em
> Burke an"are, the pair of 'em
> Out to snatch your body from you.

The main characters enter to the theme from *Steptoe and Son*, a 1960s British TV comedy about a rag and bone man (remade in the United States as *Sanford and Son*), and are quite the comic duo. Has the Bridie influence at last run its course? With its French prostitute, high-class brothel, louche young doctors, and entertaining murders, this film lies somewhere between Tod Slaughter's productions and Joe Orton's *Loot*.[13] Still, the anxious medical student who gets involved with a lovely victim-to-be, and a community of medical students and prostitutes—both eager in every way—recall Bridie's concern. The minor regrets available to comedy only highlight our shared blame.

We can trace Bridie's influence beyond this moment, too—even in a film with no visible British connections and the unlikely title *Nightmare in Blood* (1976). What relation can there be to this scenario? Four friends/lovers organize a conference/screening in celebration of the good old days of Hammer Horror (British Hammer Studios opened in 1934, and their heyday in horror was the 1960s). The honored guest is Malakai, who stars in vampire films, and vogues in the part offstage—he sleeps in a coffin. As movie makers and cinema staff all over town are sucked dry or butchered for their organs, our intrepid four figure out that Malakai is (surprise!) a real vampire. In 1828 he was starring as Macbeth in Edinburgh, where he hooked up with Burke and Hare. Today, he lives on blood, but "BB" and "Harris" need to be topped up with decoctions from body parts every couple of years to stay immortal. These are provided by Malakai—a Knoxian experimental scientist. And of course the daring four (now three, since one was lost to Burke and Hare) fight back and win. How can this plot tie to James Bridie? Apart from the bloody slaughter, it does not much resonate with our story's history in melodrama either. Again, community is everything. In a movie that overlaps with the development of urban folklore as a trend in horror cinema, a distinctly American group of city sophisticates unites against Burke and Hare and "Malakai"—but this community is sensitive to the threat because it is implicated to begin with.

Thinking that horror is merely a genre, these naïfs invite the vampire into their domestic space, the old-fashioned movie theater. Conforming to genre, but also to Bridie's philosophy, they are therefore partly responsible for what follows. At the end, the conference convener addresses a more self-aware audience: "These creatures...do exist.... Beware the monster—he walks among us." We have invited Burke and Hare in, and they reveal who we are—for better and for worse. Though we assert ourselves as the good, and expel them, they remain out there/in here.

The power of Bridie's story, visible even in a low-budget mishmash of horror themes, is best indicated, perhaps, by a remake of the melodrama. In 1960, the writer for Tod Slaughter's 1948 film scripted a second version: *The Flesh and the Fiends*, starring Peter Cushing. The film begins melodramatically: "This is the story of lost men and lost souls. It is a story of vice and murder. We make no apologies to the dead. It is all true." It features a suitably daft Jamie, a ruthless Knox, and a leering Burke and Hare: "a man could become a millionaire at this game," Hare gloats, "it gives a man pride.... Burke and Hare, members of the great medical profession." Yet this movie offers a domestic setting for Doctor Knox, complete with lovely niece and lovesick junior doctor. Indeed, there are two lovesick young men: Mitchell for niece Martha, and Jackson for Mary Paterson. Jackson, a student, is implicated in an illicit relationship. He recognizes Mary on the slab, and he is murdered for it. Mitchell questions Knox about a number of suspicious corpses. And now, an unusually contrite doctor knows that "you are an ogre, Doctor Knox.... They seemed so small in my scheme of things, but I knew how they died." Still Martha is sure he acted "For the good of humanity!" while Mitchell defends Knox on her behalf, attacking the consanguinity between all doctors: "We have all traded in death.... Ask yourselves whether you condemn each other." So in this film, despite its descent from melodrama, significance still lies in a turn toward blame for all. Even lovely Martha, and Mitchell who has saved the doctor from legal consequences and thus colluded in crime.

SCOTS AS OTHERS

Bridie was not uninvolved in this translation of his dramatic and philosophical values to the screen. He was well aware of the competition posed by film as he wrote *The Anatomist*, for in that moment, the theater and the cinema were in a pitched battle in which either might fail. Bridie jokingly warned that "until you go out for debauchery with your whole heart & soul you will never compete with the Talkies," and working toward a Scottish theater he remarked: "We shall be wired for the Talkies in case" (n.d., NLS MS8181/6; [November] 14, 1931, NLS MS8181/22). At the same time, the *Curtain* noted that the London production of *The Anatomist* was staged in "The Westminster... another theatre converted from a kinema" (*Curtain*, November 1931). Furthermore, Bridie did show interest in writing for the movies. In 1946, Hugh MacDiarmid sneered:

> Mr James Bridie has gone to Hollywood, where he would seem to have his spiritual home. It is to be hoped that he will remain there. He has certainly done nothing for drama in Scotland.... Hollywood is the proper place for a playwright who has such a lamentably—not to say ludicrously—inadequate aesthetic as to imagine that entertainment is, and should be, the Alpha and Omega of drama. Mr Bridie has, he says, no use for any propaganda of ideas, or apparently for any ideas. He is particularly opposed to the introduction of politics into plays. (MacDiarmid *Raucle*, 3:95)

Undeniably, Bridie did go to Hollywood at Hitchcock's invitation—though he missed the director, came back...and found Hitchcock waiting for him at Heathrow.[14] He wrote an unproduced screenplay for a Hitchcock movie eventually titled *The Paradine Case* (1947); he wrote the screenplay for *Under Capricorn* (1949); and he provided additional (uncredited) dialogue for *Stage Fright* (1950). Numerous of his plays were filmed.[15] But MacDiarmid here makes two mistakes. First, with his elitist notion of folk culture and art, he is deaf to the lively popular discourse of cinema. Second, with his determination to take Bridie at his word, he fails to read Bridie's work by its aesthetic—which might reveal a philosophy (even a politics) strenuously in operation.

Needless to say, Bridie was incapable of singlehandedly infusing the movies with art and with Scottishness. Besides, art and Scottishness were doing just fine there, though differently than either MacDiarmid or Bridie might have preferred. Nor did Bridie completely redirect the story of Burke and Hare and Doctor Knox. *Britannia and Eve*'s 1939 "Murder in Auld Reekie," written and illustrated by F. Matania, gave new life to the story through its voluptuous illustrations.[16] "Ghoul's Gold," an American comic (1946), showed its provenance through David Pae's Sheffield syndication of *Mary Paterson*, for it takes place in the northern town, and through the melodrama: the *Star* mentioned a sailor in Slaughter's production, and here he is (*Star* October 22, 1931). Robert Bernstein (writer) and Jack Alderman (graphic artist) give Burke and Hare a distinctly American tone that focuses the story on American-style crime and courts. And this comic rises to no heights of complexity either in presentation or in what it demands of its readers. Moreover, if Burke and Hare became shorthand for medical horror in *Nightmare in Blood*, they signified comedy in England's *Doctor in Love*, where two irresponsible and lovestruck medical students go by their names.[17] Clearly, once it had entered the forms of mass culture, the story of Burke and Hare and Doctor Knox made its own way in the world.

Nonetheless, we can confidently trace Bridie's influence in a range of later, non-Scottish dramatizations. The alternate speech Bridie provides to Knox (to allow for a faster curtain) gets reprised by Dylan Thomas (*Anatomist*, 72–73). Doctor Rock assesses the human heart, then on film he persists in not getting the point of his own lecture. Peter Cushing's doctor in *The Flesh and the Fiends* does get the point: his lecture is on the Hippocratic Oath. However he has just admitted his guilt, so the niece and students who applaud him are wilfully complicit. Most notably, even as titles turn to melodrama and horror, or the tone to triviality and comedy, and even as movies end with distinct finality, Bridie's formal innovation continues in the movies' unclosable ethos. MacFarlane gallops over the precipice in *The Body Snatcher*; Hare is thrown to the mob in *Horror Maniacs*; Knox lectures to a full house in *The Flesh and the Fiends*; McGregor gets all boxed up in his own story; Mrs. Docherty falls from a cupboard and the players resolve into a woodcut in *Horrors of Burke and Hare*—and yet these stories never end, for they have opened the implicated community. Ultimately, these tales turn to us. "Posterity," Mary Belle snapped, "will have to be very clever to judge you justly, Dr. Knox" (*Anatomist*, 67). Under Bridie's direction, "posterity" is us—and we have quite enough trouble judging ourselves.

Still, the dynamic generated by *The Anatomist* was always a tough sell. We can see the challenge Bridie posed to himself as author in the performance history of the play. Bridie balanced the potential horror and guilt of his production with mild humor. Jokes such as Amelia's claim that Mary Belle's "heart is in the right place," together with Walter's riposte "As a student of anatomy I hope so," give context for the play and cue its themes without yet taking us into any deeper concerns (*Anatomist*, 2). When Walter later gets a "corpse-reviver" (drink) from Raby even as we know his companion of last night has shuffled off her mortal coil, humor has turned to dark dramatic irony (40). And when Paterson describes the atmosphere of the dissecting room, "It's as if the deid men stirred," only to have Burke knock at the door with Mary Paterson, we are poised between laughter and tragedy (41–42). The later suggestion that a heavy piece of luggage indicates the traveling Amelia has "killed the courier and brought him home to stuff him" shows that we are all naïve whistlers caught in the graveyard (50). In this context, laughter implicates the audience. But subsequent directors of Bridie's play, less nuanced in their reading, stressed humor in its own right.

Of the 1948 London production, the *Scotsman* noted, "Comedy…is the key" (*Scotsman* November 3, 1948). Sim "softens the grimness with gawky humour and in his richly rolling period, with something of the air of a Scottish Micawber." The next celebrated Knox only carried the humor further. In 1968 the *Glasgow Herald* remarked, rather querulously:

> [This is]…the social Knox, the Knox of "cheering words and affable manner," the Knox "kind and sympathising with women." The Knox of bitter tongue and Luciferian pride…has become jolly, pawky, almost bonhomous.
> …everything goes tumbling along from laugh to laugh.…[T]he odious Davie Paterson…[is] like some one in pantomime. (*GH* February 14, 1968)

The "lamentable comedy" has become merely funny.

These performances refracted an early tendency toward caricature in the play's rendition. Even as Bridie's play challenged audiences for the first time, Henry Ainley vogued in melodramatic portraits of the doctor (*ISDN* December 5, 1931: 548, 549 and UGla). Magazines featured humorous cartoons. But at least some of these, like the ones in the *Illustrated Sporting and Dramatic News* (*ISDN* November 7, 1931) and the *News of the World* (*NW* November 15, 1931), indicated that they understood *The Anatomist* was not simply a star vehicle (see again figure 5.2). They represent the importance of the ensemble cast, and the characters' complicity in a layered plot. Moreover, the early performances enacted that complex dynamic with an uneasy audience.

OTHERS AS SCOTS

It is significant that while audiences laughed at the Sim and Fleming portrayals of a Knox now decidedly center stage, they knew something was missing in the move from fable to entertainment. In 1952 Glasgow, Bannister registered an audience "who obviously cherished their memories of the original performance…there was some headshaking" (Bannister, 70). Still, there was confusion about what, exactly, was missing. The *Stage* caught a hint of the problem in this new Doctor Knox. This critic dropped the cautious thought that "it is the hovering between [comedy and tragedy] that leaves one's emotions in a state of uncertainty"—or should do so (*Stage* November 4, 1948). That is, the audience is not there merely to be entertained. Rather, they are crucial in the dynamic of *The Anatomist*. If, however, we are not now poised between comedy and tragedy, where are we? *Blackwood's* had encouraged the mob, but Bridie kept them offstage. Now, the *Scotsman* notices the lack of a crowd to attribute blame and enact justice: "Why was the Edinburgh mob, 2000 strong, powerless to follow the students into the Disharts' drawingroom?" (*Scotsman* September 10, 1952). A comedy requires simple solutions, but Bridie's nuanced drama pointed elsewhere. The lack of the mob never mattered before because a Bridie playgoer, caught in the hall of mirrors, should not need them. In the 1930s productions, the audience itself is implicated in the role of the Edinburgh populace. The riot should be internal. So we are the thing that is missing in these comic restagings of Bridie's play. This Scottish author has taught us to expect more of the drama and of ourselves.

After a century during which authors had sought to define Doctor Knox and export him from Scottish culture, Bridie faced the issue of how to help Scots put themselves in the picture, and to help us all recognize the big picture. Walter, banished by Mary Belle and falling into drunkenness, moans what might be the Scots' post-Knoxian catchphrase: "I'm all right, but the world's all wrong" (*The Anatomist*, 30). In this respect, he is like Burke and Hare, who fear to place themselves in the mortuary where they eagerly send other people (43). Mary Belle and Amelia are like Walter and his underclass associates, for they refuse to acknowledge their relation to others. Walter needs their recognition, but it is withheld. They are "Scottish enough not to show it" (55). Bridie shows that we are all connected, whether we acknowledge it or not; we all carry baggage from our travels. The lady tourists who have managed to miss the entire Burke and Hare debacle arrive back into its midst—they need the smelling salts that they thought would support them in foreign lands, but not till they return to Edinburgh and catch the reek of their own involvement in nefarious deeds (50). Together, we make up quite a mob.

And this is our productive plight as the audience for James Bridie and his moviemaking descendants. Bridie successfully put not just Edinburgh, but us, into the picture. In a nation-building that might disturb Hugh MacDiarmid, Bridie's many audiences find themselves rewritten as Scots through the story of Burke and Hare. This story that is "not our problem"—and even less our problem than it is the concern of any of the characters—is structured by Bridie to wind us into its toils precisely where we identify with those characters who are "all right" and comfort themselves with the naïve assertion that it is the world that's "all wrong." This is the bigger picture: our supposed distance from Edinburgh's underside is what forces on us our disturbing proximity to cultural guilt. Even as—and even because—we assert our lack of involvement, and claim an absence in our memory, Bridie's play remembers us. We, too, belong in the story of Burke and Hare.

Let be, lads, I'll rise myself
—Epigraph from Norman Adams, *Dead and Buried*, 66.

6

Bringing Out the Dead

SILENT VICTIMS SPEAK IN ALASDAIR GRAY'S *POOR THINGS*

BY THE 1970S, it might seem there was nothing left to say about the scandals of 1828. From the first, the villains Burke and Hare had been confined within the narrow cells of melodrama—whether posturing in Robert Seymour's illustrations for *The Murderers of the Close* (1829; see figure 6.1), playacting in Alexander Leighton's *The Court of Cacus* (1861), terrorizing Fettes in Robert Louis Stevenson's "The Body Snatcher" (1884), or superstitiously cowering from the dead in *The Anatomist* (1931). Burke and Hare were easy marks. But Scotland's trauma had required the apportionment of blame—especially to the resistant Doctor Knox—and the Scots' own acceptance of culpability. Now, both these tasks seemed achieved. Leighton and Pae pursued Doctor Knox, then Stevenson dissected him; Bridie anatomized the audience and implicated them within the next generation of Burke and Hare plots. The Scots, as survivors of 1828, had at last expressed and thereby confined this distressing past. There was nothing left to disinter, no sin left to expiate—Scotland knew where all the bodies were buried. This chapter, however, asks about the bodies themselves—the actual victims.

These bodies now rise. Their appearance at first seems odd—more than belated, because it comes at a moment when the story seems finally over. Anxiety about individual guilt and cultural complicity had driven the story down through the years. What more could be said once blame was assigned to Knox and to Scots by the handful? For many authors the answer was: not much. Absolved of the duty to reveal wrongdoing or accept blame, these novelists and historians turned with evident relief to gathering up the loose ends of a tale that supposedly had been told, once and for all. Niggling worries are addressed, and complex plots prove rewritable because their trauma has been expunged. Some writers blithely resolve the issue of Knox's students' involvement, and even the doctor, having accepted his responsibility, can be rehabilitated. Since there are no further remains to this awful tale, indeed, it begins to dwindle. The story of Burke and Hare and Doctor Knox, lacking compulsion, often turns to repetition for its own sake: merely descriptive texts accumulate. The events of 1828 apparently cast the lure only of a retellable (if rather grisly) historical tale, one capable of eliciting a mild frisson.

Yet with the story now boxed up in prose, new readings swarm upon us. Twentieth-century issues reanimate the fading tale of Burke and Hare. In the era of cultural studies, the drive to review, retrieve, and reorient recognizes additional patterns and meanings in this Scottish past, such as those of gender and race. These new emphases, visible in writers within and beyond Scotland, manifest the period's own wide-ranging anxieties. Such uses of Burke and Hare do not sort through or ameliorate the trauma of 1828. Rather they use it to play out a present concern and address the problems of an unrelated dynamic. For writers in this moment, the past seems resolved enough in itself that it can serve to articulate and confine newer worries.

As Alasdair Gray demonstrates, however, such an overinsistence on resolution—to and through the story of Burke and Hare—actually implies that something has been left out. Something, moreover, cannot be included; something cannot even be accessed and consequently lurks as excessive. The dead, those murdered by Burke and Hare and disappeared by Doctor Knox, cannot be retrieved. Why does this matter? After all, "dead men tell no tales." Anthropologists researching mortuary rituals teach us that societies need to negotiate their relationship to the dead (Metcalf. Ancestors who lack burial rites are not firmly placed in culture. They are thus potentially disruptive. So the victims of Burke and Hare, lacking such rites and even (courtesy of Doctor Knox) a final resting place, haunt the society that has been unable to recognize them appropriately. After 1828, more so every generation, and more again when outsiders started to rewrite this tale as a matter of other places and different concerns, Scots forging a national future needed to reestablish a relationship with these dead.

Not an easy task, for as "Mister Jock" discovers in W. Gordon Smith's 1987 play by that name, the unlocatable dead inevitably resist all tidy plots and finished tales. Jock, retired from the army and now a museum keeper (like David Paterson in 1828), tells history under an epigraph from T. S. Eliot:

A people without history
Is not redeemed from time, for history is a pattern
Of timeless moments.
       (*Four Quartets*, "Little Gidding," V)

What does this mean for Mister Jock, self-assured historian of all things Scottish? Eliot's words raise questions of whether, inside or outside "history," we are always within pattern (a comfort for Scots famously posited "out of history" by Cairns Craig in 1996). Or might history stand always at the point of collapse, its patterns a delusion, because it is made of random moments? To Mister Jock, the representative Scot, the answer is, disturbingly, this last. By the case of Burke and Hare, Jock shows that history is made not in life but through death. From the unknowable instant of their death, the moment Burke and Hare's victims exited time, these people who are not just gone, but also lost, inevitably rise.

Jock performs within a tradition of gregarious Scots. His history voices itself through the couthy puns of a Harry Lauder, plots the grand sequences of national romance, and cannily deconstructs according to the Marxian discourses of Red Clydeside and Scottish postcolonialism.[1] Jock knows how to pattern Scotland's imperial plots, and how to critique them—he commands the narrative strategies of Scottishness. Mister Jock himself collapses, however, in the context of William Burke. Jock is riffing along on Scottish history:

Lights dim down, he sits "at window"

Who's this, d'you think perched at a window overlooking the Lawnmarket? Wednesday, the twentyeighth [*sic*] of January, 1829, and twenty-five thousand folk… gather to see the hanging of William Burke… [ellipsis in text]

Burke and Hare.… The hellish twins, who sold the freshest beef to the anatomists.
And the man with the grandstand seat is Sir Walter Scott.…
Burke drops through the hatch.… The corpse is put on public view then, as decreed by the judge, dissected.
They cried ballads in the streets for weeks:
Attendance give, whilst I relate
How poor Deft [sic] Jamie met his fate
'Twill make your hair stand on your head
As I unfold the horrid deed.

> You get used to most things in museums but I couldn't work in the surgeon's place in Edinburgh where they display Burke's skeleton, or in that other place where they've a wallet made out of the skin flayed off his back. (Act 2)

Jock can tell and even sing a well-known tale (complete with myth of Walter Scott). But he cannot work where Burke has fallen out of history and story into otherness, as a "thing" for the surgeon.

Jock reveals that the major problem in the tale of 1828 was not Doctor Knox, or even ourselves. Nor, in fact, was it William Burke, who fits too well into the conventions of story as the villain awaiting death in front of a righteous mob. Our obsession with stitching together these moments manifests a greater anxiety about what remains untold. The tale everyone knows, and has articulated in museums or wrapped up in prose, centers on an absence. And with stupendous irony, poised here at the moment of pain between life and dissolution, Burke mimics this lack. Carved up and passed around, he points to those both made and obliterated by the story of Burke and Hare: its actual victims. It is in the presence of this inaccessible and consequently irreducible excess that Mister Jock cannot go on. These dead will always disrupt any telling of the national tale. So now we will consider how authors strive to contain the victims of Doctor Knox, but then learn to let them live, move, and remake Scottish identity. More, as the final chapter will demonstrate, once these dead live, all tales must be retold.

The chapter at hand tracks how, just when the story of 1828 seems well and truly over, the dead demand room within the tale. Notably, writers number off victims, tidying them away by category; historians imply that everything, finally, has been told. Yet such encyclopedism speaks for the past, rather than letting it echo into the present. These tales only appear complete. Their urge toward categorization is reductive; their apparent resolution depends on omission. Thus, despite themselves, such narratives evoke the thing they cannot express—the victimhood that was manufactured and obscured by the dissecting arts of the surgeon's knife. And the consoling structures of history and story in turn collapse when disrupted by the strident voicing of the inexpressible otherness that is the dead.

Our data will stretch from the sure sequences and easy plots of history and genre fiction to Alasdair Gray's *Poor Things* (1992), with its victim made visible through the pains inscribed on her body. We will pursue how Bella Baxter's difference, rendered unmissable by her scars, both allows and disturbs the stories we contrive for our own comfort. Then we will consider how the Scottish body politic, meeting its corporeal metaphor in the instant of its un-making (and the sewn-together person of Bella), can learn to break the bounds not just of politics but of all singular identities. From 1828, the embodied metaphorics of Scotland take a problematic but now productive turn—the body of Scotland, expressed in the im/politic, cobbled together parts of its victims, can unravel all our self-satisfied inner worlds. Thus with Alasdair Gray, we may embrace the opportunities when poor things, too long neglected, inevitably rise.

DOCTORS AND STUDENTS

Despite the possibilities offered by gothic fictions and horror movies, the dead took considerable time to rise in the narrative of Burke and Hare and Doctor Knox. In 1828, only Mrs. Docherty was around to tell her tale—which was written on her body and explained at the trial of William Burke (see figure 6.1). Yet Doctor Christison, testifying for the prosecution, found even her body and bruises not revealing enough to make a certain case or describe her sufferings fully (Christison, 1:306–10). That is, Mrs. Docherty contributed to the story of Burke's conviction but Knox's escape. Daft Jamie did feature in street ballads, and Mary Paterson anchored a novel, but neither victim—as a victim—could impinge on the legal or even the imaginative narratives about criminals and doctors. Sixteen people left only the tatters of their lives to be told, and meant nothing except for those tatters. As in Doctor Knox's dissecting laboratory, after death they remained the subjects of other people's stories. There was no voicing from beyond the grave.

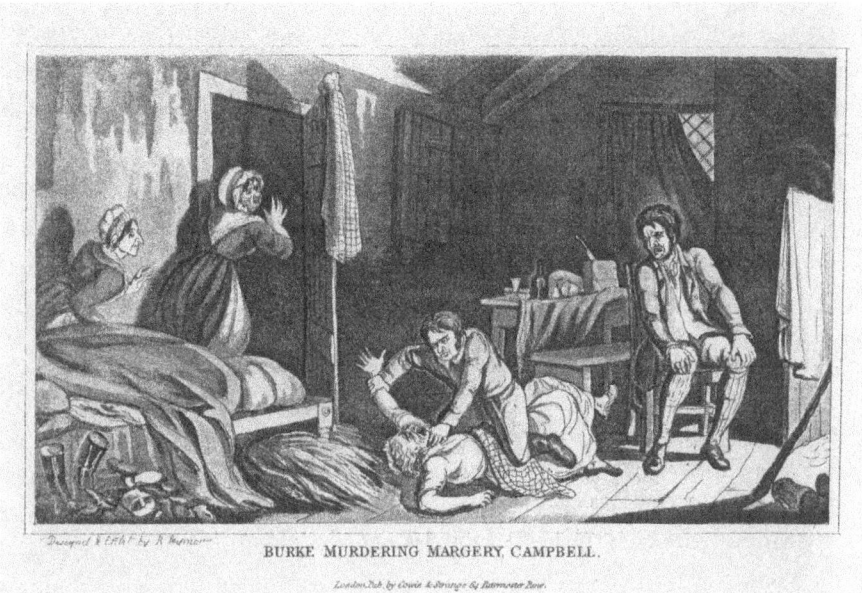

FIGURE 6.1 "Burke Murdering Margery Campbell [Mrs Docherty]." Etching by Robert Seymour, in *Murderers of the Close*. Courtesy of Edinburgh City Library and Information Services.

Worse, even when the concerns about Knox and about Scottish complicity had been addressed, authors continued to elide victimhood, with all the pain that translated person to object, and that pain's need for utterance. The years after *The Anatomist*, indeed, are notable for the way in which this history turns from anguish and anger (such as in Leighton) to apparently objective assessment, but shades into committed argument for anyone other than the victims. Isobel Rae and Hugh Douglas, scholarly and popular historians, actually recast Knox as victim. In 1964, Rae importantly seems to get beyond Scotland's trauma. Despite her Scottish descent she disinvests from nineteenth-century bias and works to depict the complexity of Robert Knox. Yet if Rae's biography advances understanding of Knox and his context, she turns toward paean at the end. When victims remain merely incidental to Knox's plot, his story swerves from objective history, taking a dramatic form. In increasingly fulsome terms, Rae concludes:

> Dr Knox's story would be one of unmitigated tragedy had he not, towards the end of his life, been able to return to the fringes, at least, of his old world. The doors of the lecture-room were for ever closed to him, but those of the laboratory and dissecting-room remained open, and in 1856 he was offered the most suitable post imaginable.... pathological anatomist to the [Cancer] hospital [in London]. He took up the position on 18 October, and continued to do excellent work there... until he was stricken by mortal illness. (Rae, 157)

Knox, in his demise, approaches the condition of poetry, such that Rae cannot resist ending with the ennobling biblical cliché: "Robert Knox, a prophet without honour in his own country" (161). Rae's history transmutes into eulogy for that erstwhile pariah, Doctor Knox.

Hugh Douglas, a Scottish newspaperman writing for a more general audience in 1973, moved further again from the traumas of his ancestors. This author does not hesitate to go for the gusto and the heroic rewrite. Douglas's preface quickly runs through the questions posed by 1828 but shares Rae's conclusion. He begins with the doggerel beloved of Burke and Hare scholars:

> Up the close and doon the stair
> Ben the hoose wi' Burke and Hare,
> Burke's the butcher, Hare's the thief,
> Knox the boy who buys the beef. (Douglas, 11)

And then he's off, racing through possibilities to a conclusion allowed by the notion that only details remain to be told:

Four scurrilous lines but an accurate enough summing up of the murders in the West Port of Edinburgh during 1827 and 1828. Mary Docherty, indeed, went up the close, and down the stair.... Fifteen others preceded her...

"Burke's the butcher"—that is what the law said with absolute truth, but was Burke the only butcher?

"Hare's the thief"—there can be no doubt about that; but the house from which he stole was "the bloody house of life". Was he in fact a greater fiend than Burke as was commonly thought at the time or did he deserve the lesser punishment?

And "Knox the boy that buys the beef"—Robert Knox bought the 'beef' all right, but did he know where it came from?... people are beginning to ask whether he was not the victim of a campaign of hate generated by the ignorant mob and jealous rivals. (Douglas, 11)

It is not that either Rae or Douglas finds the loss of life unimportant—far from it. Yet when actual victims remain absent, even Knox can fill that ennobling role.

Still, with the doctor rewritten as pilloried for his intellect, surely the stage is clear to consider true victims. But authors continue to look away—they look to Knox's students. In *The Court of Cacus*, Leighton had struggled with their role: were they "generous and well-bred youths [who] never entertained a suspicion of murder" (Leighton *Court*, 89)? Should we "estimate the turpitude of the professors and students the more lightly, in proportion to their freedom from all endearing feelings of recognition or friendship towards those whose remains came within their studies" (53)? Leighton might have set loose the incipient irony in his remarks. However, he temporized, for the most part shuffling the students off the stage to focus on the antics of Burke and Hare. But in 1952 I. Goodwin (from Germany), and in 1978 the Indian Scot Hector Bryson [Chawla], with the major concerns increasingly resolved, filled in this backstory. In and out of Scotland, writers produced opposite conclusions but under the same ethos and to the same effect. Now that the story no longer carries a freight of anxiety, students can be cast as either villains or heroes. The victims, however, remain unspoken, their sufferings unexpressed.

Goodwin casts students as villains. In *Bury Me in Lead*, her ne'er-do-well English medical student is so good-looking that (to his humiliation) he becomes the cynosure for every eye: his body serves as a model for fellow anatomy students needing practical demonstration (Goodwin, 44–45). Roland Barton to this point may be considered a victim of science, yet he is clearly set apart from Knox's actual victims:

Roland awoke on the Sunday to all the wretchedness that a bottle of inferior whisky could produce. He was also stark naked and covered with charcoal lines and ink blots. His clothes, strewn about the room, were crumpled, streaked with greasy finger-marks, smelling of sweat, whisky and tobacco....

It was hardly worth while to begin life again. He disliked his body: they had soiled it, bruised it, and poured poison into it. However, in the end one must admit that indignity was preferable to death. (45)

That is, Roland mimics victimhood, and later he even comes close to being burked…but he wakes up in the morning (145–47). The medical student remains capable of improving his own situation—an option not open to Knox's cadavers.

Nor is Roland averse to making others his victims. He begins the very night after he has paraded as "beef," joining his fellow students in grave robbing to the rollicking rhythm of:

Three days the Christian lies in's grave
And then there's just a hole—
Knox receives the body
And Christ may keep the soul! (Goodwin, 48)

This exploit produces a near murder (by the students) when they are disturbed. Then Roland becomes fascinated by the novel's Mary Paterson surrogate. But although he thinks of marrying her, when she turns up on the slab, he is one of those to sketch her.

So here you are, he thought, come to the surgeons at last. He felt no grief. In a way it was relief that he felt—relief that she was out of his way—and a malicious guilty pleasure that he should have got the better of her after all, that she should be dead, and he still alive. (120)

Not surprisingly, then, when Knox orders the premature dissection of Daft Jamie, presumably to obscure evidence of crime and complicity: "Every student who helped, in however humble a way, to render down the subject's identity, felt an obscure sense of complacency in doing the work of time and worms" (227). So when disaster strikes and "Knox whom Roland loved" stands exposed, Roland knows that "he himself was never among the innocent" (59, 228). At this point, it lends only a dubious distinction to line up beside a Knox who declares with unconscious irony: "We may have killed our patients, but we have made our discoveries" (231). Lest we should miss the point, while Roland lies devastated by the execution of William Burke, his wife gives birth, and both she and her child die of Roland's neglect. From a perspective outside Scotland, a student doctor can play quite the irresponsible young devil.

Hector Bryson [Chawla], with a complex set of cultural investments, goes to the opposite extreme. Bryson is a product of India and Scotland, and a noted eye surgeon in Edinburgh. In his *Doctors, Bodies and Snatchers*, a young man very similar to Roland (intriguingly named "Bryson," for the author) is plotted into comedy. The book begins: "My medical studies began when Father came home from Waterloo with three legs" (Bryson, 1). Mary Paterson shows up but in a moment of farce when Bryson, advised to let himself be caught in flagrante at a brothel in order to shake a clinging young woman, meets that same girl's minister father exiting a luckless prostitute's room. "There is in that room a creature. Mary Paterson is her name," the reverend McGrath fulminates (67). "Mrs Peddleclap was told about her by some wretch by the name of Hare, who lives up at the West Port. The Devil is at work in her, and I must cast him out. It is a powerful, heavy task." He blusters on, translating future horrors into "Carry On" plots: "I tried to reason with her and she laughed. I tried to mortify her flesh, and she displayed herself."[2] And Mary seems to have been enjoying a good time, for Bryson has just heard "a fierce caterwauling.... [s]ounds of...a whip, [and] female giggles" (66). That is, though young Bryson promenades his author's name through Knox's dissecting rooms, the same low dives frequented by Roland, and even into the graveyard, his story turns to roles retellable by lascivious old men and risqué females.

This writer offers a broadly positive tale alongside his raucous comedy, for he tells a wider history of Edinburgh medicine. The medical student learns much from James Hamilton (1749–1835), Professor of Midwifery, and his midwife assistants; he gives lengthy descriptions of the Infirmary, procedures, and treatments; and he sits in class beside a thoughtful young Mr. Darwin (Bryson, 29). Furthermore, this character succeeds because among the charlatans there are numerous competent and kind doctors who can save his injured lady love.

Perhaps most important, our medical student graduates before Burke and Hare come fully on the stage. His friend Deelatrumpe tries to persuade him, on the novel's last page, "to join me in just one little expedition before you become sewious" (Bryson, 189). Creepily, but in this case comically, when young Bryson demurs, Quentin declares: "Oh, no.... There is no gwave wobbing." Then he schedules for that very night:

"I have come acwoss a bwace of capital fellows. They've got their glimmers open for a swift guinea, I can tell you.... [O]ne of them wuns some sort of lodging house down near the Tanners Close—calls himself Fewwet or Wabbit or some such, or no—Hare: yes, that's it—Hare; and his colleague—ah, his colleague—if I am not much mistaken he goes by the name of Burke." (189)

With "Bryson" verging to the end of his plot, and with no one by his name figuring in the history that writers focused on Burke and Hare can presume their readers to know, this story ends with a laugh, not a tragedy. Boys will be boys. So although our outsider ends negatively, and the Scottish doctor writes positively, the one producing tragedy, the other comedy, the story takes the same trajectory for Goodwin and for Bryson. These authors would rather turn to side issues and wrap up loose ends than tangle with Knox's victims.

THE ENCYCLOPEDIA OF VICTIMHOOD

This turn to tell another side of Knox's tale, or to provide the backstory of his students, is part of a larger encyclopedic trend. With the elements of the primary and even secondary tale now assimilated, authors, popular historians, and scholars alike—and inside and beyond Scotland—started to pursue a wider range of materials for different audiences in descriptive and cumulative fashion. Readers had long been interested in the gory bodysnatching context for Burke and Hare, but now there was an upsurge of documentation, filling in every informational or conceptual gap, and addressing or invoking every level of readerly interest.

In the most obviously encyclopedic contribution, Jacques Barzun (providing a service to scholars and voyeuristic readers alike), raided the Fenwick Beekman Collection at the New York Academy of Medicine to publish *Burke and Hare: The Resurrection Men*, subtitled *A Collection of Contemporary Documents Including Broadsides, Occasional Verses, Illustrations, Polemics, and a Complete Transcript of the Testimony at the Trial* (1974). In England, Hubert Cole's *Things for the Surgeon* (1964) went back to the history of London resurrectionists, but with an interesting twist. Unlike in Bailey or Turner, Burke and Hare appear once more in the story. Cole titles his sixth chapter: "Burking Comes to London." So London's tale is not entirely separate. Burke and Hare provide a pivot for London crimes that consequently supplement their tale. Publishers, too, recognized these possibilities. In 1982 the Marlboro Press (Vermont) reissued *Murder for Profit*, written in 1926 by the South African William Bolitho [Charles William Ryall]. Bolitho's chapters progress from "The Science of William Burke" to "The Imperialism of J.—B Troppmann" and "The Self-Help of G. J. Smith." These not only locate Burke and Hare within economics, but with the perspective of 1982, show forming around them the pantheon of what had, by now, become the serial killer. As recently as 1995, working from the University of East Anglia, Tim Marshall brought a microscope to the tenuous relationship between Mary Shelley's *Frankenstein* (1818) and Burke and Hare in *Murdering to Dissect: Grave-Robbing, Frankenstein and the Anatomy Literature*. Marshall focused on Shelley's (not much revised) 1831 third edition, and thereby achieved encyclopedic effects from sparse data for a popularized academic audience.

Scotland has shared this turn toward assembling every little detail, every perspective. Kathy Stephen slotted Knox into a series of pamphlets from the History of Medicine and Science Unit at the University of Edinburgh. These booklets were "intended to populari[ze the] contributions of Scottish men of letters, medicine and science, [for the] betterment of contemporary society" (foreword). Aberdeen writer Norman Adams, in *Dead and Buried? The Horrible History of Bodysnatching* (1972), gives more evidence about the pervasiveness of Scottish bodysnatching than heretofore available. Adams multiplies the audience for Burke and Hare by carving it up according to nationality (Scotland), tone (comedy), and genre (gothic horror). This was not all, for in 2002 he published *Scottish Bodysnatchers*.

Much writing of this period is alike, whoever produced it and where. Still, medical historians will note that in my rehearsal of the encyclopedic trend I fence around Londoner Ruth Richardson's *Death, Dissection and the Destitute* (1987; 2nd ed. 2000). Richardson's magisterial text is the exception that proves the rule: although this book is a testament to the urge for completeness, with its extensive research and careful scholarship it constitutes a genuinely encyclopedic contribution to the understanding of society, medicine, and resurrection. (After twenty years, it has been joined by Lisa Rosner's *Anatomy Murders*, and A. W. Bates's *The Anatomy of Robert Knox*, which suggest a further genre of medical remembrances in process.) Using its authoritative scholarship as the standard, we can register how far, once the traumas of Burke and Hare and Doctor Knox seemed resolved, encyclopedism became a strategy and an exploitable theme for more popular authors and publishers. Such writers increasingly presumed they knew or could easily get at and express all there was to know about Burke and Hare for their niche market of the moment.

Naming the Dead?

The Irish, the Upper Class, and the Money Question in Owen Dudley Edwards

All these renditions of the events of 1828 shared one thing besides their encyclopedic ambition: they tidied up known loose ends. But with the ground cleared, new issues could arise. T. S. Eliot's suggestion that moments mean in time thus gains new meaning in the moment of cultural studies. From the 1970s on, scholars informed by theories that pointed away from the grand movements and stories of history, and toward ordinary people in their local situations, recognized hitherto invisible loose ends in stories like that of Burke and Hare. Consequently, the story showed fully for the first time as one of class, race, and gender. However, in this age at once encyclopedic, critical, and yet recuperative, I will suggest, the real victims remained voiceless.

Problems that could be identified could also be addressed, and even healed. That would stay an impossibility for those exiled beyond the grave, courtesy of Doctor Knox.

Owen Dudley Edwards provides the best example of this cultural conscience brought to bear on Scotland's murderous past. Edwards is an eminent historian, and as a faculty member at the University of Edinburgh he has applied a sophisticated sensibility to the Athens of the North. He has made two substantial contributions to the study of the West Port murders: the scholarly text *Burke and Hare* (1980; 2nd ed. 1993), and a play with the interestingly inverted title, *Hare and Burke* (1994). In today's Edinburgh he figures as an arbiter of things Burke and Harean, having penned an introduction to Raymond Burke's musical comedy *The Return of Burke and Hare* (1994), and become the go-to scholar for public lectures and sound bites.[3] Nonetheless, in Edwards we can see how the urge to encyclopedism, even in the surest hands, trends to identity politics. Such a perspective can multiply concerns without addressing those whom cultural studies would, by its ethos, most want to reconsider: the victims of Burke and Hare.

In 1980, Edwards stresses that "The Irishness of Burke and Hare was an important feature in their story" (Edwards *Burke*, 1). What role Irishness plays, however, is difficult to assess: Edwards makes a lot of Walter Scott's ability to track the economic determinism that might have produced a Burke and Hare from among the hardworking but needy Irish (39–40). Then in his 1994 preface to the play, Edwards places later Scottish anti-Irishness against his knowledge that: "what there does not seem to have been in Edinburgh in 1829 is an anti-Irish or anti-Catholic dimension to the riots, despite the religion and ethnicity of the Hares and Burke.... 25,000 yelled execrations at Burke during his execution, but they were personal, not sectarian" (Edwards *Hare*, Preface). Thus far, Edwards appropriately studies an underclass and registers the complexity of its cultural moment.

But through *Burke and Hare*, Edwards plays a precarious balancing act that leans from the few facts in hand toward more distinct possibilities. In his 1993 introduction, he remembers that he had intended to "use the facts established or asserted in connection with [the] case as revelatory of the nature of Irish immigration in Scotland" (Edwards *Burke*, x). As he researched, however, he realized that "My terms of reference had meant that I would treat Burke and Hare as being humans rather than monsters. It became evident that none of my predecessors had taken such a view" (xi). So far, so even handed. Edwards, however, wrote at the height of the Irish "Troubles" (1970s–80s), and it is interesting to find this Irish author recuperating the figure of William Burke and verging, perhaps, to a new type of bias.

Of course, writing during the formation of cultural studies, Edwards recognizes his own investments and critiques them. *Burke and Hare* features a photograph of

Edwards beside the (surprisingly small) skeleton of William Burke, and under it Edwards claims both his Irish Catholic origins and his new Scottish ties. The 1993 introduction reveals a droll author, dreaming of a visit from a "quite extraordinarily charming" William Burke, "pleasantly appreciative of my attempts to humanise his reputation," and nonetheless determined to murder "his only friend known to historiographical science" (Edwards *Burke*, xii). "I may have tried to explain he was killing a golden-egg laying goose...but he hardly needed telling that he was killing a goose" (xii).

Yet in his preface to the play, Edwards admits: "[My] first emotional commitment to research on Burke and Hare arose from rage at the racist dismissal of them in [*The Anatomist*]....*Hare and Burke*...answers the Bridie notion of the thick Mick" (Edwards *Hare*, Preface). This is a logical response for Owen Dudley Edwards—his own reasoned politics that critique current violence in Northern Ireland cannot be expected to overcome his dislike of endemic contempt for the Irish (Edwards *Burke*, 2). Still, Edwards might more accurately—and more fairly to Bridie—have tracked his concern to post-1828 readings of Burke and Hare, and especially to the 1970s Fleming production of *The Anatomist* that may have been inflected by current anxieties about events in Northern Ireland. Anti-Irish sentiment erupts in the later history of the Burke and Hare story—not at the time. Although *Murderers of the Close* comments on Irishness in 1829, it was a London text, and even more triumphantly anti-Scottish (*Murderers*, 41, 263). A Newcastle paper reports contemporary attacks on immigrant workers in protest against Burke and Hare and the "low Irish" they represented—but the violence was in Sunderland (Johnson, 409). We have to wait until James Grant's *Old and New Edinburgh* from the 1880s for a full-on Scottish assault against the duo's Irishness: "The West Port has long been degraded by the character of its inhabitants, usually Irish of the lowest class" among whom are "those terrible Irish Thugs" who occupy a "low Irish lodging-house" that serves "wretched and obscure Irish tramps" (Grant, 223, 226). Edwards, that is, may be led astray from his subject by his wide knowledge of the scandal's history, and his own moment. The imperatives of cultural studies, combined with Edwards's personal concern, color the limited facts at hand for 1828.

Edwards recognizes the problem. Not infrequently, he points out that the Irish backstory he provides for Burke and Hare (Gaelic language, military career, and so on) "really is the purest speculation" (Edwards *Burke*, 34). But even still, in 1980, he supports his argument for the racial aspects of Burke's 1820s construction by reading Knox as a racist. Edwards draws on Philip D. Curtin's *The Image of Africa*, with its quotation from Knox's *Races of Men* that through a 1980s lens certainly reads as racist—and thus as a motivating factor in Burke and his victims' Knoxian career: "Race is everything: literature, science, art—in a word, civilisation depends on it"

(136). Edwards carries on from Curtin: "The history of the world was an evolutionary struggle between the races.... Knox's opinion of the Irish was perfectly simple: they were to be eradicated from the face of the earth." However, as Evelleen Richards points out, these same writings reveal Knox as a transcendental anatomist with a surprisingly liberal politics. Today, Knox is beginning to emerge as a precursor to Darwin, not to the Social Darwinists, and seems remarkable not for his racism (common at the time) but for the complexity of his thinking (see Kidd for an in-between view). Reading on in the chapter on the Celts, we can see that Knox is building toward an argument for a more active response to hostile circumstances in Ireland—and he thought Celts could achieve it, for he was a great admirer of Napoleon (a "Celt" by his terms). Moreover, though he affirmed "the permanency of race and its... role in determining the character and behavior of the different races," he worked to prevent reductive racializing based on his theories (Richards, 401). Richards quotes: "The white races are not the more fully developed, and the negro the more imperfectly developed, species of one common natural family. The development of each is perfect in its way—equally so." And Knox fascinatingly argued that in Africa, overextended into inappropriate lands, *whites* might appropriately die out (402). This Knox appears even in the most damning quotation marshaled by Edwards: "The [Celts] must be forced from the soil.... England's safety requires it. *I speak not of the justice of the cause*" (*Burke*, 136; emphasis added). Knox could distinguish between different imperatives of transcendental anatomy, and also their morality. But this more complex doctor is, unfortunately, by the tone of the times in 1980, not recognizable. It is a noble project, certainly, to rescue William Burke from his construction by the determinations of nation and race. Edwards's argument is worth pursuing and required by his times. Yet it manifests the narrowed vision of topicality, which is the other side of encyclopedism, nevertheless.

Still, the ethics of Edwards's discipline might be seen to override his understandable concern with Burke as victim and turn him toward the truly neglected victims of Burke and Hare in his play of 1994—such as Daft Jamie (see figure 6.2). One of the major fascinations of *Hare and Burke* is that here at last we find them walking the boards. As perhaps required by his generous interest in the underclass, Edwards introduces a veritable "chorus of wraiths and ghosts" (Edwards *Hare*, 1). Even better:

> Throughout the first act, the ghosts, being ghosts, are more or less at liberty to do as they please; wandering about the theatre, onstage or off; at times coagulating in the gallery like a second audience or jury, at times jostling the principals or audience as the mood takes them.... They may even show interested individual punters their operation scars. (1)

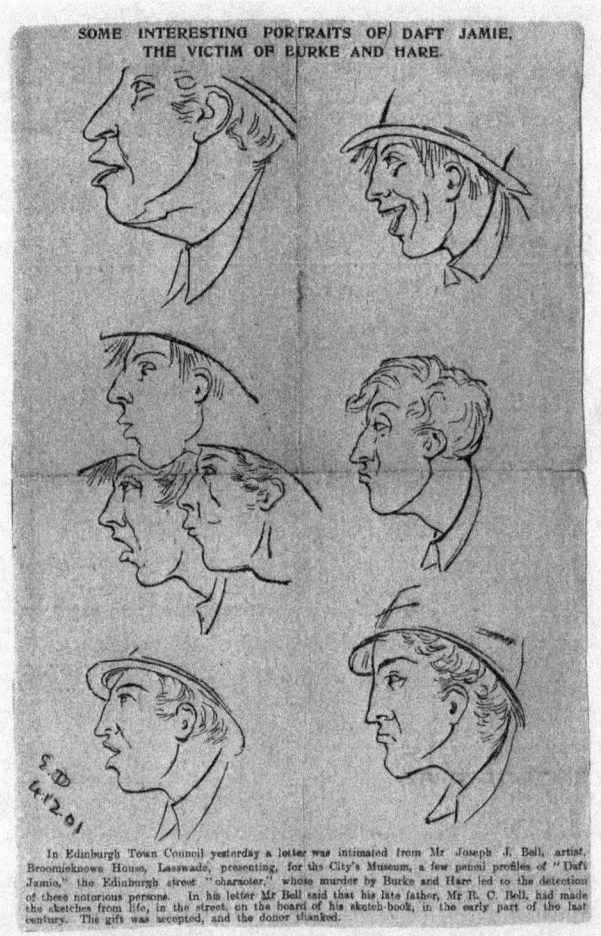

FIGURE 6.2 "Some Interesting Portraits of Daft Jamie the Victim of Burke and Hare." By R. C. Bell (circa 1820s). Newspaper copy, n.d. Courtesy of Edinburgh City Library and Information Services.

Nonetheless, where the Edwards of 1980 tracked economic, religious, and racial determinism through Burke and Hare, now his cultural studies perspective yields not those murdered at the West Port, but those who kept them voiceless: the Edinburgh lawyers and politicians who feared the mob and therefore elided the dead.

Young Archibald Alison opens the living scene, served by his man Chivas. Edwards insists: "for non-Scots... [Chivas] should be pronounced with a 'Dj' sound for 'Ch', its 'i' lengthened to an 'ee', and the 'a' elided" (Edwards *Hare*, Preface). This casts Chivas as "Jeeves," the archetypal "gentleman's gentleman" (post–P. G. Wodehouse). As a result, he and Alison, K.C. (King's Counsel; Advocate Depute of Edinburgh) figure class and authority as motivating factors in this tale. Archie is studying

Malthus. Unexpectedly, this Tory manifestation of class and law considers the theorist of population growth and its inherent and necessary controls "the pernicious 'Malt-house'" (3). But Archie's reasons themselves are perverse and limited. He aims to exhibit:

> to the public the absurdities upon which the Reverend Thomas Robert Malthus has founded his theories of the growth of population, views upon which our compatriots the Whigs… have the insolence to offer themselves in place of his grace the Duke of Wellington and his ministers who now happily rule us. (5–6)

Archie's potential nobility of mind sits askew.

Nonetheless, from the more liberal viewpoint of 1994, the Malthusian events of 1828 can be seen to test and perhaps improve Archie's sentiments. The powers of Edinburgh break in on Archie's rarefied deliberations—Lord Meadowbank literally so. Chivas has just acknowledged the instruction to "forbid you to your acquaintances" when "*Enter Lord Meadowbank,*" declaring "But not to me, good Chivas, never me!" (Edwards *Hare*, 6). Close on this party fixer's heels come Rae, the Lord Advocate, and then Margaret Hare with her attendant brace of policemen and a rather timid spouse. In the naïve Archie's chambers, these four act out the drama of power and politics. Archie presumes "there will be a full enquiry" (8). Meadowbank exclaims: "Perish that thought" (8). To Meadowbank, "Knox deserves hanging, and it is a perpetual grief to me that he shall not have it, for his damned insolence. No, they shall hang Burke. The murderer of old women so that the doctors might have their bodies!" (9). Meadowbank continues, fully demonstrating the confusion of bigotries that supports the pretense of justice: "Why the doctors should thus cherish the bodies of old women I find hard to say, but they do. Though I am told one of the bodies was a young woman, and of remarkable pulchritude. This perhaps makes more sense" (9). Small wonder that by the end of the play, Margaret Hare has run rings around these temporizing prosecutors, confessing to multiple murders under the cover of king's evidence. She has escaped judgment while telling the truth and thus undoing, as Edwards says in his preface, the notion of "thick Mick." But there is a greater wonder: at the start of the play, Archie is on the eve of being promoted to "His Majesty's Solicitor General for Scotland"; now, he resists such politics—and so becomes their victim (5). He cries out in the middle of the play, "My duty is to prevent a miscarriage of justice," leading Meadowbank to tut: "Well, well, perhaps you are not for the law after all, Archie" (39, 41). Archie is gone from the rest of the performance.

Here, Edwards's Irish and underclass counter narratives reveal the masterplot that drives cultural studies: the play of economics and power that makes victims of us all. This proved a strong complement to the story of Burke and Hare during the Thatcher era (1979–90), and it resonated into Ronald Reagan's America. As laissez-faire economics reached their zenith, the arts suffered a lack of funding—as did other humane endeavors—and translated their own and others' suffering into theater. In New York, on the eve of Reaganism, Dan Bianchi's 1980 musical *The Burke and Hare Company* built on the story as "quite conducive to making a few social commentaries.... [T]hey killed for money."[4] In Scotland, a Labour-voting nation at the time, and particularly out of step with Thatcherite politics and economics—Edwards's play stands alongside Richard Crane's *Burke and Hare*, staged at the Tron Theatre Glasgow in 1983. Crane notes his attraction to the tale as arising from "the idea of murder as business."[5] He elaborates: "it is much more tragic and disturbing, to see murder as a regular, wealth-producing activity." Chris Ballance, now a Green Party politician in Scotland, also recognized the potential for critique in the proto-Thatcherite economics of Burke and Hare. He writes of *Water of Life*, 1989: "it occurred to me that Burke and Hare were demonstrating exactly the sort of entrepreneurial spirit...championed by Margaret Thatcher."[6] Interestingly, the authors in Scotland both attribute their interest to Edwards. Edwards himself claims a dramatic trend originating with his history that pushed his perspective and in Ballance's play rose to "riveting drama"—Edwards nominated Ballance for a Fringe First award (which he duly won) (Edwards *City*, 237).

Then in 1991 Raymond Burke (acknowledging possible Burkean ancestry despite his East Kilbride home) staged *The Return of Burke and Hare*. This play focuses on the downside of rampant power in the form of medical capitalism—and conforming to what by now was itself a market imperative, the 1994 publication features an introduction by Edwards. The basic plot is brought up-to-date at the failing Hare's Hotel in Tanner's Close, and it is played in music-hall style complete with ditties like: "Bodysnatching Baby" (Burke, 74–75) and "Transplant Surgery":

Knox: Transplant surgery's what it's all about.
We're pruning the population in medicine[']s final bout.
If you want to put the kidneys in, you've got to take them out....
Heart, lungs, liver and Kidneys, hair upon your head,
Skin graft emergency to stop you being dead.
Frontal lobotomy, spare parts are brought to me....
Decomposing corpses are becoming history.
They used to go to Heaven, but now they come to me.
(95–96)

Further, in true capitalist form, victims are would-be perpetrators. Abigail, fresh off the bus from Glasgow and declaring in unabashed middle-class cliché "I might not be rich but I've got my pride," quickly segues to: "I'm not sleeping in the same place as all those old tramps.... I'd line them up, give them all a good wash, a decent set of clothes, a hot meal, and then I'd shoot the bastards! Bloody waste of public money" (60–61, 63). By the 1980s Burke and Hare have gone global yet turned into one, disturbing tale: our own, recursive story of greed and exploitation that works the same through any of its participants.

And where victims are also perpetrators (like Abigail), and perpetrators are only victims of class expectations (like Archie and perhaps Burke and Hare), even Owen Dudley Edwards's "wraiths and ghosts" must remain as they are. Though they may wander around, show their scars, and "coagulat[e] in the gallery," they cannot impinge on those around them (Edwards *Hare*, 1). Each gets to state who they were, suggest what happened, and gesture to what they lost (1–3, 21–22, 41–42). However, it really does not matter. They cannot be embodied and so cannot affect events. Though voicing uncannily through the lines of Macbeth—"When shall we sweet 17 meet again"—to a Burke caught in the toils of "Tomorrow, and tomorrow, and tomorrow," they still cannot touch him, or anyone else (Edwards includes Donald, who died naturally and gave Burke and Hare their idea; 43, 45). Maggie Hare mocks: "Ghosts, is it?... They're dead to me, and dead they'll remain" (38). The author wrestles with this problem: though the ghosts can disturb Burke, he cannot encounter them unless they transform into another, living character and no one else (except the audience) can see them (44, 46). As Edwards says, while "they might become most agitated and make low moaning noises... what they must not do is interrupt the flow of the play nor upstage any of the action" (1). Through Edwards's sympathetic approach, these dead must arise, but they cannot intervene in human events.

It might seem, then, that as times progress, authors and historians, whether Scots or strangers, can only slice the scandal of Burke and Hare and Doctor Knox into smaller and smaller pieces in service of rising narratives from elsewhere—those of niche markets or market capitalism. The encyclopedic approach, whether folding in place or power or persons, acknowledges no remains—except, perhaps, for the lingering whiff of the cadaverous Margaret Thatcher. The absent heart of the tale, the victims of Burke and Hare, remains unsought and unexpressed.

Wives, Daughters, and Tinkers in Byrd and Scarborough

Oddly, Maggie Hare points to one way of addressing this lack. In times informed by cultural change—the moment of women's liberation—the heart of the tale often turns out to be female. Though Burke and Hare were equal opportunity killers, for whom any drunk would do, their victims were predominantly women. Nonetheless, until the 1970s, the women of the story had been neglected. Only Mary Paterson figured with any regularity or prominence. Yet even in David Pae's novel that goes by her name, though her female frailties initiate the plot, she must disappear from the middle of a story that cannot, in the end, be hers. We track the ramifications of Mary's plot in the lives of others as Pae works to re-establish the idea of community. That is, as in every case so far, the story is all about us: how we relate to Robert Knox, and how we relate to one another. The dead play no part in the conversation.

Now, by contrast, women as victims move to the center of the tale—and in ways informed by the current cultural moment. We can track this gradual movement in two novels by Elizabeth Byrd: *Rest Without Peace* (1974), and *The Search for Maggie Hare* (1976). Living in Scotland and with the benefit of numerous archives and the assistance of police (Byrd *Rest*, 223), this American author focuses first on the historical tale, next on the ways in which it produces victims. In *Rest Without Peace*, she dwells particularly on Maggie Hare and Nelly MacDougal; in *The Search for Maggie Hare*, Byrd moves on to speculate about Maggie's child—the "yellow, 'yammering' infant, (the image of its father)" observed by Christopher North (*Blackwood's* March 1829: 384; see figure 6.3). Although Byrd does not neglect Burke and Hare's actual victims, detailing them one by one and including in the first novel even those who got away (which at times pushes the novel beyond encyclopedism and toward catalog), she interestingly brings together the dead and the women as all victims in their own way.

Like Owen Dudley Edwards after her, Byrd is alive to the implications of Irishness in the United Kingdom of 1828. In this context, everyone is a victim. Because of their difference, the Irish form a community in Scotland—Hare jokes to Burke, who is at his door looking for drink: "*Buy* from a fellow Irishman?" (Byrd *Rest*, 11). But this is a community of decay, where Hare tempts Burke into his nefarious schemes, and all are subject to the rot. "Log's Lodging in Tanner's Close [Maggie Hare's house] stood between rotting houses in the shadow of Edinburgh Castle.... Two and three to a straw bed, [guests] scratched and coughed, slept off the aches of a beggar's day" (9). Burke (who did have testicular cancer at the time of his death), "didn't like to think that his right testicle was eaten away—but it was. He didn't know why, and he was afraid to find out for fear a doctor would say that all of him was rotting" (77). Significantly, however, the women are in worse shape than the men.

These women are directly involved in the procurement of subjects, but their exploits reveal only their considerable neediness. Maggie confidently declares, "We've to have our wits about us. I promised Hare we'd look for a subject," but when fourteen-year-old chimney sweep Andrew Cay is lured to her lodgings, he is

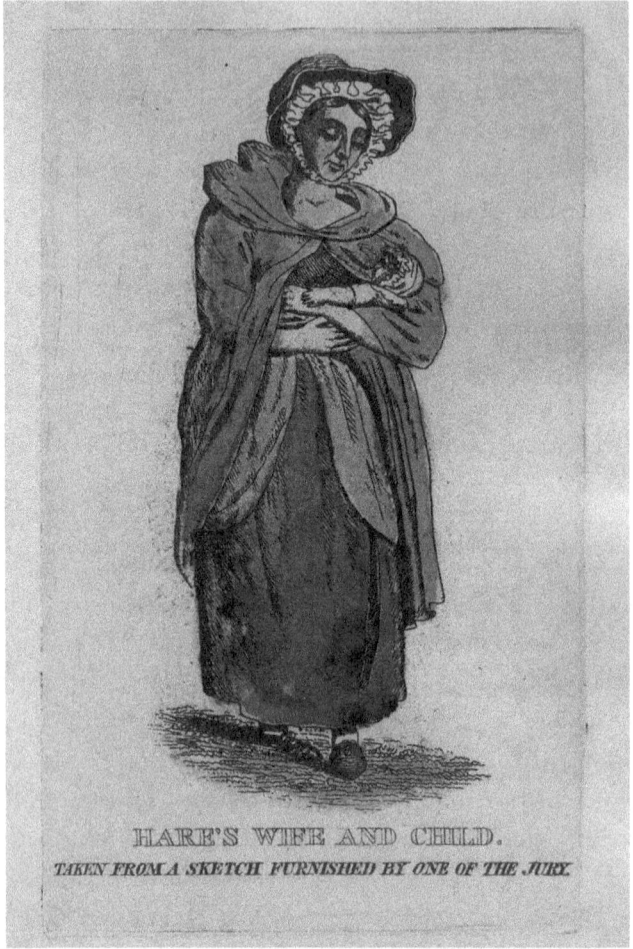

FIGURE 6.3 "Hare's Wife and Child." Contemporary print, tinted. Courtesy of the Royal College of Physicians of Edinburgh.

driven away when (unnecessarily for Knoxian purposes) Maggie starts to disrobe (29, 39):

> after another drink he found himself not shy but just happy to be here, for she was so nice.... And then—he didn't know quite how or when she did it—she had lifted her petticoat and he could see a red garter on a skinny leg.
>
> Why, she was almost an old woman—thirty, maybe—and now buttons had come undone at her bodice and she was coming towards him saying things that made him want to vomit, and then she was kneeling down at his feet with her hand on him... [ellipsis in text]
>
> He got out of there so fast he knocked her over. (39–40)

Maggie the predator, though revolting in her sexuality, is also its victim.

Helen MacDougal (Nelly) ends up in the same subjected position by a different route. Not that Nelly, too, does not attempt to fulfill her quota: she lures a blind beggar—but the beggar is not so blind:

> He watched her pour drops of something into his glass before she added the whisky—laudanum? He watched her lift [his] basket and gently remove coins into her own purse. And he sprang to his feet, snatched her purse into his basket, picked up his stick, called to the dog and left, slamming the door.
>
> It was all so quick that she couldn't believe it had happened. (Byrd *Rest*, 71–72)

In fact, the beggar points to Nelly's generally confused disposition. Later, on the brink of exposure, this Nelly (like her historical predecessor) will offer impossible bribes to the Grays to keep them from the police:

> Still on her knees, Nelly pulled at Ann's skirt. "You are like one of the family. Say nothing, and there will never be a week but you receive ten pounds...."
>
> "So you sell them," [James] Gray said.
>
> "God forbid we should be worth money with dead people," Ann said. "And you?"
>
> "I cannot help it!"
>
> "You surely can help it or you'd not stay in this house," Ann said. (187)

Ann Gray grasps the issue: Nelly is trapped in her relationships.

From early in the novel we know that Nelly is dependent on a Burke who cannot respond to her womanly needs:

> now, at thirty-three, nobody looked at her twice....
>
> It made her uneasy, for fear of losing Burke. At the drunken bouse the other night she'd caught him squeezing neighbour women.... For, at thirty-five, Burke held on well, smooth-faced, not a pox on him.... Not a handsome fellow but something about him went to her head like drink....
>
> But how long since he'd said anything like a compliment to her? (15)

And the virago Maggie is no better off, for she is in the toils of William Hare:

> Maggie admired the quickness of him, tall and muscular like a fine animal. Funny though, when he'd first come here as a lodger, before Log [her husband]

died, she'd been afraid of his looks. His face was somehow brutal.... You don't play around with this one, she decided, and yet he had fascinated her like stoats fascinated rabbits. (10–11)

Thus the trajectory of the novel implies that all are victims: the Irish are particularly victimized by economics, and their women are the victims not just of class and race but also of gender.

Yet we might question whether, whatever the imperatives of gender politics, any amount of such victimhood can ally a Maggie Hare with a Mary Paterson. Having raised this question, Byrd pursues it through her next novel. In *The Search for Maggie Hare*, Maggie's (dubious) victimhood is displaced into and given meaning through the child she neglected in *Rest Without Peace*. References to the child echo throughout the earlier book. For instance, Burke admires the child and Maggie thinks: "Och, what an oily liar, paying for his lush with compliments. The baby was puny and pasty-faced and likely wouldn't live out the winter" (Byrd *Rest*, 11). This baby poses a problem of inheritance: is it natural heir to horrors—or victim? In *Rest Without Peace*, the child is treated as an object—it almost serves as a "thing for the surgeon."

> The infant in its box made a mewing sound and Hare said, irritably, "It's waking for its feed, and Maggie over to the neighbours."
> "She don't seem much attached to it."
> "It's just a chore to her."
> "And you're not after being fond of it either?"
> "Nobody wanted it; it just came."
> Burke smiled a little and Hare began to giggle in that high-pitched way of his, "I know what you're thinking," he said, "but it's too small. I doubt it would bring a shilling. Besides, it would be stupid, like selling a piglet before it's fattened up." (21–22)

Moreover, the baby appears through the fragments of a metaphor that casts it as uncertain possibility: a jail/bird. "The baby," we are told, "wanted to move about now and hold onto people and try to talk but they kept it in its box and when friends came in at night, put a cover on top, like you keep a caged bird" (151). No contemporary record gives the baby's sex. But this child, product of murderers and yet punished by the lack of that attention they (unfortunately) lavish on others is, significantly, a girl.

The Search for Maggie Hare opens just as this girl, having fled her mother and been adopted into Edinburgh's middle class, finds herself an orphan with no sense of her actual inheritance (Maggie went incognito after the debacle of 1828). When the papers report that Maggie Hare is back in town, and "Dorothea" sees her picture sketched in the newspaper, this construct of respectability responds as one might when confronted with m/other—that awfulness bred in the bone. First she faints, and then (like Andrew Cay before her) she throws up (Byrd *Search*, 16). In the tortuous plot that follows, the apparent return of Maggie Hare prompts fear and desire in Dorothea; the daughter does not want to confirm that Maggie is her mother, but she is drawn to the woman if only to determine the truth. That truth matters because Dorothea is on the brink of marriage. She worries: "I dare not drink spirits; I even avoid wine.... Until I fled Maggie, gin was my solace when I could get it. It made me sleep; it eased the bruises. So what might my children inherit of two murderous grandparents [who] were both drunkards?" (24). Is Dorothea a victim as the descendant of perpetrators, or inherently a perpetrator because their victim in descent?

No matter how perplexed or ironic Dorothea's victimhood may be, insofar as she is a victim, unlike her predecessors she gets to fight back. Undeniably, she bears the marks of her inheritance. A brogue sporadically breaks through her elegant tones and links her through race memory to the otherness of Irishness as manifested in Maggie Hare. Maggie may be identifiable through marks on her body (we keep hearing about the warts around her mouth), and so is Dorothea. When she finally confronts Hare, he identifies his daughter by the moles under her arm—moles Hare calls "mice turds," and that link Dorothea, again in the body, to squalor and to horror (Byrd *Search*, 175). Worse, Dorothea is thereby linked to the strange sexuality of the Burke and Hare ménage. When she finds her father, she is translated into a figure of suffering and (perversely) family inheritance through the lurking threat of incest:

> Hare moved to block the window. "Stand up, I said, and undress—or is it you're wanting a lady's maid like meself?"
> Hopelessly she stood, tossed off the cloak, removed her bodice and petticoat and stood shivering.
> "Now," he said genially, sipping the drink, "you don't have the good full tits Maggie had, or the bottom." ...
> "So," he said. "Me dear daughter," and took her into his arms.
> ... how to think, with his thick, wet lips on hers? (174–75)

But Dorothea is as complex as her body and mind. The marks of her victimhood—her voice and street smarts—have allowed her to take charge of her story. By appearing to be a seamstress/prostitute, she has tracked her ne'er-do-well parents. And just as the strength of character that is *not* written on her body has allowed her to abjure drink, here she can resist William Hare even as he claims paternity and threatens a nearer relation: "She thought, if I struggle it may be my last. I mustn't rouse his temper, only hope to trick him somehow. It seemed his only weak point was conceit.... Very gently she drew back. 'It's nice to know I've a father who was so famous and all'" (175). Then she flees back to her lodgings, back to the trappings of respectability: "Now, the pretty petticoat, the hose and slippers, the decent black dress.... Never mind the past, slide into the future quickly and gracefully and thankfully" (178). Representing all those lost before her, Hare's daughter can refuse victimhood.

Still, this is an escape, not a revenge. The turn to feminism allows British director Roy Ward Baker to take a dark step toward expressing the rage of victimhood. *Doctor Jekyll and Sister Hyde* (1971) might seem many worlds away from the Edinburgh of 1828, even if we accept that Robert Louis Stevenson mapped Knoxian concerns onto his story of Henry Jekyll and Mr. Hyde. But Baker draws these worlds close: Doctor Jekyll, with the usual movie commitment to goodness for his character, is trying to concoct a universal panacea. The problem is, he might not live so long. So Jekyll turns his attention to an elixir of life: "An elixir of life! A secret that had fascinated men for centuries, but they had sought it through witchery, black magic, and superstitious nonsense. But I had science at my fingertips. I was seized and engulfed by the idea. It became my passion and obsession." So far so Jekyll. But this elixir, it turns out, will require the body parts of young women. Thus at this point, as at the time of *Jekyll and Hyde*, the story swings into alignment with Burke and Hare, and the Whitechapel murders. Jekyll is the doctor 1888 London feared: he is the experimental chemist supplied anatomically by Burke and Hare—through exploits attributed to Jack the Ripper.

Even more interestingly, once Jekyll starts to ingest his potion distilled from the generative organs of nubile young women, he produces not a monkeyish little man, but the luscious Mrs. Hyde. Though bred in the bone like Dorothea (if by chemistry, not natural means), Mrs. Hyde is less a younger, more active Jekyll than an avenging, notably female, murderer. Jekyll, as doctor, began the dissections and encouraged murder; with Burke hanged and Hare blinded (as per London myth), he combines the roles of dissector and murderer. Mrs. Hyde comes to the game late. At first, she chases women through the streets because Jekyll has realized the police are looking for a man and decides to go undercover in his female incarnation. Later, however, Mrs. Hyde goes out to procure prostitutes on her own account, because her persistence depends on female hormones. Still, although she is created through the victimization of women and repeats that victimization, as a woman she may be a victim, too. Tellingly, in this case, her great threat is not to other women, but to the doctors. Before long she has stabbed Jekyll's randy medical friend (in lieu of him). When Jekyll stabs his mirror, yelling "It was *you*—I'll be rid of you," she re-emerges to declare "It is *I* who exist Doctor Jekyll, not you. It is *I* who will be rid of *you*." And, indeed, she is. When the police finally arrive, Jekyll takes off across the roof, but Sister Hyde asserts her presence. Her weaker grasp precipitates him/her/them to the pavement beneath. That is, in a flurry of references that include *Oliver Twist* and *The Picture of Dorian Gray*, along with the Whitechapel murders, woman emerges as victim but (in the person of Mrs. Hyde), inevitably as vengeance.

In taking this trajectory, Roy Ward Baker shows the pervasiveness of the feminist ethos as it plays a part in encyclopedism—but he gets no closer to the central problem of victimhood. In *Rest Without Peace*, the story of Burke and Hare and Doctor Knox was resolved by history—following closely along the line of archival events, the story must end in particular ways, whatever discussions of generalized victimhood have been begun. In *The Search for Maggie Hare*, Byrd's clever consideration of how guilt works itself out across generations gives voice to an interestingly constructed victim. But Dorothea operates within conventional plots. No matter how much she worries that descent from the Hares might produce her as perpetrator, not victim, and exile her from respectability, her story ends with marriage: all previous agonizing notwithstanding, as the child but therefore victim of Maggie Hare, Dorothea falls back into a (very contrived) romance. As for Sister Hyde, although she enacts in full the vengeance required by a feminist reinterpretation of the victimhood perpetrated by Burke and Hare and Doctor Knox—complete with knives and gore—in so doing she becomes another perpetrator. She is still Doctor Jekyll, locked within the inevitability of Stevenson's plot.

Of course, it is a strength of this feminist moment that in bringing women to center stage, and attempting to give victims a voice, Byrd and Baker paint a complicated picture. Viragos can also be victims; the inheritances of the body can empower; victims can be avengers. Nor is it a surprise that these women emerge in the time of Margaret Thatcher, who on the one hand declared "I owe nothing to women's lib," and on the other hand fulfilled its strongest dictates.[7] But memorably for our purposes, Thatcher also asserted: "To wear your heart on your sleeve isn't a very good plan; you should wear it inside, where it functions best."[8] In this early stage of feminism, resistant stories too easily resolve into familiar plots. Perhaps the surgically excised hearts of anatomy's victims belong "inside, where [they] function best," motivating bodies that speak for themselves.

But as Elizabeth Ann Scarborough shows, though victims—however unconventional—can be ventriloquized through conventional plots, writers both inside and out of Scotland have difficulty meeting this moment's need that they speak for themselves. Scarborough is an American writer of note, and occasional collaborator with Anne McCaffrey. In her 1998 novel *The Lady in the Loch*, she recognizes the feminist drive of her story but has as much trouble as all her fellow writers in giving voice to actual victims. In Walter Scott's Edinburgh, those victimized by class, race, and gender are further victimized by the doctors. This high-gothic version of the tale features tinker women who are being stolen and dissected to support Doctor Primrose's perverse idea of romance—he is trying to produce a body to match the head of his lady love, who was guillotined in France (Scarborough invokes a tradition of "burker" tales—see Baird, 79–83, Sheila Douglas, 103–5, and *Tobar an Dualchais*). Scott, supposedly the "Sheriff of Edinburgh," has already seen the dead speak. Early in his career, assisted by highland magic, a murdered woman rose to accuse her lover. Now, the dead beseech the tinker seer Midge Margret. More, these dead walk, either by possessing Margret and speaking through her, or by animating the patchwork body assembled by Doctor Primrose. These visible remains of Primrose's victims kill his murderous henchman. Even his beloved Veronique proves unbiddable. Possessing Midge Margret, she dashes Primrose to his death in revenge for his role in her family's demise by the portable guillotine he invented.

Clearly, Scarborough's book has reached a pitch of overdetermination with regard to victimhood. Expendable through race, class, and gender, these dead *must* rise. Scarborough actually suggests a certain authorial desperation in the need to recognize all victimhoods and make them function—in whatever possible way. But still and yet, these dead may walk, but they cannot really speak. The young woman who accuses her lover is (again) dead as soon as she has uttered; the patchwork woman has no voice; others can speak only through Midge Margret. In the hands of this earnest American author, keen to address every victimhood, encyclopedism bears down the possibility of meaningful voicing. That is, the assembled emphases of the cultural studies moment cannot accomplish it.

Can a Scottish writer come closer? Notably, among all the writers about Burke and Hare, few are women, and among the women only Rae is (part) Scottish. Could it be that in the era of Liz Lochhead, Scotland's preeminent feminist writer, or looking back to Naomi Mitchison, feminist issues loomed so large that they could not be reduced to the story of Burke and Hare? Certainly Mitchison would produce *Memoirs of a Spacewoman* (1962) and *Solution Three* (1975); Muriel Spark had her Edinburgh tales, not least *The Prime of Miss Jean Brodie* (1961); and Lochhead engaged the roles of women past and present in *Mary Queen of Scots Got Her Head Chopped Off* (1989) and in poem sequences like: *True Confessions and New Clichés* (1985). It may be that whereas the events of 1828 provided a template to discuss women as victims for writers outside Scotland, Scotland's great women writers resisted such reduction into a tale that they knew had its own important imperatives. That said, there is one remarkable Scottish and feminist intervention in the Burke and Hare story so far—and it comes from a Scottish man. This story is fully feminist because it is so much more.

Among all these earnest retellings of the events of 1828, which together manifest the compounded failures of normative history and popular fiction, the absent corpse lurks, ever more insistent by its inability to voice. Alasdair Gray, artist and author, pre-postmodernist and political activist, reached beyond identity politics to express the complex dynamic between past and present from the victim's perspective. Gender helps him to articulate the necessary and productive difference that is shared by Scots and women as victims yet creators of experience.

POOR THINGS SPEAK: ALASDAIR GRAY

The corpse he swam out of the whisky
And he rattled the latch of the door
Crying, 'Fare you well, brother surgeon,
You sha'n't cut me up any more!'
        (Epigraph from Goodwin, 97)

How intense was the lack at the heart of the story of Burke and Hare, and how strong its need for voicing? We can gain some idea of the problem through Jean-Luc Nancy's theories of the body—that invisible yet excessive aspect of Knox's dissected subjects. For Nancy, though we think of mind as the essence of individuality: "Bodies are places of existence.... The body-place.... is a skin, variously folded, refolded, unfolded, multiplied, invaginated, exogastrulated, orificed, evasive, invaded, stretched, relaxed, excited, distressed, tied, untied.... [T]he body *makes room* for existence" (Nancy, 15). This necessary bodiliness proves doubly problematic at death, for "the body, the mortal spacing of the body [as dead], [registers] the fact that existence has no essence." We do not exist separately from our bodies: there's a living body, or there's not. If we extend Nancy's theory, anxiety about how and where we exist can only increase when there is no body, not even dead or buried, to mark the space in which we once were seen to live.

This is even more the case in the circumstances of silent killing and illicit dissection that produce the victims of Doctor Knox. From Nancy's perspective, all body and all being is a mystery of physiology—of spaces folded, refolded, and unfolded. We might note that this living body evokes the body as it is revealed in the anatomist's lab. So bodies made absent and thus oddly present by the fact of their dissection are even more distressing—excessive and anxiety-producing (*Trial*, 65–66). Intensely implying body and its lack, the whole problem of ex-istence, the victims of 1828 at once beseeched expression, yet for over 150 years proved impossible to embody in story. Then in 1992, Alasdair Gray figured out how to let these "poor things" speak for themselves.

Gray meets the challenge by embracing the bodily terms through which, in Nancy's parlance, we "ex-ist" (Nancy, 15). That is, avoiding the reductive categorizations of the encyclopedic urge, Gray expresses the play of bodies im/politic. Thus, Gray stands heir to Pae, Stevenson, and Bridie, with their particularly Scottish, vexed, but lively relation to 1828. Informed by recent political events that required but exaggerated Scott's image of the nation as the body undergoing hostile dissection (the failed referendum for a Scottish assembly of 1979), Gray reads anew the metaphoric connections between a body and politic troubled by the exploits of murderers and dissectors.[9] Pae and Stevenson worked to dissect the doctor, and Bridie to anatomize the audience—each to expiate public trauma. Gray, by contrast, traces the scars of the past as they are borne on the body of its victims and shows that through such visible damage, as sufferers or perpetrators, we all connect to otherness. Rather than falsely recuperating the victims through the cohesive forms of story (whether as history or romance), Gray pursues what "he," as narrator, calls "a complete tissue of facts" (Gray *Poor Things*, xii). As fragments produced by the past, the dissected body now walks, speaks, and disturbs. This absence that is really excess recasts the terms by which, as Scots and other others, we must "ex-ist."

Scottish theoretical writing from the broad period of Gray's thinking, similarly informed by Scotland's growing political and socioeconomic anxieties, assisted the author toward his strategy. In 1970, Tom Nairn recalled Scott's metaphors of medical destruction to posit the problem of contemporary Scottishness. Scotland suffered "chronic laceration of the Scots mind—most brilliantly conveyed to the world in Stevenson's fable of Jekyll and Hyde" (Nairn "Three Dreams," 32). The nation required "healing of the secular wound which has informed—and most often poisoned—Scottish consciousness ever since the Union of 1707." Nairn pointed further to the problem of national identity, medicine, and metaphor constituted by the events of 1828 when in 1977 he pondered the possible breakup of Britain. Here, he imagines Scotland as a modern Lazarus. He invokes an image poised at the cusp between life and death—but memorably finds the nation's trajectory uncertain (Nairn *Break-Up*, 116). This, in particular, he wrote in 1998 (with the Scottish Parliament in the offing), is the Janus-faced moment, looking to past and present, but unsure how to proceed (Nairn *Faces*). Yet he elaborates:

> through nationalism the dead are awakened, this is the point—seriously awakened for the first time. All cultures have been obsessed by the dead and placed them in another world. Nationalism rehouses them in this world. Through its agency the past ceases being "immemorial": it gets memorialised into time present and so acquires a future. For the first time it is meaningfully projected on to the screen of futurity. (*Faces*, 4)

Nairn reconnects body and nation in a discussion whose potential turns on the un/desirability of raising the dead. By the time he extended this theory through the modern Janus and in relation to an actual Scottish Parliament, his medical metaphorics took a new, positive turn—one that Alasdair Gray had already embodied in *Poor Things*. Perhaps it was possible to admit the dead and thereby project all Scots toward a future.

Gray was also supported, and his new discourse built, by the theories of dis/integration developed by his fellow Glaswegian, R. D. Laing. Gavin Miller has convincingly argued the direct influence from Laing to Gray (Miller, 57–66). This influence can further be recognized in compelling connections between Laing's ideas and *Poor Things*. Laing had begun his career by studying medicine—because it gave him "access to the issues of birth and death" (Ticktin). His first job took him to the West of Scotland Neurosurgical Unit, where lobotomy was the issue of the moment. That is, Laing's researches wove together mental and bodily ideas of the self, and tested them at the moment of collapse (whether by death or vivisection). Perhaps not surprisingly, from the 1960s on, Laing developed a "social phenomenology" that sees supposed mental aberration less as disease (treatable by the knife), and more as part of a social dynamic. In this dynamic, standard medical narratives are reversed. "Treatment," for Laing, becomes a matter of relationships. This shift expands into psychoanalytic and medical treatments, for treatment now refracts both the physician's in/ability to engage with the patient, and the patient's ability to impinge on those around them in mental and physical ways. Treatment, in fact, becomes a test of those delivering it, and the difficulty in meeting a patient's needs is an indication of that "victim's" productive excess—if I might be allowed here to bring Laing, Gray, and Doctor Knox's subjects into alignment.

Bella Victoria

It is by making such alignments between nation and absent person that Gray breaks the bounds of past stories and opens up a future for victims of all sorts in *Poor Things*. First and foremost, it is important to recognize that Gray's main character is, beyond all doubt, a victim. Victimized in specifically Knoxian ways, Bella stands beyond hope of recuperation. Elaine Scarry points out that pain is almost impossible to communicate: we need to externalize pain, yet it resists language, uttering itself outside our codes; voicing pain according to our linguistic conventions fails to express the pain (Scarry, 4–7). Worse, since pain exchanged between people implies a power differential (as between torturer and victim), the victim becomes visible only at the point of pain and only as lack and loss (18, 27). The victims of Burke and Hare might be considered to fit Scarry's argument in that they are constructed at the point of pain/murder, but as victims cannot express themselves (except within narratives that rewrite and diminish their situation according to reductive codes—they were Irish; they were women). But in Bella, Gray embodies absence, death, and pain: they are written on her body.

Bella has been put together from pieces by the aptly named "Godwin." Godwin Baxter's father was a vivisectionist, but Godwin's friend and the teller of this tale remarks his insistence that he himself is no such thing: "*I have never killed or hurt a living creature in my life, and neither did Sir Colin*," he shrills (Gray *Poor Things*, 20; see figure 6.4). Yet two chapters later, we are presented with Bella, a thing of visible shreds and patches. It turns out that Godwin may temporize: the marks of slicing and stitching that Bella bears on her body figure the death of her mother (by suicide), and the transposition of Bella's fetal brain to her mother's body. (So Bella enacts, in addition, the double victimization by medicine most deplored by Laing: that of mother and child.)[10] Thus bound, did Bella or her mother suffer a death or a life? At the very least, "Bella's" body is made visible as anatomized; it manifests pain both *at* and *as* the cusp of death and life. Bella is suspended at the point of victimhood. There is no previous, outer, or other side to suffering for Bella. Her presence depends on an irretrievable loss that is yet visible and never can be healed.

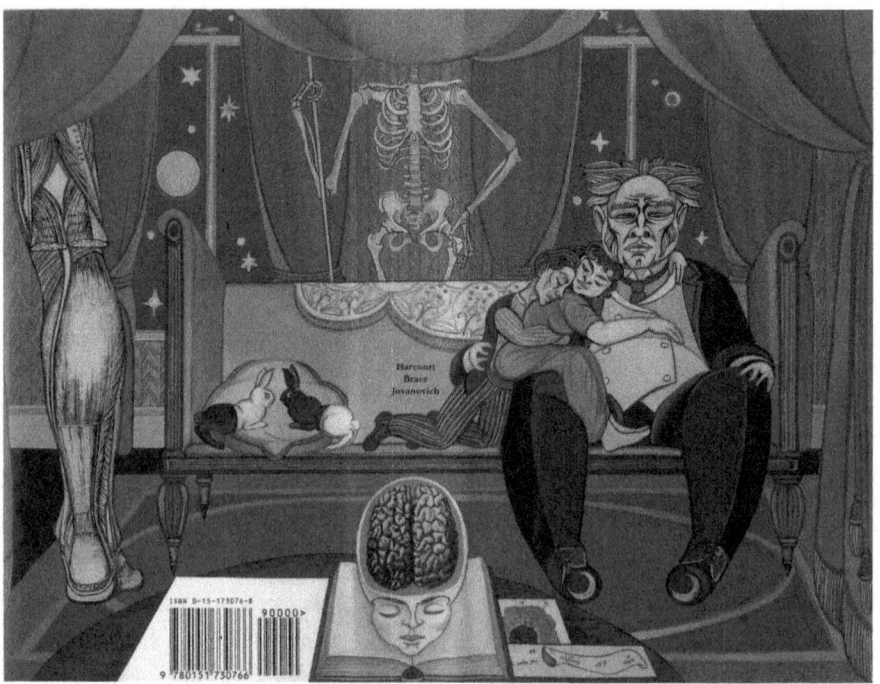

FIGURE 6.4 *Poor Things*, cover. Courtesy of Alasdair Gray.

Predictably, Bella has been recognized as descending from the creature in *Frankenstein*. Stephen Bernstein comments extensively on this theme, mentioning *Frankenstein*, the creature, Victor Frankenstein, Mary Shelley, her father William Godwin (an interesting coincidence), and Percy Shelley's first wife (who drowned herself) (109–12). (He misses the author's mother, Mary Wollstonecraft, who attempted suicide by drowning, and died as a consequence of giving birth to Mary). Gray points in that direction when he criticizes Frankenstein for "having brought [his] creature to life" but failing "to give it an education" (Bernstein, 118 and n. 20). Nor should we forget that as Tim Marshall shows, Mary Shelley wrote within the era of dissection and its accompanying nefarious practices (*Murdering to Dissect*).

But for Gray, writing in Glasgow in 1992, Bella's is still a story of Scottish anatomy and Doctor Knox. Gray himself, as his biographer tells us, through his life has been subject to the Glasgow medical profession, with a body scarified by eczema and racked by asthma (Glass). Illnesses that show the body at its point of dissolution, at the boundary of skin and in the necessity of breath, have perhaps allied Gray with the victims of science. Furthermore, Gray has studied and worked in the shadow of anatomy—and interestingly, the collections in Glasgow University's Anatomy Museum feature the work of (Glaswegian) William Hunter, with his famous molds of pregnant women (Alice Marshall, Series 48 "Gravid Uterus"). Archie McCandless, the narrator, studies medicine in Glasgow and is directed in how to become "a greater surgeon than [John] Hunter, a finer obstetrician than Simpson, a better healer than Lister" (Gray *Poor Things*, 10). That is, he is directed toward the pantheon of Scottish doctors, for John Hunter was brother to William, and both began their careers in Glasgow; Simpson was the Edinburgh obstetric anesthetist; and Lister had tested antibiotics in both cities.

And Gray is well aware, in *Poor Things*, of the doctor most identified in popular consciousness with the destruction rather than the recuperation of the suffering body. He is here—made prominent through an interesting remove. In the "Notes Critical and Historical" that close the novel, but, in the way of Gray's texts, do not necessarily ratify it, we find reference to a play by Archibald McCandless:

1892 *The Resurrectionists*.
  This five-act play about the Burke and Hare murders is no better than the many other nineteenth-century melodramas based on the same very popular theme. Robert Knox, the surgeon who bought the corpses, is treated more sympathetically than usual, so the play may have influenced Bridie's *The Anatomist*. (300)

Archie, bred an anatomist, friend to Godwin Baxter, and husband to Bella, connects Gray's story to a particularly Scottish tale and its attendant anxieties.

Most meaningfully in this context, Bella, unlike Frankenstein's creature, does get to marry and does not die—except in the normal course of human events. Bella's form of life is particularly interesting. The creature and Bella, echoing a long tradition, become uncanny because both dead and alive—on the cusp of being. As numerous scholars have indicated and popular culture proves, indeed, whether through religious concerns, misunderstandings of decay, or our fear of the abject, the corpse may be considered endowed with mysterious life (Sawday, Park, Zimmerman, Warner, Kristeva; J. H. Robinson, Bondeson). Burke and Hare's description of their victims' confusedly postmortem activity fits the pattern: "[the victims] would convulse and make a rumbling noise in their bellies for some time; after they ceased crying and making resistance, [Burke and Hare] left them to die of themselves; but their bodies would often move afterwards, and for some time they would have long breathings" (*West Port Murders*, 350). The difference in Bella, however, is that bodies animate in their graves (through premature burial), alive at the point of disinterment (in bodysnatching stories), or resurrected through medical intervention (*Frankenstein*), fulfill the conditions of abjection, threatening being—everyone runs away from Frankenstein's creature. By contrast, in Bella death in life betokens beauty and power—hence justice and opportunity.

Bella's bones move, and they also live, in the fullest sense. At first, Bella seems unpromising, lumbering in body and speech in ways reminiscent of Victor Frankenstein's invention.

> The woman stood and faced us, stepping unsteadily forward then pausing as if to keep balance. Her tall, beautiful, full-bodied figure seemed between twenty and thirty years, her facial expression looked far, far less. She gazed with the wide-open eyes and mouth which suggest alarm in an adult but in her suggested pure alert delight with an expectation of more.... She spoke carefully... and each syllable was as sweet and distinct as if piped on a flute: "Hell low God win, hell low new man." Then she flung both arms out straight toward me and kept them there. (Gray *Poor Things*, 29)

But those who meet Bella are instantly attracted (the other side of abjection)—even entranced. Archie remembers: "I grew confused as the offered hand was too high for me to shake in the conventional way. I surprised myself by stepping forward, rising on tiptoe, taking Bell's fingers in mine and kissing them" (29). Whereas the creature automatically repels, through her obtrusive body, death manifesting life and inherently excessive, Bella impels.

Bella speaks, too, in that unlike her predecessors, she is not subject to but rather disturbs the fictions by which we live. Bella is presented as Godwin's niece, but she asks questions that pry loose inconvenient truths. Eventually she devastates Godwin with "Where is my child, God[win]?" (Gray *Poor Things*, 191). Importantly, Godwin, her "creator," attributes his turn to death to such questions: "she asked a frightening question from which my neural network never recovered" (242). At the end of Archie's account, as a result:

> He put the glass down, gripped his gigantic knees with his gigantic fists, threw back his head and laughed. I had not heard him laugh before. The sound started small and swelled up huge, so huge that I flattened my hands over my ears, though the throbs and twangs of his heart-beat swelled loud too until it and the laughter stopped in a sudden sharp snap. Complete silence. He swayed neither forward nor back, but sat perfectly rigid. A moment later I stepped over and, trying hard not to peer into the huge tooth-edged cavity which gaped so horribly at the ceiling, discovered his neck was broken and that *rigor mortis* had instantly ensued. (243–44)

The doctor is dead, turned into a grotesque anatomy by Bella's question that brought him back to the moment of her grafting together as mother/child, life and death.

Bella, then, both impels attraction and accomplishes the ultimate of disruption. In the course of the book, she attracts and upsets not just the medical profession, but the law and the religious and social mores of the land. Exiled beyond the world by her death, Bella enters life as new—fulfilling Laing's call for "rebirthing" (Laing *Facts*, 66–77). Bella is a child in a woman's body. Her child's mind races to meet that body, enacting another Laingian imperative: the inescapability of experience. Laing writes, "*Only* experience is evident. Experience is the *only* evidence" (Laing *Politics*, 18). But the experiences Bella seeks test and often destroy those around her. Bella runs off and around the world with the notorious ladies' man and cad, Duncan Wedderburn the lawyer. After a day with his "Houri, a Mahomet's paradise," Wedderburn begins to tire (Gray *Poor Things*, 82). "I needed the hotel," he remembers: "I had now not slept for twenty-four hours. Bella seemed as fresh as when we left Glasgow" (83). By the next day, Wedderburn has started to babble. Reading over his letter, Baxter says, "I am going to omit several sentences here…for they are hideously over-written, even by Wedderburn's standards. All they tell us is that he and our Bella spent the night as they had spent it on the train, except that shortly before 7 a.m. he begged her to let him sleep" (85). The lawyer Wedderburn ends "in a locked ward of Glasgow Royal Lunatic Asylum" (220).

The state fares no better. When Aubrey de la Pole Blessington arrives to repossess his wife (the Victoria Blessington who was transposed into Bella), as "Thunderbolt" Blessington he cuts quite the figure of a man. He is "as popular with newspaper readers as Sir Garnet Wolseley and 'Chinese' Gordon" (Gray *Poor Things*, 206). But Blessington is well on his way to becoming a physical and also moral cadaver. He has left bits of himself across the killing fields of British imperialism, and as a consequence he is now forced to stand or lie in premature rigor mortis (208, 216). As a representative of state and religion in the institution of marriage, Sir Aubrey is accompanied by Victoria's father, a north country industrialist. The husband is given to clichés like "UNHAND ME WIFE, SIR!" and the father to sentimentalities like "Do not talk about my Vicky like that" (213, 214). Together, they represent the massed hypocrisies of family life, and the deathly state and social compromises that, historians say, produced Burke and Hare as villains of capitalism and Knox as its medical entrepreneur.

Blessington, it turns out, was inadequate for conjugal relations—though he related plenty outside his marriage. Victoria fled her husband and was failed by her father, who "explained that a wife who abandons her husband is a truant in the eyes of man and God" (Gray *Poor Things*, 231). But Bella, now renewed as Victoria, feels empowered: "I know everyone here is telling what they think is the truth," she says, "but it sounds daft. Sir Aubrey talks as if he was liable to tear women apart, but honestly, if he cut up rough with me I think I could break him over my knee like a stick" (218). And the experiences required by Bella have shown her husband in another light: abandoned by (but rather abandoning) Wedderburn, Bella enthusiastically embraced prostitution as productive labor in Paris. One client of the house turns out to have been...the prematurely ejaculating "Sir Aubrey de la Pole Spankybot V.C." (238). Of her father, Bella declares: "You are strong...fierce...cunning...but can never be kind, because you are afraid" (ellipses in text, 214). To her husband, she declares: "Fuck off, you poor daft silly queer rotten old fucker hahahahaha! Fuck off!" Bella/Victoria, fully living because factually dead, is only educated, strengthened, and given devastating speech by the medical, legal, and cultural oppositions embedded in patriarchy.

When Bella returns from exhausting Wedderburn, we see that her lively trajectory goes even against the grave:

> Bella demolished most of a cold boiled ham with bread, cheese, pickles and two or three pints of sweet milky tea.... Her face lost the thin haggard look, her cheeks grew rounder, her brow smoother and softer, the tiny lines and wrinkles faded from her freshening skin. From looking any age between twenty-five and forty she became any age between twenty-five and fifteen. (194)

Against the rigidity and decay of the state and its killing institutions, Bella is vital enough to withstand a bullet in the foot and win the game. She manifests in full

Cixous's idea of the opportunistic other. Because fragmented, she impugns the limitations of systems and societies: through death, she attains the movement that is life. In victimhood, Bella stands victorious.

How wide is Bella's victory? Bella is inherently deconstructive. She brings into question not just the narratives conventionally deployed to express and contain victimhood, but even her own story. This story comes to us in bits, through "Gray's" introduction of a discarded text. Archibald McCandless's *Episodes from the Early Life of a Scottish Public Health Officer* in turn contains documents such as Wedderburn's letter, Blessington's entry in *Who's Who*, and Bella's anguished facsimile scrawl. Gray follows up with "Notes Critical and Historical." The story, like Bella, bears the marks of its making. Consequently, it implicates readers as perpetrators in the violence of suturing this text into some sort of whole. At the same time, the book makes a map of misreading (in Wedderburn and Blessington, for example). Bella is simply too much for the text that seeks to contain her. In fact, Bella deliberately pulls apart the tale we have read. In her letter (placed between text and notes), as Victoria McCandless M.D. she details an ordinary life and brings into question her husband's knowledge, veracity, and intelligence.

Bella Caledonia

This means, of course, that when late twentieth-century Scotland was fighting for the idea of wholeness through an assembly, and fearing the Frankensteinian effects of remaining stitched any old how within the Union, Gray's metaphor seems to be running the wrong way. We can only read a certain irony in Bella's cheerful farewell to Wedderburn as she packs him off home on the train: "GIVE MY LOVE TO BONNY SCOTLAND!" (Gray *Poor Things*, 94). The body at last made visible seems not to operate as Nairn's Lazarus—for good or ill. It is not coherently reborn, not uncritical, not in service of the nation that (by its sins of 1828) animated the suffering body as national metaphor. Yet Bella's body proves unhelpful only to the degree that it refuses to participate in straightforward critique or sentimental reconstruction of the body politic. Alasdair Gray was fully aware of and participated in the Scottish and British politics of this time. He might well have echoed his character Jock MacLeish's cry: "POLITICS WILL NOT LET ME ALONE" (Gray *1982 Janine*, 231–32). Moreover, *Poor Things* locates itself squarely within Scotland's 1970s anxieties as they were visited upon Glasgow. Gray cites the loss of industry and destruction of history that were the late capitalist results of centralized government on the eve of Thatcherism (Gray *Poor Things*, vii). And of course, Gray is well known for his direct intervention in political discourse, the 1997 *Why Scots Should Rule Scotland*, published just before Scotland's successful vote for devolution. In essays running

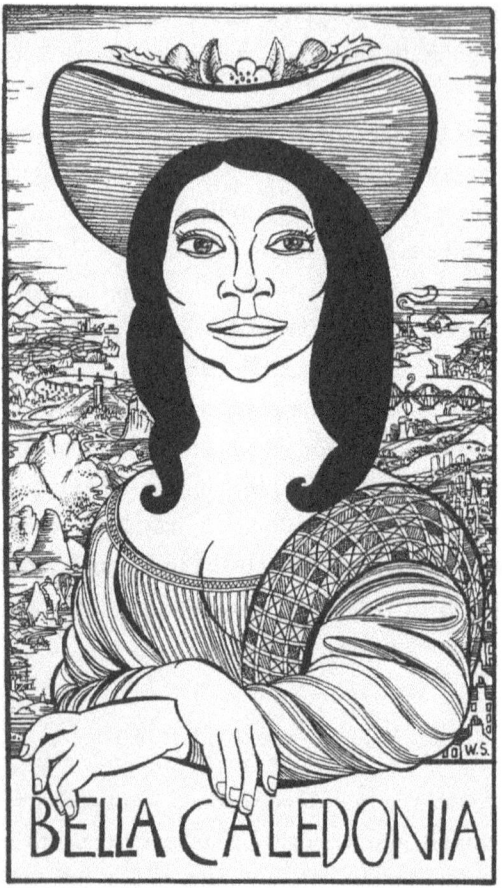

FIGURE 6.5 "Bella Caledonia." From *Poor Things*. Courtesy of Alasdair Gray.

through the period of Gray's concern, Cairns Craig recommended stepping *Out of History*; Bill Forsythe provided recuperative romances like *Gregory's Girl* (1981) and *Local Hero* (1983) to displace anxiety. Alasdair Gray, informed by Nairn and Laing and the fractured metaphorics of an impossible past, strove for more. Perhaps the body of Scotland, so long a fiction sustained by limited tales, should revisit one of its de/formative moments—and there find not comforting meanings, but energizing difference.

This is the wider function of Bella Caledonia: Alasdair Gray lets Lazarus speak and thereby lets Caledonia rise (see figure 6.5). Gray had already tried to address the contemporary fragmentation of Scotland. In *Lanark*, embracing the grotesquery that Frantz Fanon considers the result of the postcolonial condition, Gray depicted a Duncan Thaw who, living much of Alasdair Gray's life, transforms through bodily pain and social failure into a dragon-hide being. Thaw/Lanark suffers under and rejects the mantra "man is the pie that bakes and eats himself" for which the recipe is the deathly "separation" (Gray *Lanark*, 411). But ultimately he must participate in a suspect politics that can be attained only by means of transportation that consumes its passenger's future (466). Through his embrace of "poor things," however, Gray manages to move beyond mere grotesquery and its inevitable degeneracy. Paradoxically, following the lines of Bella's victorious body, the ruptures and scars that mark the other in *Poor Things* transform into opportunity. That opportunity is noted not by its Scottish separateness, but by the way the adjusted metaphor and adventurous processes of a Bella Baxter suture difference to all her readers.

Trauma like that of 1828 is considered to scar a pathway that translates later anxieties into repetitions of the prior experience. This causes more damage to the victim.

Gray turns such pain toward possibility. On the one hand, Gray directs the scarring outward. The damage is not to Bella Caledonia, but to the beholder. Thus, the self-satisfied Wedderburn becomes part of an attack on "Acts of Union," when he is done in by Bella's insistent "wedding" (Gray *Poor Things*, 83, 107). Wedderburn's body and sanity together dissolve into incoherence through metaphor: his letter stutters to a halt through his lack of adequate remaining identity to figure as a signature. He closes:

I am Faithfully and Forever,
Bella's Outcast Welter Weight
Bleeding Waistcoat Hearted
Duncan McNab Wed Wed Wedder
(Writer to the Signet and Auld Jessy's Big Tumshie). (98)

So Gray does offer an effective (and obvious) critique of British master narrative.

But on the other hand, Bella points to the impossibility of any coherence—and not just in the telling of her tale. She is not alone in her patchwork existence. McCandless is illegitimate, a thing literally of shreds and patches—whether of intelligence and insight, or threadbare trousers (Gray *Poor Things*, 9–11). Godwin, who was never small, whose voice does not match his stature, whose size belies his proportions, and who seems a preparation of potions and doses, hints for himself an origin not unlike Bella's, courtesy of his doctor father (19, 20; cover illus. and 25, 19). And of course, Bella's origin as mother and child implies that fragmentation and incoherence—damage—is the condition of the Scots.

Yet here it is worth observing that Bella is a patchwork of all sorts of parts, and that some of those parts are not Scottish. In fact, she is only made in Scotland. Her body is English; her education is expansive; she is the product of world travel (never mind travel through the social classes right down to the brothel); her mind is evaluated by Charcot in Paris; and on and on. Damage, the condition of Scotland, expressed through Bella's body and her fragmented story, thus becomes the condition of all readers.

Is this condition necessarily a bad thing? Does Gray compose through Bella another attack on our master narratives? Or could Bella constitute one more sacrifice of Scottishness to the service of Britishness? Gray, through the many complexities visited on Scotland by the complicities of 1828, achieves something better. Retelling the story of Burke and Hare and the doctors yet again, hugging it to Scottish culture but this time letting its victims speak, Gray rewrites the world along the lines of this Scottish story. Approaching *Poor Things* across Bella's fractured body and Gray's disrupted prose, we uneasy readers stand as Scots in the moment of unimaginable victimhood; we participate in Bella's voicing, her speech from an absence made visible by the pain that was the dissection and regrafting of her body. Thus in Bella's im/politic tale, Scotland's scandal is recast. At the cusp of its own destruction, Scottishness speaks the productive code of us all: difference and disruption. Our life is "an agitation in something essentially dead"—a phrase Nancy might appreciate (Gray *Poor Things*, 17). As such, life is peculiarly "Scottish."

It is, then, appropriate that Alasdair Gray has willed his body to Glasgow University, and Bella Victoria ends as a family doctor (Glass, 247). Bella is neither a Doctor Knox nor the sentimentalized country doctor of Scottish legend. Rather, she specializes in family planning: she prescribes relations *without* generation—a new way of making community from its otherness. Indeed, wielding no knives but suspected of illegal abortions, Bella practices medicine amid a purgative patch of rhubarb (Gray *Poor Things*, 313). Her treatments will bring the inside out, but not as we might expect. The victim, remade as doctor, is in, and all bodies, which can only be impolitic, must be the better under her rigorously cleansing regimen.

7

Resting in Pieces?

PRESENT COMFORTS OR RESTLESS FUTURES
IN IAN RANKIN'S SCOTLAND

IN 2009, CELEBRATING Robert Burns's 250th birthday but coinciding with their own tenth anniversary, the Scottish Parliament launched "Homecoming Scotland." Edinburgh met the challenge by adding to its usual round of tourist frolics a "Winter Festival." Frequenters of the Tattoo and the International Festival may have been surprised, however, by the Illuminated Art Car Parade. This "spectacular cavalcade" applauded "Scotland's history of invention and culture." Ads touted a "Robert Burns Poetry van... a golf car, a whisky truck... a bagpipe truck"—and a "Burke and Hare barrow."[1] One might wonder whether the infamous duo featured for their efforts to convert murder to a fine art, or for their innovations in time and motion. In either case, Burke and Hare seem a strange couple to "come home" to. Yet if they make odd partners for the sentimentalized signs of Scotland's tourist economy, they do belong in this oblique celebration of self-determination. This book has tracked how over time the events of 1828 compromised, challenged, and sometimes energized Scottish identity. Ever since Walter Scott likened the nation under English law to "a subject in a common dissecting-room," dissection and devolution have been conjoined in Scottish sensibility ("Malachi," 1:10–11). They were laid out together for the generations when Scott refused to heal the wound that Doctor Knox (see figure 7.1) had opened in Scottish culture and thus forced later Scots to keep an anxious finger to the pulse of their national pathology (in all senses of that term).

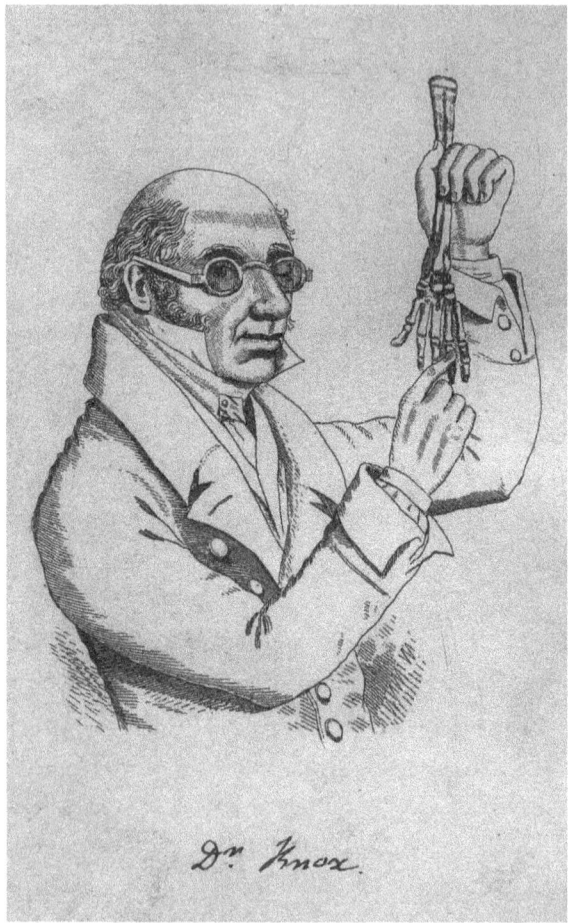

FIGURE 7.1 "Dr. Knox." Courtesy of the Royal College of Physicians of Edinburgh.

Still, by 1999, Scott's medical metaphor appeared to have run its course both as politics and as literature. The body politic, once dissected into its component parts, now looked to be in recovery. When Members of the Scottish Parliament first took their oath on May 12, 1999, Winnie Ewing of the Scottish National Party declared the Parliament "reconvened" (Ritchie, 163). The past was connected to the present, the politic once more whole, the body healthy. So if Scottish culture had had to work through a trauma horribly refigured by Burke and Hare and Doctor Knox, that work might be considered complete. In almost textbook sequence, David Pae rebuilt community around the gap opened by Knox and his silence; Robert Louis Stevenson thrust the Doctor into that gap; James Bridie addressed complicity; and Alasdair Gray let victims speak. Past scandals had been more than recuperated within the national tale—they had been co-opted and inverted, with victims now functioning as agents in the testing and new construction of a culture. That is, the Scotland disrupted by trauma had now worked out its anxieties through literature: this story might be considered at an end.

Nonetheless, the story of Burke and Hare had always been driven by its commercial potential, too. The *Courant* piled up ads: the Weekly Chronicle "will contain a sketch of Burke's life, with the fullest report of his trial" and other delights, necessitating orders "to be given as early as possible" to meet demand; Buchanan's *Trial* is "illustrated by striking likenesses," and doubly worth buying for its "original and curious introductory matter" (*Courant* December 29, 1829). David Pae may have argued a religious case, but his evangelical disposition both met and required the mass audience that he built yet further for the *People's Journal*; it was no accident, too, that Stevenson took his "Body Snatcher" to London in the person of Doctor Jekyll, and thereby made Mr. Hyde pay worldwide. Even as Burke and Hare and Doctor Knox offered Scots a site wherein to critique the irresponsible pursuit of profit (Burke and Hare) and intellect (Doctor Knox), they equally served the dominant narrative of our—and Victorian—times. As popular authors outside Scotland have been only too happy to demonstrate, they may have undermined the traffic in bodies and the market of ideas, but they proved quite the money spinner. Even Northern Ireland, home to Burke and Hare, is at last jumping on the bandwagon and trying to steal back its notorious sons. To serve the media market that is popular history, BBC Scotland and BBC Northern Ireland in 2009 developed "A Necessary Evil."

We might wonder, then, whether the Scottish Executive paraded Burke and Hare as colorful remnant of a story now told, or as commercial supplement to twenty-first-century Scotland's economic ambitions. But these may be the same thing: Michael S. Roth reminds us that to one school of historiography, "history writing... indicates that collective memory is in the process of disappearing" (Roth, 10). Perhaps Burke and Hare can be situated within the dubious historicism of Scotland's tourist culture because they no longer carry the load of meaning they have borne for almost two hundred years. Could it be that the Parliament can now write Burke and Hare into their story of return and economic completeness because they no longer understand the criminal partnership's darker significances?

There is another possibility, however. John Frow focuses not on meaning but on telling. To Frow, "The time of textuality is not the linear, before-and-after, cause-and-effect time embedded in the logic of the archive" (Rossington, 154). The past does not simply lead to the present, whether it is remembered or forgotten. Instead, "[the past's] meaning and its truth are constituted retroactively and repeatedly... alternative stories are always possible" (154). Frow here describes a dynamic in which the past is productive of the present, but always different when viewed from the perspective of the present (as we have seen in chapters so far).

Frow's statement carries further implications: "Forgetting is...an integral principle of this model," for "the orderliness and the teleological drive of narrative" "[involve] at once selection and rejection" (Rossington, 154). Our interpretation's "relation to the past" is, thereby, "not that of truth but of desire." We connect what does not go together. Thus, I suggest, any moment remembered from the past is both linked and disparate—a fragment. That fragment may not only rewrite the past, it can destabilize the very idea of a coherent or completed time and tale. In this way, Burke and Hare cut loose from their evil deeds may appear to serve Scotland's tourism project; they may even look naturalized and domesticated as they steer their barrow around whisky trucks and poetry wagons. Yet in the same instant they may run against all pasts and presents—even those of a self-satisfied Scottish Executive.

This chapter begins with the fact that the Burke and Hare story has been thoroughly worked through according to the stages of trauma, then translated into economics. But we will consider how far these compelling narratives have produced the story, today, as remnant and supplement and thereby, inevitably, as a fragment. In this context, neither an originary moment nor a current discourse should rest easy. Though a "Burke and Hare barrow" may seem a comic leftover from a resolved tragedy or a minor contribution to a global economy, it is at the same time a symptom of the unpredictable, irreducible, and undigestible. So a society eating up its own past in service of a consumer economy may be inviting—even forcing—a gag reflex to follow.

The fragment, in fact, is the major new manifestation of the Burke and Hare story. Bella Baxter may have been made up of bits and pieces in *Poor Things*, but today, the fragment stands in jagged isolation; fragmentary is the mode of its telling; and fragmentation is the source of its agency. Prickly remnants cannot be mixed into the general hodgepodge of culture, or swallowed into its grand narratives. Rather, in post-Parliamentary works by Scotland's authors—from tour guide Robin Mitchell, to postmodernist Christopher Wallace, and Ian Rankin the detective writer extraordinaire—they stick, catch, cause discomfort, invite probing. They evoke in characters and readers alike an "odd, subjective disturbance" that is at once reminiscent of Mr. Hyde and a symptom of individual heartburn and generalized cultural indigestion (*Jekyll and Hyde*, 54).

What follows will consider whether this situation is an accident produced by the decline of master narratives—the postmodern predicament—or whether it also manifests a new strategy of difference allowed to Scottish authors by the ongoing challenge to identity posed through Burke and Hare and Doctor Knox. Specifically, we will consider how, as the new Parliament settles in to its story of homecoming, with the body politic once again made whole, Scotland's authors show a more schizophrenic sensibility. Scottish manifestations of the Burke and Hare story today privilege either tales of control or instances of disruption—in the form of the fragment. Tales of control signal a presumed completeness and complacency in Scottish culture, but tales that erupt unpredictably with mementoes of Burke and Hare may gesture toward a less naïve and optimistic but more edgy and active culture. The Scotland that can embrace the unimaginable—and that insists on doing so even when the culture's unimaginable otherness is reduced to the choking fragment—is one that is oddly replete, because never thoughtlessly and emptily at ease.

FOREIGN BODIES: FROM MOVIES TO MANGA

Culture, of course, is littered with and even made up of fragments. Certainly, bits of Burke and Hare and Doctor Knox have landed far from their Scottish home. In recent years and months, they have come to earth on American TV in Smallville, terrestrial home of Clark Kent ("The Cure"); they have erupted in Hollywood as gory in-joke (*Hannibal* and *Ravenous*) and gothic comedy (*I Sell the Dead*); plotted video games ("The Dr. K——Project," "Mind's Eye," and "Stitch, Cut & Dye"); filtered into manga and anime (*Fullmetal Alchemist*); and perhaps named rock bands (*The Body Snatchers* and the Leeds hip-hop indie band *DR Knox*—complete with vertebra for album cover). They continue to motivate novels outside Scotland such as Matthew Kneale's *English Passengers*, which takes Knox and his racial theories on his own "voyage of the Beagle" (2000), and Sheri Holman's *The Dress Lodger*, which follows Knox's student through later crises of the personal and social body in plague-entrapped Sunderland (2000). They echo in plays like Shelagh Stephenson's North Country drama *An Experiment with an Air Pump* (2000). And they rattle around in trade paperbacks by the handful. For instance, in American Mark Graham's *The Resurrectionist*, set in Philadelphia (1999); Australian James Bradley's *The Resurrectionist*, which extends the story down under (2006); army brat James McGee's *Resurrectionist*, which develops the concept as a case for his retired military/proto-detective hero (2007); and (giving us momentary titular relief) American Hal McDonald's *The Anatomists*, which aims for authenticity in resurrection-era London (sponsored by TruTV, 2008). But in every case, their work as fragment serves the purpose of completeness, not disjunction and critique.

Smallville, in the episode "The Cure" (2007), shows the pattern. Doctor Knox (who dates all the way back to the Mongol horde) has been operating on those contaminated by kryptonite to make them "forget"—an interesting intervention in our discourse of history and memory. But ultimately, their memory loss is complete, because fatal. Knox follows up initial treatment with murder (linking to Frankensteinian plots as he seeks to make his lady love immortal through transplant surgery). Knox is the caricature of old when he declares "Mankind's greatest advances would never have seen the light of day had the genius minds behind them been scrutinized under a microscope." And Knox's acts are so egregious that even his employer—even Lex Luthor—decides (rather bathetically) that "your practices deeply concern me." However this is *Smallville*, and Superman saves the day—as he must, and as he always does. In other words, fragments of the Burke and Hare story inflect a plot itself made up of bits and pieces from Shelley to Superman, but all serve the same tale of recuperation that is typically demanded by American television.

I Sell the Dead (2008), touted as gothic comedy, is more predictable again. On the eve of execution, Blake the bodysnatcher confesses to Father Duffy. In bumbling partnership with Willie Grimes, and in service of "the demented Dr. Vernon Quint...a twisted old coot who uses fresh corpses for his clandestine medical research," he has disturbed corpses that have proved only too eager to fight back—hence the tagline, "Never Trust a Corpse."[2] The Philadelphia Film Festival website whips up business thus: "Vampires, ghouls and vicious rivalries are just part of the fantastical adventures in this devilishly mischievous horror film that slayed audiences at Slamdance '09 and the Toronto After Dark Film Festival."[3] The writer anticipates that, topped off with "an appearance by horror icon Angus Scrimm...*I Sell the Dead* will achieve a rabid cult following." The film matches its hype, notably ending with the recursion of its plot. Having "resurrected" the undead, our duo continue to circulate in Pythonesque terms as "Not Dead Yet": Blake is broken from prison by partner Willie, now a zombie himself. Although aligned with the rotten fragments of zombiedom, Burke and Hare serve, again, to support a narrative with its own conventions and cohesiveness—this time they feed the tongue-in-cheek plots of comic horror.

The Dress Lodger, American author Sheri Holman's tightly woven story of prostitution, medicine, courage, and inadequacy also refracts Knoxian plots. In 1831, Gustine the prostitute (she who rents the dress), courts Dr. Knox's erstwhile assistant, Henry Chiver. She needs his help for her child, born with its heart beating outside its chest. But Dr. Chiver, though traumatized by his Edinburgh experiences, still can take only an anatomical interest. In a city under threat of plague, contamination runs along the lines of perplexed human interaction. Here, the dissolution of Chiver's identity initiated by Burke and Hare turns out to foreshadow—but perhaps not to cause—the damage he inevitably deals to the child, to Gustine, to his wife. In this inventive and challenging novel, the remains of Burke and Hare again serve a plot not their own.

Video games demonstrate what is at stake. On the one hand, they show the sheer reach of the tale—who would have thought that Burke and Hare and Doctor Knox could resonate into gaming? Clearly, the story is pervasive. But to what effect, or at what cost? We might at first assume our tale, with its historical determinations, must clash with the imperatives of this unpredictable genre. Video game maven Chris Crawford sees "The Dr. K——Project" (designed pre-1999) as offering a "bizarre approach to the whole problem of interactive storytelling."[4] Inventor Brandon Rickman forgoes narrative sequencing in favor of serendipity and contingency, claiming: "any fragment of the story can be selected" to a "lurching and discontinuous" effect.[5] Crawford describes a typical moment in the game:

> A place. A tea chest. A body bag. A scrap of paper. An assassin. A character. Something happens.
> [User selects "A character".]
> A place. A tea chest. A body bag. Some scenery. An assassin. A rascal. Something happens. (Chris Crawford, 320)

Crawford applauds Rickman's antinarrative innovation, with its "unfolding vignette" effect—"If you're wondering where the story is, well, there isn't any" (320). Yet as mere remnants, Burke and Hare are perfectly suited to the fragmentation thematized in this game. That is the problem: here, Burke and Hare fit, rather than disturb, the purposes and practices of the game.

Still, "Dr. K——" was developed as an experiment in narrative for an M.F.A. Perhaps a more conventional game shows and suffers from the disruptiveness of Burke and Hare. "Mind's Eye" (c. 2005), which its creator Shane Stevens admits he cannily developed for Halloween release, turns out much the same.[6] It includes "Dr Knox, Burke and Hare... actual people in England's [*sic*] shadowy past," and a reviewer for the Girl Scouts easily draws (closer) connections in plot and theme between game and history:

> the infamous duo... procured fresh corpses—often killed by Burke and Hare themselves—for Dr. Knox, an eminent professor... of anatomical study at the University of Edinburgh, who some argue to this day was aware of the murders and ignored them for his personal benefit. [Stevens's] Dr. Knox [similarly] ignores [a character's brutality].[7]

On the one hand, Stevens says: "I wanted to implement Delirium Mode," but equally, "I just thought it would be fun to create a game where the protagonist is unreliable and the player has to figure out for themselves what is real." What might disrupt instead seamlessly meshes with the postmodern dynamic of electronic gaming.

And "Stitch, Cut & Dye," developed at Newark School of the Arts as a nonviolent video game (c. 2007), likewise turns Burke and Hare to its own mixed purposes. This concept piece links global trafficking of bodies and a plastination factory in China to the war in Iraq. The player, as journalist, assembles evidence that constructs a graphic novel. In level one, that data includes "Burke & Hare, two young and disillusioned soldiers out to profit from a war that's dragging on too long"; in level two, players meet "Dr. Von Knox" (a naming that folds in Gunther von Hagens of *Bodyworlds* fame), "an infamous scientist and inventor, known for his highly specular public dissection. He invented plastination, and his work is shown all around the world."[8] This game intends to pose moral challenges and thereby to produce thoughtful responses, yet here too a player is encouraged to dart off in any direction. No matter how fragmentary the appearance of Burke and Hare and Doctor Knox, and however strangely and randomly the three seem aligned with historically disparate characters and events, again they serve an experience paradoxically motivated through its own mobility. These outcasts add only a hint at history, lend only a flicker of authenticity to a deliberately unpredictable genre.

Our trio do not even have to be recognized or published in English to provide this gloss of local color. If in video games they constitute no disruption, provide the site for no subjective disturbance, today they similarly serve convention even in Japanese manga. The comic/anime *Fullmetal Alchemist* features a recognizable Knox—a pathologist who "kills people [as test subjects] instead of saving them."[9] This Knox, with his hidden past, merits much discussion in the online community, but he also gets a fan page and instantiates no critique.

Dorian Wiszniewski and Richard Coyne ponder the dynamics of masking in video games, and outline the effects and opportunities for a developing identity, whether ironic and productive, or solipsistic and limiting. Ultimately, they conclude, possibility lies in "practice," through which they hope for "a more playful critique that reveals the prejudicial ground, background, and foreground."[10] Such a critique depends on "many games, serious and flippant, and... various apparatuses of conversation." In other words, the more games and the more versions of a character the better, for the more critical and productive the discourse. Perhaps gamers have not yet masqueraded enough as Burke and Hare and Doctor Knox for our notorious characters to accomplish the disruption they promise. At the moment, they only participate in and express the randomness of modern "communication," meaning anything to anybody.

A further opportunity to make a difference looms: *I Sell the Dead* encloses a comic book with its DVD which concludes: "Guard the Wakes! Watch the Cemeteries!! Look after your Dearly Departed! Keep your Eyes Peeled for... *The Further Adventures of Grimes and Blake*." Can the online multiverse be far behind? Surely the gaming community will find some morsel of Scotland's unsavory past that even they cannot swallow, and that will make them ponder the story they so easily consume. But until that moment, perhaps Scotland, where the range of Burkes and Hares burgeons day to day for audiences as diverse as early readers and Festival goers, allows these fragments more play to accomplish generative possibility—to critique and to change.

BODIES OF EVIDENCE: FRAGMENTS OF SCOTTISHNESS

In Scotland, the discourse of Burke and Hare and Doctor Knox oddly seems fallen into fragments at the moment when the story of the nation culminates in the new Parliament. The tale of Scotland's "return" is fulfilled: there is no lost ideal to mourn, and no story of future national completion for which to prepare the way. Is there any remaining anxiety to express through Burke and Hare and their tale of death and dissection? Lacking such motivation, the story of 1828 seems to lose momentum and meaning. Essential elements collapse into discrete units serving an audience that can now relax into the enjoyment of fragmentation: with no urgent tale to resolve or create, perhaps Scots can allow themselves to be randomly entertained—just like the international audience that meets across television shows and interactive gaming. As stories for children, plays at the Edinburgh Festival, and detective novels by Ian Rankin (all of which suddenly surged toward Burke and Hare in the moment of the Scottish Parliament), these remains of 1828 overtly serve the niche markets of a society now driven only by commerce. Furthermore, in the era of the Scottish Parliament the market, ironically, is global. So we might expect our story to meet the same, supplementary purposes as it does elsewhere.

We should remember, however, that especially where the history in question is our own, rather than some abstract source of plot elements, any instance of a tale can support but equally call into question the possibility of consolidating or fixing that tale. Roth points out that Richard Rorty finds history both "something that can be used to construct forms of solidarity" and "a disruptive force...a reservoir of stories that can underscore contingency, multiplicity, and possibility" (Roth, 5). Any utterance of history is by necessity fragmentary and disruptive even as it derives from a past or articulates a present.

Bodies Politic: Bedtime Detective Stories for Children Strange and Scottish

At first glance, children's stories stand at odds with the possibility that a fragmented tale might disturb the master narratives of modernity. "Horrible histories" abound in Britain, but they take as their context the predictabilities of their young readers' current circumstances. The children who make up the audience for Terry Deary and Martin Brown's *Measly Middle Ages* or *Awesome Egyptians* (*Horrible Histories*,

Scholastic UK) do not gnaw turnips beneath a castle wall; they will not be sacrificed to accompany the pharaoh beyond the grave; they benefit from today's medicine. So at most, the strange prevalence of children's versions of Burke and Hare (including one by *Horrible Histories*) may indicate only the fragmentation of the market into adult, adolescent, and "early readers," and set the past against a comfortable, book-buying, middle-class present.

Moreover, whether by Scots or strangers, these children's stories all are narratives of control. Their young protagonists turn detective, and in plots hailing back to Enid Blyton or (in America) Nancy Drew, they persistently save the day. But there is a difference between stories written inside and beyond Scotland. English writer Mary Hooper makes all-embracing gestures in the direction of sentimentalized Scottish history. *Bodies for Sale* presents a hero, the red-haired Jack, who encounters villainous bodysnatchers, the grotesque Doctor Knox, and is accompanied by a Greyfriars Bobby substitute by the name (truly) of "Braveheart" (Hooper, 6, 16). Nothing too unusual here. Committed to the service of medicine (Jack scatters sawdust in the operating theater and collects leeches), our hero pursues and, with Braveheart's help, nabs the bodysnatchers. There is not a murderer in sight, but there is "a large reward"—something that was unavailable to the honest, impoverished Grays in 1829 (57). Their fund produced little, and when James Gray died soon after, Ann had to beg support (letter in Sharpe, ECL). So young Jack enjoys all the triumphs of narrative closure, even as the story of Burke and Hare is fragmented into unfamiliarity.

Hooper's 1999 book, aimed at Key Stage Two readers (ages 7–11), seems positively complex beside John Townsend's *Burke and Hare: The Body Snatchers* (2001), written for an English publisher as part of the New Spirals series for "reluctant readers" of 7–8. Townsend offers six books under this imprint, with titles that show no particular pattern other than mild horror: *Back on the Prowl, Beware the Morris Minor, Night Beast, A Minute to Kill,* and *Snow Beast*. His *Burke and Hare* is advertised as nonfiction and rehearses many of the events of 1828. Again, however, we are in the presence of "grave robbers," and no one is ever "murdered" or even "killed"—this is hardly a complete account (Townsend, 8). Rather, "The pillow came down" on Daft Jamie, and a little boy "struggled for a minute. Then his body fell to the floor" (20, 19). Interestingly, here, we lack a detecting protagonist—in such accidental circumstances, what is there, really, to detect? Yet what we lose in character, we gain through a remarkably declarative style. No doubt this is part of the publisher's strategy for early readers, but as with Hooper's detecting hero, the effect is to simplify and to solidify. When an author summarizes: "Two grave robbers saw a way to make quick money. They have gone down in history as two of the most evil men in Scotland. What they did shook the world," the style advertises that however horrid, these two will get their just deserts (8). It is small surprise, then, to learn that "Crime didn't pay" (30).

Nor is it strange to find the story of Burke and Hare, however fragmented, taking a turn toward the children's market outside Scotland. Moreover, it does well here—well enough that Townsend has also emulated the *Horrible History* genre with *A Painful History of Medicine: Scalpels, Stitches and Scars* (2006). Most recently, it shows up in its own *Horrible History* as (anachronistically) *The Vile Victorians*, and also in Terry Deary's *Horrible History* tour of Edinburgh for children. For non-Scots, this has always been a story contained by distance and tellable for distant purposes. Not to mention that today's children's market is ready for gore.

In Scotland, we would expect this urge to retell the stories of 1828 for children to spring from a different but converging phenomenon—the feeling that the events of the past have run their course. They have been contained and so can be shown to be contained within the discourse of successful detection, and the language of children. Certainly, in Scottish representations of the past, even child victims have spoken—and not just as the mother/daughter Bella Baxter. In 1991 Owen Dudley Edwards remembered an unusually thoughtful production from Hazelhead Academy, Aberdeen, with its:

> pre-teen schoolboy actor, playing the part of Daft Jamie.... [He] alone had realised the truth... but [was] unable to convince anyone in the cast until his message got through to Burke. Jamie stammers out a Burke and Hare rhyme, Burke replies savagely with 'Wee Willie Winkie.' (Edwards *City*, 238)

A story of detection but not of control (for Jamie ends up dead) shows that as presented through Scottish children, too, the trauma had played out—from naming the guilty to voicing the dead. Apparently "complete," the story should now be a fragment of its former self, but not one that can disturb. It stands available for market manipulation.

Of course, where Hooper and Townsend build reading skills as you might build bones in a sort of "Got Milk?"/"Got History?" mode, recent Scottish stories should be better informed (and the *Vile Victorians* version is, disappointingly, uninformed). This is the case in Karen Doherty's *Murderers!* (2004). Doherty clearly aims at the market for "horrid" and historical children's books, for *Murderers!* is one in a series with *Threat! A Story of Mary Slessor* (the missionary) and *Cannibals! A Story of Sawney Bean* (by Helen Walsh). Doherty also negotiates toward the control desired by young readers, but she hides no information. Young Calum keeps encountering Burke and Hare, and is a friend to Daft Jamie. Calum thinks Burke and Hare are bodysnatchers or thieves; however, his suspicions expand when his friend disappears, and Janet Brown searches vainly for Mary Paterson. Inevitably, Calum takes to detecting, and it is he who implicates Burke and Hare in murder. Thus far, this is a more accurate retelling, though still one defined within the parameters of children's literature.

But here the similarities stop between outsider and Scottish versions of the tale. Calum's Edinburgh is full of threat: the child is starving; every other turn brings him cheek by jowl with Burke and Hare; Daft Jamie is his friend and support, and must be lost; and the police will pay Calum no mind. No wonder that even with Burke about to swing:

> Surrounded by a huge angry mob Calum felt as if he was underwater. None of this felt real to him. He wasn't sure about anything any more. Why did Hare go unpunished? What about doctor Knox? Why Jamie?... Calum felt nothing but sadness and a longing for an end to his nightmares. (Doherty, 52)

Evidently, Doherty has purposes for her tale that run beyond mere entertainment of young readers. Indeed, she writes for Gallus Publications, who advertise under a banner touting "Citizenship and Values-based Education" with the motto: "If you want something done, do it yourself."[11] And this Scottish writer brings her audience into unsettling proximity with the past.

Still, genre and audience seem to prevail: Calum ends in a warm bed, under the care of a motherly woman, and after the author has comfortably run forward the history of William and Margaret Hare: Hare "died penniless. His wife...died a miserable death" (Doherty, 53). Yet even as the story wraps up with full, and childlike justice, this fictive fragment for an impressionable audience points away from narrative completeness and personal safety. Calum "was warm, well fed, and safe. Maybe now that it was all over he might sleep properly again." "'Nighty night, Jamie' he whisper[s]. 'Sleep well'" (53). The author attempts closure, but the ending allowed by childhood drags Calum's sympathetic reader at once into the land of nod and the nightmare of irony. Those who remember the text and appreciate a metaphor will find it hard to "Sleep well."

Written from Scotland, a thoughtfully questioned and carefully controlled story for children finds itself disrupted by what it would contain. Nicola Morgan's *Fleshmarket* (2003) struggles with the same tensions between audience need and the implications of her telling. The resolved trauma that was Burke and Hare allows their story to be recast for the younger audience. But writing for young adults, this onetime Chair for the Society of Authors in Scotland is not afraid to reactivate the anxieties of 1828. Morgan's fourteen-year-old hero, Robbie, runs through all the stages of Scotland's trauma. Morgan points back to the grand certainties of George IV's visit to Scotland: "August 1822. [Robbie] would never forget it. The city swarming with excitement" (Morgan, 29). This is the moment of Robbie's happiness: his mother, father, and sister all healthy and well, the family about to graduate into the middle class. But then his mother dies; his father drinks and disappears. Robbie's life turns around that moment in 1822 when, returning from the festivities, his mother "brushed against the doorway.... She winced, stopped, breathed hard" (41). She has breast cancer. Robbie, waiting outside during her operation at the hands of Doctor Knox, hears her scream, then watches her die of septicemia. His life thereafter becomes one of hating and dogging the doctor—like that of Scots from Sir Walter to Robert Louis Stevenson. Knox, to Robbie, is evil: "Yellow gas-light fell on Knox's face as he turned. He looked like a corpse himself. Robbie's hatred was something hard and physical inside him. It seemed to grow, feeding off itself. He let it grow, needing it to create a meaning for what he was doing" (141). But to pursue the doctor, Robbie aligns himself with Burke and Hare. He stands in the shadows watching because he has served as their lookout. He and James Bridie's guilty community stand not far apart. Worse, he takes to drink, and falls into cadaver-like victimhood: "[The rat's] eyes tiny circular beads.... yellow teeth bared.... [It] landed on Robbie's chest.... [H]e stumbled, fell backwards.... [S]omething slice[d] into his hand" (163). However, this is a recuperative text, still aiming at the cohesiveness required in children's fiction: Robbie realizes that Burke and Hare's merchandise is not found, but made, separates himself from their business, and though he is their victim, stitched up like Bella Baxter, ultimately, he proves instrumental in their demise (194–95, 227–28). Robbie chooses to end the story of Burke and Hare and Doctor Knox. He thus enacts trauma but also resolves it as he passes through the set pieces of our well-established narrative.

This boy has suffered the horrors of medicine; been implicated in their production; spoken out, though a victim; brought them to an end, and even forced an apology from Doctor Knox (Morgan, 257). Morgan has hauled her audience through the stages of trauma but also supported them through the age-appropriate satisfactions of detection and resolution. Yet Morgan, too, inadvertently enacts the uncontrollability for Scots of even the remnants of Burke and Hare and Doctor Knox. She takes the story one iteration further, that proves to be a step too far. Robbie abandoned the bodysnatching business before he fully realized what was going on. Thereby, he appeared to fulfill the insistent theme of the book and did so proactively: "In some things we have no choice. In others we do. It is telling the difference that matters. You cannot choose what happens to you. But you can choose how to live. You can choose who to be" (257). In particular, Robbie chooses not to hate Doctor Knox. More, he moves on knowing that "It was hatred of this man which had almost destroyed him before.... He must move forward and wipe the man away" (210). But it is precisely on these grounds (and at the same time) that Robbie again connects with the doctor. Paradoxically, separating Robbie from his hatred—or characterizing it as adolescent overreaction—and tying him to the doctor, Knox saves Robbie not once but twice. In the process, he explains to Robbie that he, too, has had to make choices for the greater good (208–10, 256–57). So Robbie's choice is to end as an elderly surgeon, educated by James Young Simpson in anesthetics, and regretting the demise of "Someone I knew, a long time ago.... [Knox] became a good friend" (262).

That is, to conclude her tale Morgan plays her story forward through medical history. And this is a thoroughly concluded tale, complete with words (about choice) from a dead mother echoed by Knox and ratified in Robbie's memory (Morgan, 253, 256, 257). We even hear heavenly music from the dead doctor: "As Robbie sliced smoothly into the soft flesh, calmly, carefully, holding the razor-thin blade firmly, strongly, he heard it: floating somewhere above the woman's faraway dreaming, rising and falling, like the last song a swan might sing, the distant arpeggio sound of a violin" (262–63). Robbie, in the end, should not forget because his is a story of unexpected coherence. But neither can we forget, nor avoid the attendant incoherence precipitated by a Knoxian tale. Morgan's overinsistence on providing an uplifting end puts her carefully crafted story with its conflicting conclusions under pressure from its own sophistication. This story cannot be told once and for all precisely because it is now interwoven with others. Placed on a continuum, the story of Burke and Hare may lead to pain-free surgery, but Simpson's anesthesia and Robbie's translation into doctor are consequently both ends to and unstable fragments of a much more troubling story. This "choice" of an ending can lead equally to heroic medicine or to murder.

Bodies at Play: The Edinburgh Festival

If Scottish authors have trouble containing the supposedly concluded and decayed story of Burke and Hare even within the reductive parameters of children's literature, the Edinburgh Festival presents an oddly different experience for strangers and Scots alike. A double compulsion motivates the plays that litter Edinburgh every summer: a Scottish story... should sell well. The many and different writers for the Festival meet this international yet local discourse with no difficulty, for now that its threat has been evacuated, our story is easily repackaged for Edinburgh's apotheosis of the tourist economy.

At the same time, place seems more compelling than mere pennies in these plays' construction. Again and again, outsiders speak of visiting a museum, taking a tour, or simply finding themselves in Edinburgh. Robert Stocks remembers:

> I had just left drama school and didn't have much work, so I happened to also be looking for a subject to write a play about.... [We] ended up spending our

first night in this great city of culture on a ghost tour. And for the next hour and a half we became the ultimate tourists.... One of the last stories we heard was of Burke and Hare.... The drama of [their] journey was fascinating to me. I then started to research the subject more.[12]

Jonny Berliner's stage biography recounts: "In the years 2001–2002, the Jonny Berliner Band racked up more than 300 gigs and the band did a season of shows at the Edinburgh Festival."[13] Soon Stocks and Berliner each were back with a play. Overwhelmed by the experience, these authors inevitably (as they tell it) turn to Burke and Hare.

We might question whether this is the savvy discourse of a theater informed by public relations, or whether we see in operation the surplus Frow implies when he talks of the past producing the present—even if it was not our own. Stocks suggests it is a bit of both: "There was an element of strategy for bringing this story to the Edinburgh festival, but...the festival was chosen because it was appropriate for the subject matter rather than the subject matter being chosen for the festival."[14] Edinburgh produced the play, and the play required Edinburgh. Stocks's experience aligns interestingly with that of insider Ben Harrison. Educated at the University of Edinburgh, Harrison now co-directs the Edinburgh-based company Grid Iron and collaborates with the new National Theatre of Scotland. He tracks his investment in site-specific work to an Edinburgh and Knoxian production early in his directing career (Edwards's *Hare and Burke*):

> At the close of the first act...[the cast ushered] the audience...into Greyfriar's Kirkyard....[D]uring the speech of the prostitute Mary Patterson [*sic*] [Edwards's "5th Ghost"]...the castle behind her turned red, drenched in floodlights. The audience gasped. In fact, the organisers of the Edinburgh Tattoo were simply testing the lights, but what stage set could have conveyed the epic nature of this coincidence, as the character seemed to conjure the entire city of Edinburgh to act in her defence?[15]

Building from such claims, I suggest that Edinburgh and the Festival together constitute a major site of containment for foreign and native authors alike: at the notoriously unpredictable Fringe, everyone has a Scottish play, and that play is Burke and Hare. Moreover, no matter how different they may or should be (for, also according to Frow, every present moment changes the past), in important ways they all look alike.

Hugh MacDiarmid would have been surprised. Upon the Festival's inception, he railed against James Bridie and those who invented it for importing a foreign Culture.

Scotland through the Edinburgh International Festival has gained the whole world with the usual effect on its own soul. I have always been opposed to the notion that cultural advance can be secured by giving any body of people all the culture of the world on tap—and none of their own....

This false eclecticism is perhaps the outstanding fault of the Edinburgh Festival....

When this sort of fashionable cosmopolitanism is prostituted by commercialism... [excluding] the mass of the people... the thing becomes simply a disgusting ramp [*sic*]. (*Raucle*, 3:151–53)

Today's Festival seems suitably eclectic—full of local and foreign color. Furthermore, much of the local color hails from elsewhere. The Scots would appear to be giving their own culture at last and to have made it into a currency of some value. But the arbiter of Scottishness might be equally dismayed to find that now, everyone at the Festival is an Edinbourgeois. And in these many renditions of Burke and Hare, Scottish difference, whether purveyed by Scots or strangers, turns out the same.

This is not to say that, individually, these recent plays lack innovation or quality. For instance, Robert Stocks and Tommy Luther stand out for *The Butcher and the Thief* (2005). Researched and workshopped over a year, this piece challenges many boundaries of theater and story. The performance opens with Burke considering paring an apple (knowledge?) but carving out his own stomach instead—littering the stage with entrails. It tells its story through only two actors (the creators) and the inventive use of puppets. Puppetry can easily descend into cuteness and gimmickry. Here, however, as actors and puppets fluidly shift roles, making the plot run through victims and villains alike, Stocks and Luther enact a disturbing idea of community and imply a critique. None of this could be expected or taken for granted. The issue, then, is not whether such plays are the same—they cannot be. Rather, our concern is how they merge together in the discourse of the Edinburgh Festival.

A character in *One Good Turn*, by Edinburgh immigrant Kate Atkinson (2006), generalizes about "middle-class wankers discussing some pretentious piece of fringe theater" (Atkinson, 3). The implication is that the Fringe to the Festival, supposedly celebrating the randomness of creativity that just piles up in Edinburgh every August beyond the headline events, is itself pretentious. For us the fascinating subtext is that criticism, supposedly aiming to distinguish quality among innovation, sees everything as the same. Of course, productions of Burke and Hare must share basic details: Edinburgh; 1828; Burke and Hare. But more notably, critics observe and also draw patterns in these plays—such as comedy. Terry Newman's 2003 *Burke and Hare* (Skullduggery Theatre Company) "turned the story of Scotland's two infamous bodysnatchers into a comedy"—indeed, "If the state were more enlightened we would be provided with uniforms, says Hare, and a hat replies Burke, women like men in hats."[16] In 2008, Brian G. Cooper, writing for the *Edinburgh Stage*, sees the Bridewell Theatre Company's *Greyfriars Twisted Tales* as "a hilarious musical expedition.... the grisly crimes of Burke and Hare reenacted with gruesome gusto."[17] Critics observe and affirm patterns of sympathy, too: the local *Blood on the Stones* (by Peter Robinson for Carpe Diem) presents Burke as "a simple labouring man, whose only crime (other than the murders) is trying to earn an honest day's wage"; in Skullduggery's production, "About midway through the play, the tone changes. Burke suddenly finds he has a conscience."[18]

Even when disagreeing with a production decision, critic Stuart Simpson treats plays by the handful (see notes 16 and 18 above). For instance, Simpson finds these shifts in motivation unconvincing: in his reviews, Skullduggery does well with the themes of justice and morality, but they "don't sit well with the slapstick sitcom style humour of the first half"; Carpe Diem is better able to "carry off this strange feat." Simpson does notice the oddity of similarity between the two plays: "is it now controversial to hold that Burke was a selfish murdering shit?" But as he queries, he coalesces. Furthermore, all plays are alike in one important degree: even where a critic actually critiques, the discourse is not disturbed by the question motivating MacDiarmid. Though Scottish plays jostle with those from elsewhere, none evoke what we might expect: a discussion of authenticity or ownership. Rather, Stocks's and Luther's puppets (from England), Robinson's musical from Fife, and George Young's production with Lochaber High School (2009) merge together. For each production, criticism turns to one note: to Simpson, Skullduggery may be a bit confused, but the play is "enjoyable"; *Blood on the Stones* crucially ends with the audience-pleasing number "Hang him High!"; to Rory Ford in the *Scotsman*, *Greyfriars Twisted Tales* are "great fun"; Lochaber's musical is "entertaining in a somewhat dark way."[19] Although these productions individually break conceptual or theatrical boundaries, they look oddly familiar in the critic's eye. This is Festival discourse, where even Stocks and Luther, with their "ghoulish, gory spectacle," and the "sack dummies whose limbs are hinged in such a way as to make them horribly life-like," translate for Zoe Green into "an excellent evening's entertainment" (*Scotsman* August 23, 2005). Johanna Payton sees here "a worthy theatrical experience and a visual treat."[20] Burke and Hare, paradoxically, at the Edinburgh Fringe provide "a good night out!"

What is happening here to the now fragmented tale of Burke and Hare and Doctor Knox? In some respects, the Edinburgh Fringe, operating in a global economy, invites further fragmentation. In the search for novelty, every play asserts something new and different, whether puppetry, the recuperation of villainy, or comedy. But that is the determining factor: because the Fringe requires innovation from its productions and thereby exacerbates fragmentation in its tales, fragmentation becomes thematic and manifests a strange, unifying coherence whose keynote is "entertainment."

Bodies out of Time: Doctor Who and Doctor von Hagens Critique the Festival

We might see Burke and Hare in today's Edinburgh as epitomizing the Festival dynamic. A completed tale, cracking apart, can serve the cause of novelty for the assembled local and foreign audience of a global economy. But this is where things get interesting: by displaying the overinsistences of the Festival through its multiplicity and sameness, the story of Burke and Hare points to the oddly recursive nature of the Festival itself. It thereby opens a space for critique of both the Edinburgh jollifications and its own current retelling.

Tim Luckhurst, writing from within the Edinburgh Festival but with a Glasgow eye, notes a temporal disturbance that maintains the Festival as a moment out of time:

> We are at that point in the calendar when Edinburgh is spoken of in Islington and eulogised on Radio 4. Like the mythical city in the fairy tale, this Edinburgh is impermanent. It exists for one month per year.
>
> The Edinburgh of festival time has little in common with the "city of extraordinary and sordid contrasts" described 70 years ago in Edwin Muir's *Scottish Journey*....
>
> My plea is simple. Do not confuse those feelings with the reality of contemporary Scotland.[21]

In this moment of time, everything is different and special; therefore, everything looks unthreateningly the same. This is a moment in time, but time out of memory.

Yet every story initiates an alternative, and such is the case here. The Festival's overemphasis on cohesion through the fragments of Burke and Hare brings Edinburgh's major cultural and commercial event itself into contention for its delimiting effect on memory in time. Writing of Holocaust memorials, James E. Young suggests that we cannot have the monumental experience without the crack (Young, ch. 12). The coherence of institutional memorialization may actually produce cracks in a wilfully unified expression. In such a fashion, the overdetermining edifice that is Festival and Fringe—a space out of time and with limited perception—has fractured out a new type of Knoxian tale.

Perhaps least to be expected, in 2004, *Doctor Who* came to Edinburgh. The BBC's iconic time traveler arrived by TARDIS (the time machine that looks like a police box) and by audiobook. In *Medicinal Purposes*, scripted by Robert Ross, Colin Baker's Doctor and assistant Evelyn find themselves in 1828. The Doctor, incorrigible scientist, hopes to meet Burke—to congratulate him for his contributions to medicine. For a Time Lord, in fact, this Doctor seems to be suddenly and unpleasantly predictable. Small wonder that Knox will claim to be "Jekyll to [Doctor Who's] Hyde." Evelyn, a historian, immediately starts to challenge the conventions of the series, never mind these newly visible clichés of Doctor Who's intellect. She steps into Edinburgh pondering: "I never quite understand. If the scanner sets your suspicious radar off, why oh why do we always get out of the Tardis and have a look anyway?" And she mocks: "When in a cliff-hanging situation, always go for the cliché, that's my motto." It is the link between "always" and "cliché" that ties together Doctor and Knox, past time and this time. We learn that "Knox," too, has a Tardis. He has caught the Edinburgh of 1828 in a time loop: Burke and Hare are constantly murdering, and Mary Paterson endlessly dying. This story cannot proceed in its appropriate sequence—as the random yet essential events of history—because confined within a temporal pinfold. In this respect, it is not unlike the same story retold to the point of cliché within the Edinburgh Fringe.

But the story as retold again and again produces those who will undo it: "The Doctor," who staggers through time every which way, and Daft Jamie, who cannot rise to the coherent memories allowed by normal forgetfulness. In a society capable of memory and subject to lapse, thus blithely able to tie together loose ends even when the plot is weirdly repeated—like Edinburgh in Festival time—Jamie does not belong. Impressively played by David Tennant (who later acted Doctor Who on TV), Jamie hints toward inconsistencies, fissures, and odd connections. When events recur or sequences get interrupted, he cannot control this excess. His mind cannot tie them unproblematically together because it lacks the drive toward narrative that is part of comfortable forgetfulness and the delusion of cohesiveness. Received by Jamie's fragmentary and unruly mind as scraps and repetitions, events fall outside their sequence and point to strangeness. As a result, Jamie senses that Burke "comes and goes," and Doctor Who, from this apparently random perception, can map the recurrence of a moment in time. Then Jamie, dying at last at his appointed hour, performs the essential work of reorienting history and memory within their natural patterns—both unpredictable and incoherent. So stories again progress as times change.

What requires such reorientation? "Doctor Knox" participates in a double plot: on the one hand, he breeds antibodies for aliens from the doomed victims of Burke and Hare—and can breed more by recycling these unfortunates time and again; on the other hand, these repetitions with their enforced coherence supply the voyeurism of an entertainment economy spun out across the galaxy—they offer the future and universal equivalent of reality TV. Through the events of 1828, this Knox expresses the parasitism of commerce everywhere and everywhen. Evidently, the recursive oddities of Festival Edinburgh can provoke a critical response across the time-space continuum, reaching even Doctor Who!

Jonny Berliner and Fintan O'Higgins bring a different doctor to the Fringe in *Corpus* (2003). Their musical never directly references Doctor Knox or Burke and Hare, but its resonances between medicine, money, and entertainment similarly activate memory when played out in Edinburgh. The co-writers offer a tongue-in-cheek disclaimer: "This musical is in no way based on truth and any similarity of the characters to real people, is purely coincidental…honestly" (Berliner, MS 1; emphasis in text). But it follows the statement that "This musical was inspired by the work of Professor Gunther Van [*sic*] Hagens and his Body Worlds Exhibition." More, not only does the plot tell of Doctor Archibald Integer, "the crazed genius" of plastination (MS 1), von Hagens timed an exhibition of his own plastinates in Edinburgh alongside Berliner's production (venues ranged from Princes Street Gardens to the "Burke and Hare" strip club), and rumor circulated that he would take up his violin within the play.[22] It is not hard to catch echoes, here, of controversial dissections, the circulation of bodies in inappropriate spaces, and Knox's flute playing (scripted into notoriety by Bridie).[23] Integer, moreover, waxes poetic in the artistic and anatomical terms his predecessor used to obviate criticism in nineteenth-century Edinburgh:

> My illustrious forbears in art and in science
> Allow me to stand on the shoulders of giants
> But da Vinci, Vesalius were amateurs, failures
> Compared with the glory of me.
>
> If only you realised how special you are
> If only you realised how proud
> It makes me to flay you shape and display you
> Attracting one hell of a crowd. (MS 9)

These are terms that von Hagens has applied to himself. He defended his sanity in a BBC forum: "we would have also called Leonardo da Vinci.…in which tradition I see myself[,] as fully unbalanced…[he] opened up medical science for us.…I am one who breaches taboos."[24] Again, we narrow in not on mere similarity, but on persistence and even recursion.

Not surprisingly, then, this production begins by inviting us to dissect the ways in which art consumes life consumes art consumes life. Sally the television journalist puns on camera:

Most people here tonight... might not know their art from their elbow, but they're paying good *Monet* to see *Corpus*, the gruesome new exhibition.... The exhibition, put together by Dr Archibald Integer, uses new techniques in *flesh-preservation* to create almost literally an alarming *body* of work. (Berliner, MS 3)

And it turns out that in order to produce his art/anatomy (a duality that has long troubled von Hagens), Integer has been committing murder.[25] Yet this is murder with a difference: Integer's victims are willing—they just have no idea of the deadness of eternal life, the forgetfulness enforced by their persistence as art. Herbert, newly plastinated and renamed "Spike," celebrates that "Free of pain I rejoice in this body,... I want time" (MS 29). But time only means with feeling. Losing the one itch remaining to him, he laments:

My God [...] lack of pain, I mean, lack of anything [...] I wasn't—until she scratched it, I could ignore it. That ghost pain, that reminder of my life and sensation. But it's gone... for the time being. I can't feel...... I'm dead!... Pure physical pleasure. Oh God and never again to feel. (MS 29; bracketed ellipsis added)

As "Pallas," another plastinate, points out: "Time's pretty meaningless when you live forever" (MS 10). That is, Berliner and O'Higgins parody the notion of dissection as producing life through its manifestation as repetitive entertainment. The recursions of Festival performance connect obliquely with von Hagens's showmanship to evoke a critique of the temporal looping (or stasis, in the case of plastinates) that so misunderstands the lively meanings possible through the randomness of memory.

Still, this clever, ironic play points also to the deadening that lurks within the recursions of critique. Sally figures out Integer's scheme, destroys/releases the plastinates, and entombs the doctor as one of his own artifacts. Nevertheless, the play ends with her thinking about taking a new and improved potion herself. Although it would not imprison Sally in place, it would still catch her in time—a more advanced plastinate, she would move, but, in the terms now established by the play, she would not truly live. If we consider that Sally has critiqued but not escaped the story she tells, and that her tale is itself an entertainment of the Festival Fringe, then we might wonder whether the disruptions and new connections forced by the overdeterminations of the Festival narrative have cracked that monument at all.

Michael Roth would say no. Roth's major concern, as memory gives way to history and we become capable of seeing how history is made, is that we thereby entrap ourselves within "the ironist's cage" (Roth ch. 4 and 8). We are capable of critiquing our constructions, but not changing them. And certainly, though *Medicinal Purposes* and *Corpus* map a rift in the Edinburgh Festival as monument to Burke and Hare that reaches all the way to other galaxies and postmodern times, in each case we end with the same old story and the same investment in entertainment values above all.

Other Bodies: The Public Relations of Festivals and Freak Shows from *Bodyworlds* to the Body Politic

Corpus broke the mold for Burke and Hare productions. It too, however, was folded into Festival discourse as a successful event.[26] But the crack it opened runs through the edifice, for Edinburgh preferred not to integrate von Hagens himself. Festival Edinburgh is replete with inappropriate exhibitions, but the Edinburgh Council found *Bodyworlds* too much. The *Evening News*, channeling Edinburgh's disgust in a piece lusciously titled "Over Our Dead Body," declared with satisfaction: "A controversial professor planning to bring an exhibition of skinned corpses to the Capital during the Fringe festival has been refused a licence to set up his gruesome show in Princes Street Gardens."[27] Lothian and Borders police stood ready to "respond to any complaints from the public and take 'appropriate action depending on the circumstances.'"[28] Did official Edinburgh imagine that public feelings would be offended when anatomy and local history conjoined too intimately in city spaces? Or was it rather that von Hagens challenged Scots at last to consider who can appropriately tell this tale, who has the responsibility to critique it, and whether—fragmented and contained though it might be—this story might still make a difference in Scottish culture? Anyone can tell or even enact a Knoxian tale of memory lost and money flowing in via the Edinburgh Festival (and Raymond Burke already had in 1994). But once that story cut close to the bone in the over-the-top persona of von Hagens, reactivating memory through pain and disgust in the way of Walter Scott, Scots remembered it was their story to tell—and that it had to be told aright.

Von Hagens, by his brassy willingness to figure Edinburgh's anxieties about medicine, memory, and money, only brought to the fore concerns that had been growing for Scottish authors since the institution of their Parliament and the afflux of Burke and Hare productions to a new Scotland. Donald P. Spence warns that "the very coherence of an account may lead us to believe that we are making contact with an actual happening" (Spence, 27). He adds: "Narrative truth can be defined as the criterion we use to decide when a certain experience has been captured to our satisfaction; it depends on continuity and closure and the extent to which the fit of the pieces takes on an aesthetic finality" (31). The stories of the Fringe, within the story of the Festival, might be seen to gesture to "narrative truth." However different, they participate in the Festival narrative upon which everyone agrees. Thus von Hagens's eruptions as showman, violinist, and disturber of the local peace can actually fit within the story of a lively Festival experience. Yet even as Scotland's grand narrative of summer japes feeds on its own critique, some authors have figured out how to follow the rifts opened by art beyond the routes of mere irony.

An odd assemblage of writers, from tour guide Robin Mitchell to Ian Rankin, have gradually verged toward a more productive use of the Burke and Hare story. These authors presume on its fall from living memory into history, recognize its decay, understand its role as moneymaker, and grasp its limited function as critique. Yet they also know that this tale, because it is fragmented, can stimulate ongoing reconstruction of the self as Scottish.

Paul Johnston's *Body Politic* (1997), published as Scotland conceptualized its new Parliament, situates itself in a devolutionary world: England has subsided into drug wars; Edinburgh, saved by its second Enlightenment, bears uncomfortable similarities to a police state. But only the locals know that, for the economy is Festival driven, and anxiously protected. Edinburgh, in fact, is in a permanent state of Festival, with all the accoutrements of licensed prostitution, twenty-four-hour celebration, and historic "hangings" on a daily basis.

The novel's disillusioned son of Enlightenment, in a nice touch of symbolism turned sanitation worker and private detective, opens the novel at such a hanging:

> there was a hush as the condemned man was led up to the scaffold by guards in period costume....
>
> The guides started speaking again. The bearded man was explaining to the Americans that this was Deacon William Brodie, the city's most notorious villain.
>
> "Here, in the heart of the city where crime no longer exists... Brodie committed his outrages." (Paul Johnston, 5)

All is not as it seems. Our hero wonders:

> wheeling my bike past the tartan and whisky shops.... that maybe the execution wasn't just a piece of theatre for the tourists. I mean, staging mock hangings in a city where capital punishment has been abolished and violence of any kind supposedly eradicated is cynical enough. Actually getting rid of the small number of murderers serving life with hard labour in the city's one remaining prison would be seriously hypocritical. But with the Council you never know. (6)

So of course this detective is about to stumble into a case involving corpses with excised body parts, eager and implicated pathologists, and patients in need of transplants—notably, his mother, the head of the Council of Guardians.

Festival Edinburgh falls apart (the mother, fittingly, suffers from a degenerative disease). And Edinburgh collapses along the lines of its enforced historicism and its official forgetfulness. Supposedly this is a city of no crime; indeed, it is a place of no names. "Our hero" is Bell (for the barracks to which he belongs) number 03, and has to struggle to remain Quintilian Dalrymple (Paul Johnston, 18). However, Dalrymple's detective work requires memory; though he is separated from society by his own failures and bad memories, he holds on to the fact of himself, asserting his name, and even a preferred nickname that disturbs naming while yet hinting at secret meaning: "Quint." So it is he alone who can decode from a past which is supposedly now a mere entertainment the signs of dissection and medication. He alone can bring them home to matria and patria: mother and state. That is, in *Body Politic*, Johnston recognizes the power of the past, however much it is commodified, and perhaps because it is considered coin of the realm, to disturb the present in destructive ways. Events connect to past dissection and present devolution. They reconnect into meaning for this moment. Problematically, however, they no doubt will be reconnected again, for the state retains the data of its past even as it lacks memory. The fragments of Burke and Hare, then, thematize a present, pose a challenge to that present, but point to its repetition through the future. Johnson understands the complex represented by the conjunction of money and memory in Festival Edinburgh, and posits an active engagement with it, but he cannot change its operations.

Robin Mitchell, too, recognizes but seems unable to redirect Burke and Hare's recursive and thus deathly Festival dynamic. *Grave Robbers* (1999) is an uneven book, jerking from low comedy to guidebook information and back. For instance, researching in the Central Library, Adam is at once distracted by his neighbors, and by history:

> the fetid smell of BO instantly disappeared from the room, courtesy of the bearded man's tea breaks. Adam became engrossed in a book dealing with grave robbing.... [I]n the early 1800s the study of anatomy in Edinburgh surged forward thanks to surgeons like Dr Robert Knox who attracted up to five hundred people to his class.... Suspicious characters, sometimes the medical students themselves, became well known at the time, masquerading under the title of 'The Resurrectionists'. In city graveyards on dark moonless nights, shadowy figures were seen flitting amongst the gravestones, going about their gory pursuit.
>
> Burke and Hare were different, missing out the middleman.... Nobody to this day knows exactly how many people disappeared....
>
> Adam was altogether self-satisfied with his library achievements to date. (Robin Mitchell, 62)

Yet although it is no great literature, this book demonstrates Scottish authors' pervasive and growing unease with Edinburgh and Festival as enacted in Burke and Hare.

Why is Adam satisfied? Here, Mitchell brings us close to significance: Adam and his partner have been digging up the past—ever since they discovered that Edinburgh residents like to take it with them. Adam's researches have helped him identify graves "where wine, gold goblets, and buckled shoes were buried. Details of two Highland swords, a silver walking stick and a man who'd been buried in a full set of armour" (Robin Mitchell, 61). He ponders digging up "a famous individual. ... I'd be famous if I robbed from Sir Walter Scott, Robert Burns or Robert Louis Stevenson" (61). Adam is thoroughly caught up in the cycle of nostalgia, with all its saleable swords, sticks, and famous men—notably, writers. Endlessly recycled through the marketplace, this past smells.

Adam's friend Cammy initiated their new venture. Cammy is a gravedigger and, filling in a grave, he accidentally cracked a coffin, discovering untold wealth. Now Adam and Cammy toy with names for their business. Cammy suggests: "How about something similar to Burke and Hare? How does Burt and Player sound? Kurt and Dare? Or, em...Lurk and Bare?" (Robin Mitchell, 55). But the joke is thin. Not everything is an entertainment, especially when haunted by Burke and Hare. Cammy is in love with a tour guide—traveling on her bus and getting misrecognized as a tourist while she narrates her way around Edinburgh for the Festival crowd is one of his major enjoyments. But repetition for Festival cash again turns deadly. By the end of the book, it turns out that Cammy has unwittingly robbed his girlfriend's parents' grave, and the girlfriend now is dead. That is, in this unsteady novel, Burke and Hare lurk and dare, but they also challenge identities and manifest unpleasant truths. There is always a twist in their tale.

This is remarkable, for Robin Mitchell is thoroughly implicated in the tourist project that is the Edinburgh Festival (Robin Mitchell, author's note). He claims credit as inventor of the Edinburgh Ghost Tour, having set up the Cadies and Witchery Tours which walk tourists around haunted and criminal Edinburgh, and he anchors Witchery Tours in his role as "Adam Lyal" (supposedly executed as a highwayman in the Grassmarket in 1811). Not only does Mitchell retell Knoxian stories on a daily basis, but he has also written them down in *Witchery Tales* (1988) and boasts of owning his very own Burkean attraction: a card case made from the skin of the unfortunate William. Moreover in 1999, Mitchell made Adam Lyal walk as a spoof candidate for the Parliament. So in *Grave Robbers*, which coincided with the opening of Scotland's Parliament, Mitchell both serves his paying customers and pursues some timely questions about Scottish uses of the past—and his own.

As for Johnston, however, in Mitchell's book this seems a necessary game, with a zero sum. These novels show how the past has been bowdlerized for Festival cash and reinstall its threat. Yet at most they can observe and report. They cannot yet activate the Burke and Hare story to stimulate a more productive telling of Scotland.

The turning point may lie in Christopher Wallace's *The Resurrection Club* (1999)—which pushes the past in this present to the point of destruction. Wallace is German, living in Edinburgh. From his insider/outsider perspective, Edinburgh manifests the past as public relations coup:

> OKAY. THE WORD ON EDINBURGH....
>
> *Edinburgh. The Festival city. A city of unparalleled beauty and elegance. A refined city of culture and history. An overwhelming city. The Athens of the North.*
>
> All true, or at least based on part-truth. The pioneers in the black art of Public Relations certainly did their job here—every fault has become a charming eccentricity, a ghoulish past has been successfully repositioned as the kitsch of the present. A city where ghost tours wait for night to fall and the coach-loads of gullible Americans to join. A professional job, worthy of an industry award if the culprits could be found. A presentation that misses, purposefully, the vital part. (Wallace, 13)

What is the vital part? Kate Atkinson observes in her Festival novel that for Edinburgh, performance and reality become indistinguishable in the immediacy of the present moment. Witnessing a vicious assault, "Martin had wondered at first if it was another show—a faux-impromptu piece intended either to shock or to reveal our immunity to being shocked because we lived in a global media community where we had become passive voyeurs of violence (and so on)" (Atkinson, 7). In Wallace's Edinburgh, characters are similarly disconnected. As with Mitchell, we are all tourists, all caught in the gaze exchanged by present and past across performance, and thereby prevented from seeing their deathly connection or achieving any difference. We have lost our vital part—we don't even know what it is.

Wallace's deconstructive text places a fractured narrative of the past alongside a present both mystical and confused. In so doing it tests the coherence between the two and puts them under pressure from their relations and recursions, exposing the "vital part." At the heart of *The Resurrection Club* lies a Festival "happening." One survivor of that event ("survivor" is the correct term) recalls:

> I'd heard that something a bit...weird was taking place...or being planned. Nobody knew at the start whether it was all just hype though...happens all the time at the Festival...'the most outrageous show ever!' kind of thing. (Wallace, 8; ellipses original)

In the disjunctive chapter structure of the text, this disparate (thus conventional) event jostles against a well-known past. Alongside statements from those who have survived the "event," we learn of "Doctor Brodie." Renamed from the catalog of Edinburgh villains (Deacon Brodie the notorious city father and robber from the eighteenth century) and retimed by just a year (1827 rather than 1828), Brodie is a shadow cast by Doctor Knox (55). Wallace's protagonist is a famed surgeon and teacher whose exploits produce "an inflationary spiral as [he finds] himself bidding against rival schools for the best specimens" (55, 56). Like Knox, Brodie is the ultimate anatomist—just taking one literary step further: he dissects in search of the inaccessible soul. Keeping in step with Knox as retold through history and Festival, Brodie follows where his intellect demands, taking a route from bodysnatchers and murder to Daft Jamie, that favorite of the melodrama (101, 57). Fulfilling the narrative of Knox as villain, Brodie carves open Jamie's living body on the operating table, looking for his soul (57–59).

The Festival "event," meanwhile, is orchestrated by Peter Dexter/Pablo Dextrus. Dextrus, notable for an interest in local history (particularly medical and mortuary) that amounts to a fetish, works with a publicity agent to construct the "Resurrectionist Expression" and the event that centers the novel, "Proscribed" (Wallace, 112, 10). These expressions are at once symbolized (and enacted) as a load of manure: "Henry Hughes of Standard Mutual [a sponsor] was quite forthright when he spoke to me," Charlie the publicity man remembers. "'Art?' he said. 'This isn't art. It's a pile of shit.'" "Unfortunately," Charlie concludes, "he was absolutely right—it *was* a pile of shit, literally" (170). Such events are also dangerous. The ultimate happening involves copious amounts of alcohol (in memory of Burke and Hare perhaps) and the staged loss of all bodily inhibitions—sexual, medical, and mortal. For Festival pleasure, the participants ingest "snuff," "[an] original blend of invigorating spices mixed with the powdered bones of some of Edinburgh's finest" that invokes gentlemanly nicotine addictions and urban legends of sensation movies centered on actual murder. They then dig up graves (that of de Quincey the addict and admirer of Burke and Hare's Fine Arts), disport themselves in unseemly fashion—and end up as good as dead (116, 197).

What removes their vital part? They have been amusing themselves to death through the memories of the past and the cheap thrills of the present. The result of Brodie's experiments, for which he killed Daft Jamie, is a prosthetic device at once stimulating and killing. Producing excitement but lacking a soul, it has been a soul stealer over generations—from when Brodie fled Edinburgh and reinvented himself as a vaudeville entertainer, until he showed up at today's Festival as Pablo Dextrus. Within the Festival, where it is appropriately recognized as a sex toy, it provides the ultimate cultural orgasm. But it brings no "little death": it wipes out memory as it wipes out soul.

This novel, then, points to the soullessness of Edinburgh's economic obsession with its past as entertainment. But perhaps, informed by a new devolutionary and deconstructive sensibility, Edinburgh had had enough and was ready to move on. Importantly for our own narrative of the story of Burke and Hare, advertisers, policemen, and long-ago city fathers who look like "two old codgers in period costume straight from the set of a Sir Walter Scott novel" together invade the graveyard/venue; all Edinburgh at last pushes this past to the other side of self-indulgent pleasure (Wallace, 219, 219–227). Cultural orgasm, Wallace suggests, equals destruction. And it is destruction. As the survivor recalls:

> Pablo's eyes flicker with electricity like the lights in a pinball machine about to go 'tilt'... and then his arms... flapping [...] until he is lifted clear off the ground [....] Then there was the explosion [....] I staggered back up and out of the grave [....] as the sparks rained down on us. It was like World War Three in there. These firework displays can look fantastic, but take it from me, they are best admired from a distance [....] I had to dodge my way out as if I was under sniper attack, using the headstones for cover [...] until I was out of there and I was free. And that's how I felt, free. (228; bracketed ellipses mine)

Can there now be no going back?

BODIES IMPOLITIC: IAN RANKIN

Have Scots played with Burke and Hare to the point of orgasmic collapse, where the past is gone and they are free? Or might such freedom prove delusional? Scotland's pasts, however well resolved or beaten down, seldom go far away. Even now, the Edinburgh Dungeon advertises its new Burke and Hare exhibit to capitalize on the release of John Landis's film: "Burke and Hare are back again and open for business" from February 2010.[29] And Scots are lining up to donate their bones—postmortem. Two nurses, keen to foreground today's need for cadavers, point to the trauma's expiation by common sense, but, says the Dungeon's manager, "there are probably several people out there who would relish the prospect of hanging around and scaring people for years after they've died."[30] We have only to think of tartanry with its remnant of Jacobitism, still alive in Princes Street and cannily embraced by skeptical Scots, to realize that the unimaginable horrors of Burke and Hare are likely to continue to lurk alongside more colorful and less threatening cultural imaginations in the making of tomorrow's Scotland. But then, for negative and positive imaginations, as for past and present, we might wonder with Wallace's ad man: "The old and the new,

Resting in Pieces?

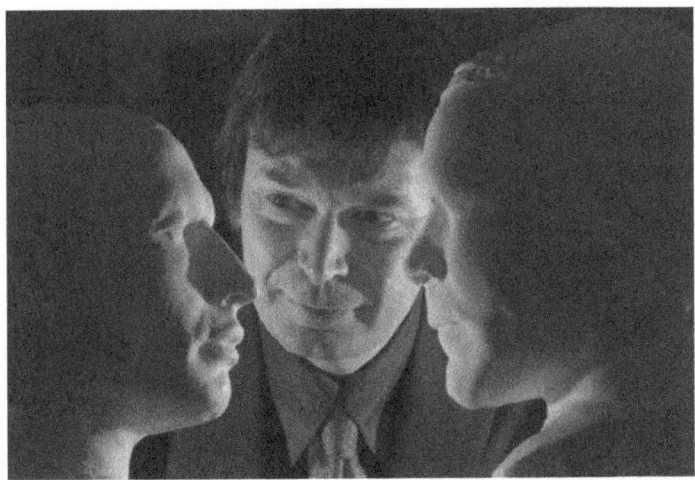

FIGURE 7.2. Ian Rankin meets the life and death masks of Hare and Burke at the Museum of the University of St. Andrews, November 25, 2008. Photo by Alan Richardson. Courtesy of the University of St. Andrews.

reinventing themselves, reinventing the past, then as now. Where is the difference?" (Wallace, 15).

Ian Rankin has figured out a difference, and a way to move on. Over the years Scottish authors have worked to resolve the story of Burke and Hare, and then to resist the seductions of this often told tale when it offers only a reductive route to addressing the problems of identity politics, or when its fragments serve the commercial narrative of their new society. Today, authors observe and report, even push and destroy. Yet there are more productive options. In *Set in Darkness* (2000), *The Falls* (2000), and *Resurrection Men* (2001), Rankin works his way through the issues underlying the national metaphor posed by Scott and enacted through Burke and Hare. By his third try, he has constructed a possibility at once ironic and strategic: a critical way to embrace the past but escape the zero sum (see figure 7.2). John Rebus demonstrates new uses for Burke and Hare in the place that is today's Scotland. He does so by living within a space in story that no one else suspects.

Set in Darkness is Rankin's Parliamentary novel. In very obvious ways, it interrogates the metaphor of the body politic at a time when Scotland seems recently embodied in the persons of its MSPs (Member of the Scottish Parliament). As Edinburgh prepares for devolved government, a body looms at the site of the previous parliament's demise and the new institution's birth. Before long, MSPs are dropping like flies. Rebus, Rankin's perennial antihero, himself embodies the problem of this politic stuck between haunting past and doubtful present. In 1979, during the first referendum, Rebus's wife was a committed campaigner for devolution. But Rebus's work made him a doubter:

They argued politics at the kitchen table until Rebus became bored by it all....

"I really can't be scunnered [bothered]," he'd say when she finished, and she'd start hitting him with a cushion....

Maybe it was because he was getting a reaction. Whatever, his intransigence grew. He wore a "Scotland Says NO" badge home one night. (Rankin *Set in Darkness*, 89)

In the end, he doesn't vote. What's worse, he remembers to forget:

He could blame work, the weather, any number of things. But really, it was to make Rhona suffer. He knew this as he watched the office clock, watched the hands pass the referendum's close. With minutes left, he almost dashed for his car, but told himself it was too late. It was too late.

Felt like hell on the drive home. (90)

Rebus is tied to a guilty past.

This book constantly draws connections between Rebus and the past. Watching archaeologists at work, Rebus hears one declare: "'What an extraordinary find'... beaming at his young co-worker. She grinned back at him. It was nice to see people so happy in their work. Digging up the past, uncovering secrets... it struck Rebus that they weren't so unlike detectives" (Rankin *Set in Darkness*, 13; ellipsis in text). Yet is Rebus stuck in the past? Rankin provides us with an important context to work this out. Those who assertively embrace the future turn out to be criminals. Rebus finds himself in a moment of patriotic karaoke. He hears:

What force or guile could not subdue,
Through many warlike ages,
Is wrought now by a coward few,
For hireling traitors' wages....

And then the singer took a step forward, and now Rebus saw who it was.

Cafferty [his criminal nemesis, capable of constant self-resurrection].

The English steel we could disdain,
Secure in valour's station,
But English gold has been our bane—
Such a parcel of rogues in a nation. (317; italics original)

Cafferty assures Rebus, "The old ways don't work any more" (321). Later he adds: "this parliament will put us in charge of our own destinies.... [I]t's maybe a time for looking forward" (427). Cafferty chooses nostalgia but not memory or history. He claims modernity while singing Robert Burns's lament for a nation betrayed by the money and "progress" he himself so desires.

We can work this out—and so can Rebus. Although Rebus for a moment considers looking only forward, "selling the flat, finding somewhere with fewer ghosts," he tends toward a new awareness neither controlled by the past nor unduly high on the present (Rankin *Set in Darkness*, 24). Cafferty officially despises Rebus because "you just can't leave the past alone, can you" (427). Quite. Rebus reads backwards through the ironies of Cafferty's sentimentality: "Plenty of rogues in Scotland.... I can't see how independence would mean less of them" (318). Thus in face of Cafferty's taunt that "We'll have our parliament... [and] this will all be history," Rebus can assert a new understanding of time and of the efforts of memory: "I don't care how long it takes" (444). The past, whatever it is, leads to work in the present. Rebus is neither deterred nor determined by times present or times past. The same strategist he proved to be when he remembered to forget to vote—but with less guilt—he knows he can make meaning through both together.

This is the more important because *Set in Darkness* offers a plot that looks like purpose but that turns out to be accidental. The present is not necessarily connected to the past, but they can nonetheless be understood to mean together. Notably, Rankin tests this insight in what we might term his "Burke and Hare" novel: *The Falls* (2000). *Set in Darkness* hinted at the medicalized aspects of the body politic. Investigating the demise of an MSP, Rebus travels to St. Andrews. The last police visit to the university was to pursue the case of "The severed hand." It was "Some student joke," initiated in the anatomy lab (Rankin *Set in Darkness*, 180). Now, Rebus is overwhelmed with hints at Knoxian meanings. An Edinburgh student is missing, and someone has found a miniature coffin near her family home. The coffin is not unlike those in actuality on display in the new Museum of Scotland, which may be connected to Burke and Hare—present seems doubly linked to past.[31]

The thrust of Rebus's work is to connect that past to this present. To such an end, Rebus is coached in history. A curator walks him through the basics:

> "It's a mortsafe," she said, then, seeing his lack of comprehension: "The families of the deceased would lock the coffin inside a mortsafe for the first six months to deter the resurrectionists."
>
> "Meaning body-snatchers?" Now this was a piece of history he knew. "Like Burke and Hare? Digging up corpses and selling them to the university?"

> She peered at him like a teacher with a stubborn pupil. "Burke and Hare didn't dig up anything." (Rankin *Falls*, 95)

And this is where the story takes a turn. Jean, the historian, corrects Rebus, but gets her own facts wrong: she goes on to insist that "a dissected corpse could not enter heaven"—a common statement, but not always supported by the discourse of 1828 (98; see ch.1 in this book). Later, Jean researches to determine the provenance of the museum coffins. She checks to see whether the doctor who flayed Burke's corpse, and was a noted cabinet maker, could have constructed them (Fergusson, Knox's student, was in reality a gifted carpenter; DNB). But she is forced to admit that "the Arthur's Seat case [where the original coffins were found] was a blind alley" (327). Worse, an obsession with the coffins was "a trap into which you could fall. This was history—ancient history, compared to the [current] case."

Throughout *The Falls*, ancient history pops up: the victim's boyfriend has a neighbor who used to be a pathologist; the pathologist has an interest in Knox and a table designed by the doctor who flayed Burke; the victim's friend is related to that long-ago doctor; miniature coffins abound. Everything seems too connected, when Devlin, the retired pathologist, sums up:

> "Lovell was one of the anatomists charged with the dissection of William Burke. It's even likely that he pronounced Burke dead after the hanging. Less than a month later, he sat for this portrait."
>
> "He looks pretty happy with his lot," Rebus commented.
>
> Devlin's eyes sparkled. "Doesn't he? Kennet was a craftsman too. He worked with wood, as did Deacon William Brodie, of whom you will have heard."
>
> "Gentleman by day, housebreaker by night," Rebus acknowledged.
>
> "And perhaps the model for Stevenson's *Jekyll and Hyde*. As a child, Stevenson had a wardrobe in his room, one of Brodie's creations." (Rankin *Falls*, 139)

None of these connections mean anything—and yet they mean everything.

Rebus's strategy of moving between past and present requires good data. But Burke and Hare are a mobile signifier that can mislead—and can be used to deceive. It emerges that the novel's coffins are a hoax, designed to drum up custom for a local Scottish business (and we certainly have heard that before, in Festival time). The friend did not channel her ancestor; Kennet Lovell did not speak down the years out of the drawers of his table! But the retired pathologist assists the murderous boyfriend by spreading rumor because he himself emulates Lovell as he imagines him to be. In fact, he is responsible for now "ancient" killings, each marked with their own little coffin. That is, Rankin suggests the past can actively mislead, yet it can still mean. What makes the difference is Rebus's willingness to live between past and present. Seemingly lost in the blind alleys of the past as Jean feared, Rebus connects apparently random pieces across time to achieve an understanding in the present that is new for his case, and for Burke and Hare.

Rankin has demonstrated the constructive meaning making that is possible despite the compulsions of either the past or the present. Rebus's sampling among fragments leveled together as data produces new realities. It suggests that in a postmodern world, amid the clash of grand narratives and fragmented, even spurious tales, we can always strategize, reorient, move on.

Resurrection Men (2001) completes the case. This novel arises in an interestingly fragmented way. In *The Falls*, Rebus and his colleague and friend Siobhan visit the University of Edinburgh's medical school. A professor coaches them, much as Jean coached Rebus:

> "[Old College is] where they took Burke's body?" Rebus added.
> "Yes, after he was hanged. A tunnel led into Old College. The bodies were all brought in that way—by dead of night in some cases." [The doctor] looked to Siobhan. "The Resurrection Men."
> "Good name for a band."
> He graced her flippancy with a scowl. "Body snatchers." (Rankin *Falls*, 292)

Of course, "The Bodysnatchers" is already a name for a band (the ska/rocksteady girl group formed in 1979). But Rankin's next novel does feature a band of "Resurrection Men." Only this time, in nicely self-reflexive fashion, the resurrection men are policemen undergoing disciplinary retraining. Rebus, with a full dose of irony directed back to this moment in *The Falls*, makes one of our happy band of brothers.

The detective, however, is a spy. Some of his colleagues are suspected not just of bad behavior, but of criminal deeds. On the verge of retirement, they are now likely to escape punishment, having hidden their reality in a delusive present. So Rebus is here for his detecting virtues, his ability to move between today and the past, and realign presents and futures. Tellingly, again, the villains maintain a distinction between what has been, and what is. "I think some tombs are best left undisturbed," says the ringleader. "Don't you, John? What do you say? Do we call it a draw?" (Rankin *Resurrection*, 464). But these crooked cops don't know enough about the present or the past. On a visit to Edinburgh, the fragments of Burke and Hare poke through the apparent camaraderie:

> "It's John Knox's house," Rebus said....
> "Bloody right, it is," Gray said.... "*Our* history."

> Rebus wanted to say something about how women and Catholics might not agree....
>
> "Knoxland," Gray said, stretching out his arms. "That's what Edinburgh is, wouldn't you agree, John?"
>
> Rebus felt he was being tested.... "Which Knox, though?" he asked, causing Gray to frown. "There was another: Doctor Robert Knox. He brought bodies from Burke and Hare. Maybe we're more like him..." [ellipsis in text]
>
> Gray thought about this, then smiled. "Archie Tennant delivered us the body of Rico Lomax [the cold case upon which they supposedly retrain], and we're cutting it open." He began to nod slowly. "That's very good, John. Very good."
>
> Rebus wasn't sure it was exactly what he'd meant, but he accepted the compliment anyway. (135)

Rebus can move strategically between extremes. He does not have to settle in the past, or presume on control in the present.

Indeed, Rebus is such a creature of mobility that for much of the novel, he does not know if he is a plant (though he has been told as much) or under investigation himself. Both in the plot he interrogates and in the plot that he inhabits, Rebus finds himself adrift between certainties and grasping at fragments, but always working toward meanings that will change apparent realities. Gray, the villain, taunted: "*When it comes to Edinburgh, John knows where the bodies are buried*" (Rankin *Resurrection*, 293; italics original). Gray does not know the half of it. If the literary career of Burke and Hare and Doctor Knox is anything to go by, bodies seldom remain where they are buried. But Rebus the detective shows that by triangulating between them, you can make a different place for yourself in support, at least in possibility, of a better Scotland.

BODIES IN MOTION: THE FUTURES OF BURKE AND HARE

Critics of national cultures have worried that nations are imaginary constructs. Cairns Craig wondered for Scotland whether a nation constructed through literary imagination both manifested and ensured its own distance from political power. In *Out of History*, Craig considered that, if there was a gain to be had in the imagined nation, it must be realized somewhere beyond the concerns of "history" and "progress." Frantz Fanon has worried that subject to colonial imaginings, nations and peoples can see themselves only as grotesque, other, maybe powerless. But the unlikely case of Burke and Hare and Doctor Knox points to imagination as the much more down and dirty work of culture, and offers enlivening possibilities.

We have tracked how the trauma of 1828 needed to be worked out through culture over generations as the community first healed itself, then disciplined the doctor, became strong enough to accept some responsibility, and finally recognized the rights of real victims to speak even against the nation. We have seen how this tale, once told, decayed into fragments that could be appropriated for a very different, commercial national tale. Along the way, we have developed a new understanding of the imagined community. On the one hand, the trauma of 1828 needed to be resolved; on the other hand, the retelling that often marks traumatic compulsion equally points to a strategic deconstruction of the society as imagined. Beside the grand narrative of nostalgia that culminates in a Scottish Parliament runs a counter tale of violence, blame, and guilt.

This is not an accident. So now that the counter tale itself has become a grand narrative and moved to the stage of recuperation through the market place, making money in the Edinburgh Festival, authors have struggled to activate once more the narrative of the "unimaginable community." Even as the remnants of our twice-told tale were absorbed to support that epitome of the imagined Edinburgh, the Festival, Scottish authors found themselves disturbed by fragmentary echoes of a negative tale and preferred not to resolve or ignore it, but to embrace it and live within it. Children's writers felt the strain; Festival authors like Johnston and Wallace recognized it for what it was: the essential other story that queries the nation as imagined. And Ian Rankin has demonstrated how Scots might live between the fragments of tales both negative and positive in a more self-aware national space. Scotland seems to need and even to want to posit against its own imaginings the unimaginable horrors crystallized into the story of Burke and Hare.

Cairns Craig worries that uncritical imaginings deaden or displace a culture, and Michael Roth laments that critical historicizing leads only to the stasis of irony. We might view these options according to Dominic LaCapra's opposition between "acting-out" and "working-through" (Rossington, 208). In a way, they are both types of "acting out." By contrast, though the sequences of trauma, with their own imperatives, might possibly be seen as "acting-out," they must equally be understood as "working through." LaCapra specifies:

> working-through need not be understood to imply the integration or transformation of past trauma into a seamless narrative memory and total meaning or knowledge. Narrative at best helps one not to change the past through a dubious rewriting of history but to work through posttraumatic symptoms in the present in a manner that opens possible futures. It also enables one to recount events and perhaps to evoke experience, typically through nonlinear

movements that allow trauma to register in language and its hesitations, indirections, pauses, and silences. And, particularly by bearing witness and giving testimony, narrative may help performatively to create openings in existence that did not exist before. (Rossington, 208)

Fittingly, by LaCapra's terms, in Scotland's experience that tendency to "work through" seems only exacerbated once trauma appears resolved and irony becomes possible. That is, the imagined community may take its official tone from its positive tales, but it draws its life from working through its negatives. As Scottish responses to the Festival iterations of Doctor Knox may show, successful imaginings provide no self-satisfying entertainment and offer no self-aggrandizing irony. They spring from Scots' productive labor as they wrestle energetically and wilfully between their positive and negative tales.

The events of 1828, therefore, are a work in progress—consider, for instance, Martin Conaghan and Will Pickering's 2009 comic book (see figure 7.3). Thus even now, this book cannot offer a last word on Burke and Hare, and cannot posit a future trajectory for the "unimaginable community." Indeed, its work so far cannot be complete. Even if I were not suspicious of casting Burke and Hare as participants in a "grand narrative" of their own, I have to admit gaps in my text where stories of 1828 fall too far away from my concerns. For this reason, I have had to pass over Elizabeth Bagby's musical *Practical Anatomy* (2006), which recasts Burke and Helen as romantic couple in order (perhaps) to consider more narrowly the issues of race and ethnicity that appeal to the writer's Chicago audience. I have not dwelt on Shelagh Stevenson's *An Experiment with an Airpump* (staged in Manchester, 1998), which interrogates issues of cloning and genetics across a play craftily split between present and past. Nor have I included the Scottish writer Evelyn Hood's one-act, *A Wake for Donald* (1996), though Hood ingeniously shows a potential victim planting in Burke and Hare the idea for future evil deeds. This is because Hood's play appeared some time after the moment when Scotland first turns attention to victimhood in the sequences of trauma, in the work of Owen Dudley Edwards and Alasdair Gray. Also, plots that center on current problems in medical ethics (for Hood, euthanasia, 14) fall outside the concerns of this book.

I have had to ignore a group of texts that provide challenging reconsiderations of the body politic through its metaphors of dissection, but not through our trio. Readers interested in how the Scottish Parliament's inception activates medical imagery should review the "Destiny" episodes of *Hamish Macbeth* (1997). These feature a jealous sibling who has abandoned Scotland, and with every step further away, suffered the loss of one, then another part of his body. Alan Warner's *The Man Who Walks* (2002), with its recurrent diatribes on the Parliament and hints at characters'

Resting in Pieces? 229

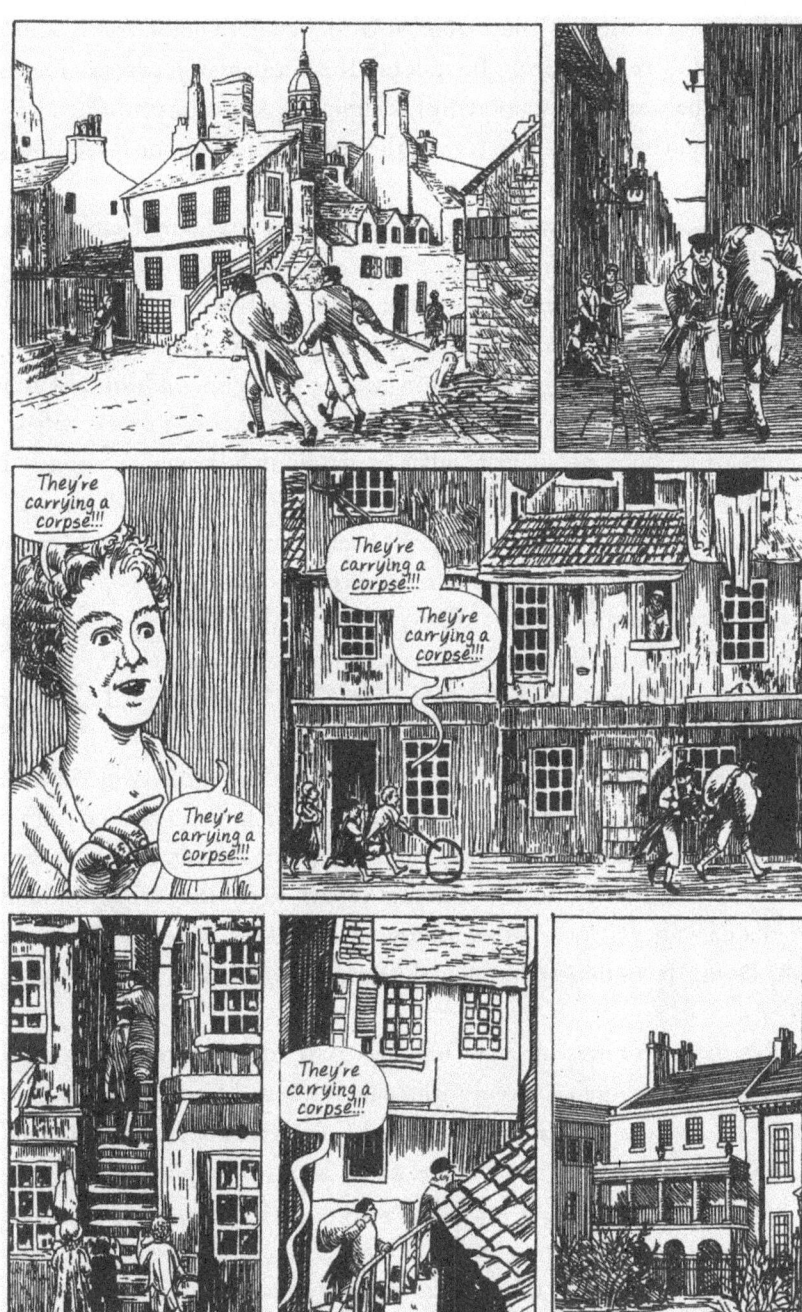

FIGURE 7.3 Page from Martin Conaghan and Will Pickering, *Burke and Hare* (2009). Courtesy of Martin Conaghan and Will Pickering.

mutual dissection is another "must read," as is Andrew Drummond's *Elephantina: A Huge Misunderstanding* (2008). This tale of "The Accidental Death of an Elephant in Dundee in the year 1706," supposedly told from the year 1830, performs a Rebus-type reorientation between Union (1707), the scandals of dissection (1828), and the present Parliament—with great hilarity.

It is impossible, too, to keep up with the histories streaming from 1828. Lisa Rosner's *The Anatomy Murders: Being the True yet Spectacular History of Edinburgh's Notorious Burke and Hare and of the Man of Science Who Abetted Them in the Commission of Their Most Heinous Crimes* (2009), and A. W. Bates's *The Anatomy of Robert Knox* (2010), seek to correct our inaccurate perception of historical events, accumulated over many generations, and inform this book. Rosner, indeed, is attempting to produce a shift in popular understanding through a website. But I have had to let fall by the wayside Deborah Symonds's *Notorious Murders, Black Lanterns, & Moveable Goods* (2006), which focuses on the underground economy that produced Burke and Hare, and crime writer Alanna Knight's popular history *Burke and Hare* for the "Crime Archive" (2007). And there are always more commercial products in the offing, such as the History Channel's "In Search of Burke and Hare," or John Landis's *Burke and Hare* with Simon Pegg and Andy Serkis (currently pending release in America).

So when *will* the retelling of Burke and Hare come to an end, and why? This book is predicated on the idea that a tale not told aright and at the right time will rattle around through popular consciousness, reminding, threatening, damaging, stimulating, and creating. Walter Scott was the author not to tell the tale. Now I hold in my hand a flier for *The Resurrectionists*, touted as "A Lost Waverley Novel—Back from the Dead!" It continues (dropping the exclamation marks):

> *The Resurrectionists* was strongly influenced by Scott's involvement with Dr Knox, the Edinburgh anatomist who paid Burke and Hare to rob graves to provide his dissection specimens. Scott and Knox were both members of the Royal Society of Edinburgh and at one point Scott had to postpone a sitting for his portrait to attend a special inquiry into Knox's misconduct. *The Resurrectionists* can be seen as Scott's comment on Knox's iniquitous behaviour: but its flights of fancy take it into *Frankenstein* territory. A bizarre Gothic tale—considered too disturbing for publication when it was written—this is a magnificent addition to the Edinburgh Edition of the Waverley Novels.

Unfortunately, however, this is only a masterly spoof from the pen of an erstwhile Edinburgh University Press editor, Douglas McNaughton.

We can never know what would have happened had Scott penned a tale; and if we now found a tale, it would make no difference. Nor do we know what trajectory our story will take when it has passed the Parliament and become part of Scotland's working discourse. In an amnesiac world that occasionally needs a jolt, we can only wait eagerly for Irvine Welsh's film *The Meat Trade* (starring Robert Carlyle—presumably in his incarnation as Begbie, rather than Hamish Macbeth).[32] Or we can ponder whether it has been burked by Landis's version. Has the tale gone global and lost its Scottishness, or even the possibility to speak itself from Scotland?

This book should have taught us to be darkly optimistic. Today, we can map the story's migration to YouTube, where it already lurks as "Burke and Hare—The Musical," on "Shadowplay." And we can speculate on what circumstances might bring the events of 1828 to Edinburgh's poetry wall. What if, on the edifice that is the Scottish Parliament, we could read alongside Scott's nationally constructive lines from *The Lay of the Last Minstrel* (1805) a rather different bit of doggerel? What might have happened, and what would happen, if we were to read: "Breathes there the man, with soul so dead, / Who never to himself hath said, / 'This is my own, my native land!'" in a mashup with a more disturbing refrain?

> Up the close and doon the stair,
> But an' ben wi' Burke and Hare.
> Burke's the butcher, Hare's the thief,
> Knox the boy that buys the beef.

I nominate for the wall Edwin Morgan's "Caledonian Antisyzygy," for it speaks to Scotland the possibilities of signs long circulating and full of perverse possibility—the argument of this book:

> – Knock knock. – Who's there? – Doctor. – Doctor Who? – No, just Doctor. – What's up Doc? – Stop, that's all cock. O.K. – Knock knock. – Who's there? – Doctor Who. – Doctor Who who? – Doctor, who's a silly schmo?
> – Right. Out! – Aw. – Well, last chance, come on. – Knock knock. – Who's there? – Doctor Jekyll. – Doctor Jekyll who? – Doctor, 'd ye kill Mr Hyde? – Pig-swill! Nada! Rubbish! Lies! Garbage! Never! Schlock!
> – Calm down, your turn. – Knock knock. – Who's there? – Doctor Knox. – Doctor Knox who? – Doctor Knocks Box Talks.

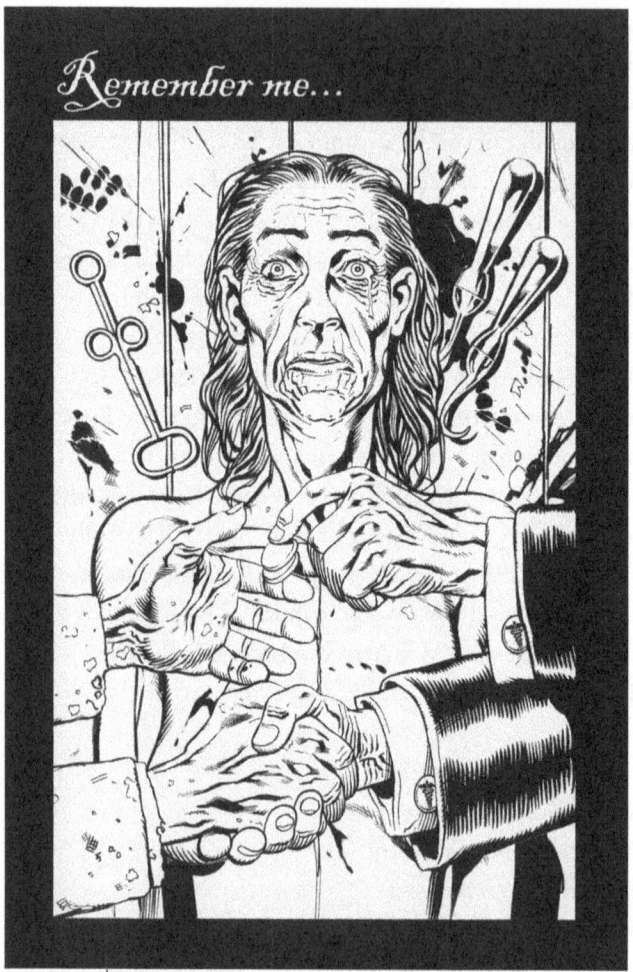

FIGURE 7.4 "Remember me…" By Gary Erskine, in Martin Conaghan and Will Pickering, *Burke and Hare* (2009). Courtesy of Gary Erskine, Martin Conaghan, and Will Pickering.

Claims T.V. Favours Grim Duo, Burke, Hare.
– Right, join hands. Make sure the door is locked, or
nothing will happen. – Dark yet? – Cover clocks.
– Knock. – Listen! – Is there anybody there?

And I close confident that, in line with Gary Erskine's plaint (see figure 7.4), Doctor Knox will continue to pound on Scotland's memory, victims will beseech an audience, Burke and Hare will walk. On such a past, Scots can never quite shut the door.

NOTES

CHAPTER I

Medicine, Murder, and Scottish Story: Doctor Knox and Burke and Hare

1. Thomas Hood's poem appeared in *Whims and Oddities, Second Series*, 1827, then was set to music by Jonathan Blewitt, and published about 1829 as No. 1 of *The Ballad Singer*. See *Complete Thomas Hood*, 77 n. Hood was of Scottish descent and spent time in Dundee.

2. Charles Darwin named Cuvier one of the "two gods," after Aristotle, that inspired him. See his letter, February 22, 1822, to William Ogle, reprinted and given in facsimile by Allan Gotthelf, "Darwin on Aristotle," *Journal of the History of Biology* 32 (1999): 4–7. Darwin studied in Edinburgh just before the scandal that entrapped Knox.

3. Adrian Desmond and James Moore, *Darwin: The Life of a Tormented Evolutionist* (New York: Norton, 1991), 26.

4. Knox's 1837 letter refers to the "winter session of 1828–29." The session at Edinburgh typically began in early to mid October. In March 1829, he numbers his current class as "above 400" students; in 1832, he gives 504 for his current class (Bates, 88).

5. Hood refers to Vyse, Bell (Guy's Hospital), Carpue (St. George's), and Astley Cooper (Guy's). St. Clair Thomson's Presidential Address to the Medical Society of London in 1917 mentions a family of Vyses, beginning with "Mr. William Vyse, Surgeon, at Spalding in Lincolnshire," running through to "Dr. Christopher Vise, of Tunbridge Wells. . . . the sixth generation of medical men in one family."

6. For examples online, visit the *GlasgowSculpture* website, and also Scotlandsplaces.gov.uk.

7. In 1832, Southwood Smith dissected Jeremy Bentham, producing the famous auto-icon. See Marmoy.

8. Owen Dudley Edwards notes: "Ireland, who had published the first two parts of his *West Port Murders* before New Year's Day 1829...had to keep up his instalments until the accounts of the execution and the texts of the authorised confessions would be at his disposal.... It was perhaps inevitable that bogus confessions of Burke were soon in circulation.... Ireland's inclusion of such matter gave it a permanent status.... Ireland's text of the trial was unsatisfactory in the extreme" (Edwards *Burke*, 94).

9. For *The Flesh and the Fiends*, IMDb also gives *Der Arzt und die Teufel* (West Germany), *Kalmankauppiaat* (Finland), *L'impasse aux violences* (France), *La carn I el dimoni* (Spain—Catalan), *La carne y el demonio* (Spain), *Le jene di Edimburgo* (Italy), *Parantava veitsi* (Finland), and *Sadistai tou eglimatos* (Greece).

10. Owen Dudley Edwards, interviewed by Linda Summerhayes, "Dark deeds inspire a series of grisly events," *Scotsman* May 20, 2008. Online, available at living.scotsman.com/people/Dark-deeds-inspire-a-series.3643967.jp, accessed May 19, 2008.

11. "Perlman in Burke and Hare Story." Online, available at filmstalker.co.uk/archives/2007/03/perlman_in_burke_and_hare_stor.html, accessed June 9, 2008.

12. "Legendary Landis" at SRQ Magazine.com, srqmagazine.com/issues/IssueDetail.cfm?iteID=1357, accessed July 13, 2010.

13. "The Meat Trade (2008)." Online, available at imdb.com/title/tt0466235/, accessed March 28, 2008.

14. Robert Carlyle's explanation to indielondon confirms the point: "Are you familiar with Burke and Hare?" he asks his London interviewer. A Scottish audience can make the connections on its own. See "The Meat Trade," under *Rumored Productions*. Online, available at firth.com/rumor.html, accessed June 9, 2008.

15. Much theory of trauma is developed in the context of the Holocaust. Massive degrees of magnitude separate the Holocaust from a local scandal perpetrated by three people in Scotland. Nonetheless, these theories help us to understand 1828 and its aftermath.

16. Robert Carlyle's frustrated claim that "the power of the story isn't there any more" seems an understandable gripe rather than a compelling analysis, given Landis's success and the ongoing energy of Festival productions. See "Interview: Robert Carlyle—Carlyle to Canada," at *Living Scotsman*. Online, available at living.scotsman.com/features/Interview-Robert-Carlyle-Carlyle.5661538.jp, accessed May 9, 2011.

CHAPTER 2

The Story Begins: The Law versus the Press, and the Doctor versus Walter Scott

1. Maria Edgeworth to Sir Walter Scott (n.d.), NLS MS3908, 19–22. Owen Dudley Edwards foregrounds Burke and Hare as Irish Catholics (*Burke and Hare*). *Blackwood's* calls Hare "an Irishman" who produced "a couple of semi-Catholic cubs" (March 1829: 371), and the English *Sun* claimed that the Scottish papers "[hasten] *to prove*... that Burke and his wife are both Irish," but the perpetrators' Irishness does not dominate Edinburgh's early response (qtd. *Mercury* December 29, 1829: 3).

2. This refinement was not unusual in celebrated cases. As late as 1881, it was suffered by the Wyoming robber and murderer "Big-Nose George." The doctor who dissected him later ran for office—wearing "Big-Nose George" shoes. Carbon County Museum website. Online, available at carboncountymuseum.com, accessed July 14, 2010.

3. Stone was not successful: George Combe replied that Stone mistakenly focused on length and ignored breadth (Combe, 3–4); W. R. Greg addressed Stone's "ignorance" by explaining that "the organs of Benevolence and Destructiveness, both powerful, are successively called into action, and sway the sceptre of the mind in turn" (Greg, 10). See also Roger Cooter, *The Cultural Meaning of Popular Science*, and *Phrenology in the British Isles*.

4. Lonsdale, 141. Knox was an inveterate paper-giver. For example, the General Minute Book for the Royal Society of Edinburgh, January 1824–May 1843, lists papers on March 15 and June 7, 1824, then May 16, 1825. In 1830, Knox gave papers on February 15, March 1, and March 15.

5. Knox tried to discourage their gift, though with his own feelings in mind: "the connection of my establishment with the late atrocities, however accidental, is a very severe misfortune… [T]he very recollection of these shocking occurrences must be ever painful to me" (Rae, 101, from *Scotsman* March 25, 1829).

6. Anne Scott to C. K. Sharpe, autograph letter in ECL Sharpe, West Port Murders.

7. On January 3, 1829, the paper noted that the *Sun*'s editor disavowed authorship of the article, and claimed it was a spoof in the style of de Quincey's "Murder Considered as One of the Fine Arts." The *Mercury* suggested the editor "ought to have distinguished between a bad joke and a virulent libel on the character of his countrymen" (3).

8. See McCracken-Flesher *Possible*, 73–113. *West Port Murders* describes the crowd at Burke's execution as unparalleled "excepting perhaps at the king's visit" (231).

9. See *Mercury* January 17, 1829: 2, for Paterson's first letter to the paper, and the paper's sharp response—accusations that he had been double-dealing between doctors, and that he had been dismissed by Knox. See a reply from Knox's assistants on January 24: 3, and Paterson's second letter and the paper's second response on January 26: 3. See also MacGregor, 157–63.

10. Anne Scott wrote to Sharpe: "Papa…is much inclined to share a window with you" (ECL Sharpe, West Port Murders, MS n.d.). Robert Seton wrote with the offer to share on January 14, 1829 (see NLS L.C. Folio 62 MS1791). Scholars have presumed this to mean that Scott attended. See Currie, and even Ruth Richardson, 133. Scott may have been in town, as a letter from J. Stevenson to Sharpe indicates (January 30, 1829, ECL Sharpe, West Port Murders, MS). Scott did specify, "I did not go to [the trial or the West Port], although the newspapers reported me one of the visitors" (*Letters*, 11:103; 71).

11. G. Gregory Smith identified a "caledonian antisyzygy" in *Scottish Literature: Character and Influence* (London: Macmillan, 1919). Today, scholars question his binary approach, but recognize the fragmented and fractious quality of Scottish culture.

12. Maulitz notes that "Normal anatomy gradually came into its own in the wake of the Parliamentary inquiries of 1828 and 1833. Pathological anatomy…now became displaced" (200). See chapter 3 in this book for Knox's arguments over the General Pathology Chair at Edinburgh.

13. This folkloric tale lacks a reliable source. See Adams *Dead*, 29.

14. Madame Tussaud modeled Burke during his trial; her sons modeled Hare. They got a cast of Burke's head three hours after his execution (Pilbeam, 102).

15. Ghost Tours, websites, and blog spots evidence the confusion. For the conservative version, see the-grassmarket.com/history/maggie-dickson.html and edinburghsdarkside.blogspot.com/2006/07/maggie-dickson-half-hangit-maggie.html, accessed May 10, 2009. See Bishop for the version including rioting students (123).

CHAPTER 3

Enlightened System versus Religious Sympathy: The Sensational Tales of Alexander Leighton and David Pae

1. Lisa Rosner analyzes *Murderers*' publisher, Cowie and Strange, for their role in supporting the Anatomy Act, refracted through this novel (256–60). From our perspective, they sought to replace the current "system" with another.

2. See [John Mackay Wilson], *Wilson's Historical, Traditionary, and Imaginative Tales of the Borders, and of Scotland*, vol. 2 (New York: Robert T. Shannon, 1848).

3. See [William Banks], *Life in Heaven* (Edinburgh: Ballantyne, n.d.), 265.

4. Graham Law notes that in the 1860 book, "the final brief paragraph of the serial version was replaced by a new forty-second chapter" (*Lucy*, xv–xvi).

5. Rosner disputes aspects of this story: Was Mary conventionally a prostitute? Why did Knox's assistants recognize her? Was she actually sketched at the time (*Anatomy*, ch. 5)? But fact or fiction, the elements of this tale had entered general circulation by 1864.

6. The story was tagged as by "the Author of 'The Factory Girl.'" It was reprinted in book form, with slight changes each time, in Dundee and then London. It appears as *The Fatal Error* in the *Sheffield Daily Telegraph* October 28, 1865–August 4, 1866. The Dundee book does not carry the newspaper preface, and the closing chapters are differently divided. The *Sheffield* serialization and the London volume share some revisions. Refs. are to the Dundee book. In 2013/14 *Mary Paterson* will be published as an Association for Scottish Literary Studies annual volume.

7. Quoted from "A weekly newspaper, published in Yorkshire," in *The Newspaper Press* (London: E. W. Allen, 1867), 177. The story ran its course in the *Sheffield Daily Telegraph*, so the claim is either apocryphal, or refers to another, untraced serialization.

8. Dr. [John] Thomas, *The Coming Struggle among the Nations of the Earth: or The Political Events of the Next Thirteen Years, Described in Accordance with Prophecies in Ezekiel, Daniel, and the Apocalypse. Shewing Also the Important Position Britain Will Occupy during, and at the End of, the Awful Conflict*. A New Edition, Revised and Corrected by the Original Author, Dr. Thomas (Toronto: Thomas MacLear, 1853), iii–iv.

9. David King, "A Glance at the History and Mystery of Christadelphianism." *Ecclesiastical Observer*, 1881. Online, available at members.aol.com/eusebos/zpayne1/christad.htm, accessed August 21, 2008.

10. For the coincidence in names for the typically anonymous Pae, see Law, 48.

CHAPTER 4

Dissecting the Doctor: Mr. Jekyll, Dr. Hyde, and Robert Knox

1. *PMG* begins advertising the Christmas Extra on December 5, and by December 9 is naming "The Body Snatcher."

2. "Style" was still the preferred aspect of Stevenson for many critics. See reviews of *Across the Plains*, which focus not on the striking emigrant experience, but on its style (Maixner, 377–95).

3. Rosner questions whether Mary was a habitual prostitute, and whether the students may have known her not from the streets but from hospital rounds (*Anatomy*, ch. 5). Edwards credits

the popular version, and settles on Fergusson as the student to recognize Mary (*Burke*, 89 and 249). Stevenson echoes this story, whether fact or fiction.

4. Rae credits the letter to John Goodsir, Knox's "most distinguished pupil in anatomy" (150–51). However, he died in 1867. The statement may come from his brother, Joseph Goodsir, a minister and also a friend of Knox, who lived to 1893. Ross details Knox's relationships with the Goodsirs ("Robert Knox's Catalogue").

5. The original shows numerous excisions and insertions as Goodsir decides whether to attack the story's focus on Knox, or on his assistants. See 4–8.

6. For example Veeder and Hirsch; also Janice Doane and Devon Hodges, "Demonic Disturbances of Sexual Identity: The Strange Case of Dr. Jekyll and Mr/s Hyde," *Novel* 23.1 (Fall 1989): 63–74; and Patrick Scott, "Anatomizing Professionalism: Medicine, Authorship, and R. L. Stevenson's 'The Body Snatcher,'" *Victorians Institute Journal* 27: 113–30.

7. Stevenson hated Act IV, with its "cracksman business and...pasteboard murders" (Stevenson *Letters*, 4:80). To Charles Baxter he admitted, "I count the Deacon dead as mud....a dead rat" (4:139). When the play faltered in America, in part because of its unreliable lead, he wrote: "all I try to do for W. E....by writing these plays, is burked by this inopportune lad" (6:93). Two months later, it was make or break: "if [the play does not come off] this time, the Deacon is dead and buried; mind that" (6:116).

8. Mrs. Stevenson later made it known that she too recognized a story when she saw one, thinking Clark's opinion "a put-up thing" (Stevenson *Letters*, 2:3).

9. Richards, 393. Knox's blend of theories produced a racist idea about the physical and moral separation of races into species—which was nonetheless radical. In their appropriate locales, he found each race superior.

10. *Davos-Platz: A New Alpine Resort for Sick and Sound in Summer and Winter by One Who Knows It Well* (London: Edward Stanford, 1878), 12–13.

11. Hilary Marland tracks the growth of chemistry as a medical field, as chemists became distinct from apothecaries and their roles were regulated by the Apothecaries' Act (1815) and the Pharmacy Act (1868).

12. To W. E. Henley, [Late December 1884], Stevenson *Letters*, 5:52–53. For the change in medical understanding, see *Webster's Revised Unabridged Dictionary* of 1913.

13. A. Gordon Salamon, "Pasteur's Researches in Rabies," *PMG* January 20, 1885: 4–5; letter from Anna Kingsford, M. D., "The Alleged Cure for Hydrophobia," *PMG* January 28, 1885: 2.

14. Wells's story is bound with Burke and Hare plots in the film *Corridors of Blood*, featuring Boris Karloff (1958).

15. Louis Goodman and Alfred Gilman, eds., *The Pharmacological Basis of Therapeutics* (New York: Macmillan, 1970), 43. Horace Wells was inspired by the events of this performance.

16. Knox opposed vivisection, but given "a wider, popular view in the early-modern period: that death was, in some measure, a liminal state," maintained by Winslow, and given the mode of manufacture for Knox's cadavers, public attitudes would not admit as much (Patrizio and Kemp, 7).

17. Lonsdale, too, featured a girl who exposes the doctor: "Only once...did Knox exhibit any emotion on account of the connection of his name with the Burke and Hare atrocities, and his freely alleged complicity in the transaction....[A] pretty little girl about six years of age caught his notice....At length he gave her a penny, and said, 'Now, my dear, you and I will be friends. Would you come and live with me if you got a whole penny every day?' 'No,' said the child; 'you would, may be, sell me to Dr. Knox'" (115).

18. See Lazare, and Kevin Sack, "Doctors Say 'I'm Sorry' Before 'See You in Court,'" *New York Times* May 18, 2008. Online, available at nytimes.com/2008/05/18/us/18apology.html, accessed May 18, 2008.

CHAPTER 5

Anatomizing the Audience: James Bridie, Melodrama, and the Movies

1. See *McLevy: The Edinburgh Detective*, ed. Quintin Jardine (Edinburgh: Mercat, 2001), 20–30; *The McGovan Casebook* (Edinburgh: Mercat, 2003), 1–11.
2. Oliver Wendell Holmes, "Mechanism in Thought and Morals," Phi Beta Kappa address, Harvard, June 29, 1870 (Boston: Ticknor and Fields, 1871), 46. Edward M. Brecher et al., *Licit and Illicit Drugs* (Boston: Little, Brown, 1972), 316 n.19.
3. MS in Royal College of Surgeons (London). The archive credits the diary to Joshua Naples, active 1811–32. It was presented to the college by Sir Thomas Longmore, dresser for Bransby Cooper (nephew to Sir Astley).
4. "Moral," [sic] Carruthers logically corrects to "morale" (45), but I have not found MS or other evidence of a misprint.
5. Alfred Wilde premiered the part; it was suggested as a vehicle for Charles Laughton, and Seymour Hicks was rumored to be interested (NLS MS8181/8); W. G. Fay, cofounder of the Abbey Theatre in Dublin, recommended the part to Henry Ainley, who pursued it aggressively and performed it at the Westminster Theatre in London, 1931 (NLS MS8181/12); Sim played Knox in numerous productions: 1948, 1952, and the film of 1961.
6. RCSEd holds a Bridie letter to [Mr. Noel?], representing a Knox descendant, September 30, 1931; letter to Mr. Knox, December 1, 1931; letter from G. Kerr Pringle to Henry Ainley, November 16, 1931; letter from [illegible: notepaper of Francis Caird Inglis, Photographer to His Majesty the King] to Henry Ainley, October 16, 1931. The *Glasgow Bulletin* July 16, 1930 mentions a letter from an old lady who claims her uncle, Dr. Tibbets, drew the well-known illustrations of Daft Jamie and of a medical student.
7. By the time of MacDiarmid's review, Bridie had done well with *Tobias and the Angel* (1930), *The Girl Who Did Not Want to Go to Kuala Lumpur* (1930), *The Dancing Bear* (1931), *Jonah and the Whale* (1932), *The Amazed Evangelist* (1932), *A Sleeping Clergyman* (1933), *Marriage Is No Joke* (February 6, 1934), and *Colonel Wotherspoon* (March 23, 1934). Five were first staged in England. See chronology in Luyben, 173–75.
8. For a full sense of MacDiarmid and Bridie's occasionally heated opposition, see MacDiarmid *Raucle*, 3:95, 151–53, 202–6. For Bridie, see *Dramaturgy*, and "The Blighted Flyting" (NLS Acc11309/18). See also Bridie's response to MacDiarmid's criticism of the Edinburgh Festival that begins "Good (as they say) God! If this is Nationalistic Communism, give me Flat-earthism or Christian Science any day…this stuff is merely nasty raving" (NLS Acc11309/32), and Bridie's newspaper articles "The Raucle Scot" and "A Lucky Poet" (*GEN* February 26, 1943 and October 15, 1948).
9. Milton. I am indebted to Ann Featherstone for references to Burke and Hare in portable theater and penny geggies. Dr. Featherstone confirms that such plays "were so popular, so frequently performed, that a script wasn't needed, because performers could 'gag' the play (improvise it). I'm sure this was the case with Sweeney Todd and Maria Marten. Burke and Hare seems to fall into the same category" (e-mail, November 2008). See also *World's Fair* April 6, 1957: 14; December 3, 1955.

10. Bates cites an 1860s version as the earliest, but the 1839 reference implies earlier productions (Bates, 194 and n. 15).

11. Fyffe was father to Will Fyffe, known for later film roles and "I Belong to Glasgow."

12. David J. Skal, *Hollywood Gothic: The Tangled Web of Dracula from Novel to Stage to Screen*, describes the advertising hype for *Dracula*: packets of henbane, the threat of fainting, the presence of nurses (New York: Norton, 1990).

13. Joe Orton's black comedy was staged in 1965, then made into a film. Prod. Arthur Lewis, dir. Silvio Narizzano, Performing Arts, 1970. DVD Studio Canal 20.

14. Patrick McGilligan, *Alfred Hitchcock: A Life in Darkness and Light* (New York: HarperCollins, 2003), 387–88.

15. Bridie's filmography is a work in progress at IMDb.com.

16. The Italian Matania had been a war artist; *Britannia and Eve* occupied the market between women's and art magazine. Matania favored well-endowed, lightly draped figures.

17. *Doctor in Love* belonged in a series of "Doctor" movies (*Doctor in Trouble, Doctor at Large*, and so on). The films used a stock cast.

CHAPTER 6

Bringing Out the Dead: Silent Victims Speak in Alasdair Gray's Poor Things

1. Harry Lauder (1870–1950) was an internationally famous Scottish comedian. His best-known songs are "Roamin' in the Gloamin'," "I Love a Lassie," "A Wee Deoch and Doris," and "Keep Right on to the End of the Road." He is reputedly the first artist to sell a million records, but not beloved by Scottish cultural critics, who have thought he contributed to the sentimentalizing of Scottishness. See David Goldie, "Hugh MacDiarmid, Harry Lauder and Scottish Popular Culture," *International Journal of Scottish Literature* 1 (Autumn 2006). Online, available at ijsl.stir.ac.uk/issue1/goldie.htm, accessed May 23, 2009. "Red Clydeside" describes the 1910s–1930s political radicalism of Glasgow enacted through labor and rent strikes, and antiwar activism.

2. The twenty-nine "Carry On" movies were filmed from 1958 to 1978 at Pinewood Studios. They were notable for risqué humor and farcical plotting from an ensemble cast anchored by Sid James (the dirty old man) and Barbara Windsor (the over-endowed ingenue).

3. Edwards gave the lecture for the National Library of Scotland's "Burke and Hare, Rebus and Friends" exhibition. See "Auld Creepy," *The List* January 7, 2008. Online, available at list.co.uk/article/5926-burke-and-hare-themed-events/, accessed May 19, 2008. A *Scotsman* journalist reports: "To historian Owen Dudley Edwards, a Burke and Hare expert, it is no surprise the grisly case continues to fascinate." See "Dark deeds inspire a series of grisly events," *Living.Scotsman.com* January 5, 2008. Online, available at living.scotsman.com/people/Dark-deeds-inspire-a-series.3643967.jp, accessed May 19, 2008.

4. E-mail to Caroline McCracken-Flesher, June 11, 2008. Bianchi adds: "In true Brechtian...fashion, I presented the thesis: mankind must advance...and the antithesis: man murders man...and the synthesis of these two premises is left to the audience to decide."

5. E-mail to Caroline McCracken-Flesher, July 16, 2008. Crane adds: "the play was site-specific, with street songs, Irish ballads, grand guignol and human tragedy. The poor and down-and-out unwittingly giving their lives for the future health of the nation has a powerful modern ring."

6. E-mail to Caroline McCracken-Flesher, February 9, 2009.

7. The *Observer* December 1, 1974.

8. Margaret Thatcher, interview with Barbara Walters ABC, March 18, 1987.

9. The Scotland Act 1978 offered the possibility of a Scottish Assembly. The referendum required a majority to ratify the Act. Two conditions contributed to a negative result. First, the Assembly would have few powers; it was thus viewed not as an initial step in Scottish self-determination, but as an inadequate step. The only way to articulate reservations on these or other matters was by voting "no." Second, though 60% of registered voters did vote, the Act unusually required that 40% of registered voters (not of the turnout) had to vote "yes."

10. Laing counts as victims "The unborn, mothers and babies in childbirth, people deemed to have lost their minds…[They] are often entirely at the mercy of, in the complete power of, others" ("Notes").

CHAPTER 7

Resting in Pieces? Present Comforts or Restless Futures in Ian Rankin's Scotland

1. Press release, "First Minister applauds Edinburgh Festivals' plans for national Homecoming celebrations in 2009," *Homecoming Scotland*. Online, available at homecomingscotland2009.com/media-centre/festivals_release.html, accessed April 18, 2009.

2. Review of *I Sell the Dead*, at *The Film Fiend*. Online, available at thefilmfiend.com/2009/03/i-sell-dead.html, accessed April 24, 2009.

3. Lewis Tice, review of *I Sell the Dead*, *Philadelphia Film Festival*. Online, available at phillycinefest.com/film-details.cfm?id=8682, accessed April 24, 2009.

4. Chris Crawford, *Chris Crawford on Interactive Storytelling* (Berkeley: New Riders, 2005), 319.

5. Rickman describes his project at http://www.aaai.org/Papers/Symposia/Fall/1999/FS-99-01/FS99-01-021.pdf, accessed July 5, 2010; and also in Mateas and Sengers, eds., *Narrative Intelligence* (Philadelphia: John Benjamins, 2002), 131–42; see 134.

6. Shane Stevens on the website *Reloaded*: http://www.reloaded.org/interview.php?IntID=27&PID=287, accessed July 5, 2010.

7. Review of "Mind's Eye," *AGS wiki*. Online, available at americangirlscouts.org/agswiki/Mind's_Eye, accessed January 2, 2009. To get a sense of the game, see http://gamesolutions.efzeven.nl/minds-eye-walkthrough-shane-stevens2005/ and http://www.reloaded.org/interview.php?IntID=27&PID=287, accessed July 5, 2010.

8. "Stitch, Cut and Dye," and "humaneGames," *City without Walls*. Online, available at cwow.org/see/feature.php?f_id=142&s_id=2&c_id=5 and cwow.org/cwowfiles/NNM/StitchCutDye.pdf, accessed April 24, 2009.

9. See the *Fullmetal Alchemist* wiki: http://fma.wikia.com/wiki/Knox. *Fullmetal Alchemist* began as a serial for the *Shōnen Gangan* magazine (Tokyo: Square Enix, August 2001 to June 2010), and takes up twenty-five books. It developed into an anime, running for fifty-one episodes (October 4, 2003 to October 2, 2004), and produced a film sequel. It gave way to a second series, *Fullmetal Alchemist: Brotherhood*. There are spin-off novels, animations, audio-dramas, soundtracks and video games, also collectors cards and action figures. See: http://en.wikipedia.org/wiki/Fullmetal_Alchemist. Both sites accessed June 25, 2010.

10. Dorian Wiszniewski and Richard Coyne, "Mask and Identity: The Hermeneutics of Self-Construction in the Information Age," in K. Ann Renninger and Wesley Shumar, eds., *Building

Virtual Communities: Learning and Change in Cyberspace (Cambridge: Cambridge University Press, 2002), 191–214; see 211.

11. See Gallus website: galluspublications.co.uk/contact.htm.

12. E-mail to Caroline McCracken-Flesher, August 18, 2008.

13. *Ca$h in Christ*. Online, available at wisepart.com/CashinChrist/about.html, accessed March 29, 2008.

14. E-mail to Caroline McCracken-Flesher, August 18, 2008.

15. Ben Harrison, "Why I Do Site Specific Work." Online, available at benharrison.info/articles/sitespecific.htm, accessed June 9, 2008.

16. Stuart Simpson, "Burke and Hare," *CultureWars*. Online, available at culturewars.org.uk/edinburgh2003/morbid.burke.htm, accessed June 9, 2008.

17. Brian G. Cooper, "Greyfriars Twisted Tales," *Edinburgh Stage* August 11, 2008. Online, available at ed.thestage.co.uk/reviews/155, accessed May 26, 2009. Ophaboom's *Burke and Hare* (2004) may belong in this argument, but it is not referenced at the Festival. It reflects the ethos of such productions as they circulate through and beyond Edinburgh, featuring "Burke and Hare, the Laurel and Hardy of the morgues." See "Ophaboom Present World Premiere," *British Theatre Guide* February 8, 2004. Online, available at britishtheatreguide.info/news/burkeandhare.htm, accessed June 9, 2008.

18. Stuart Simpson, "Blood on the Stones," *CultureWars*. Online, available at culturewars.org.uk/edinburgh 2003/morbid/blood/htm, accessed June 9, 2008, also "Burke and Hare," above.

19. Rory Ford, "Twisted Tales," *Scotsman* August 6, 2008. Online, available at living.scotsman.com/music/Musical-review-Greyfriars-Twisted-Tales.4360981.jp, accessed May 26, 2009. For Lochaber, see BroadwayBaby.com: http://www.broadwaybaby.com/index.php?option=com_content&view=article&catid=46:current-edinburgh-festival&id=3308:burke-and-hare-a-musical-play&Itemid=66, accessed July 6, 2010.

20. Johanna Payton, "Burke and Hare Return to Edinburgh," *Garbled Communications*. Online, available at garbledonline.net/butcherthief.html, accessed April 27, 2009.

21. Tim Luckhurst, "Beware the Fantasies of Festival Edinburgh," *The Independent* August 23, 2004. Online, available at independent.co.uk/opinion/commentators/tim–luckhurst–beware–the–fantasies–of–festival–edinburgh–557469.html, accessed April 20, 2009.

22. Jeanette Oldham, "Council Decision 'Will Not Stop Exhibition of Skinless Corpses,'" *Scotsman* July 30, 2003. Online, available at news.scotsman.com/topics.cfm?tid=943&id=820012003, accessed September 1, 2005; Fiachra Gibbons, "Dr Death's Morgue Show Is Body Blow to Council," *Guardian* August 1, 2003. Online, available at guardian.co.uk/uk/2003/aug/01/edinburgh2003.arts, accessed April 18, 2009. Berliner says von Hagens did not play: "he felt he hadn't practiced enough"; O'Higgins remembers the strip club possibility. E-mail to McCracken-Flesher, September 28, 2010.

23. Elizabeth A. J. Scott confirms that Knox played the violin: "The Anatomist's Violin," *Hektoen International: A Journal of Medical Humanities* 1.3 (2009). Online, available at http://www.hektoeninternational.org/Journal_The_Anatomist.html, accessed September 4, 2009.

24. "Body Part Show: Prof Gunther von Hagens," *BBC* March 27, 2002. Online, available at news.bbc.co.uk/1/hi/talking_point/forum/1888662.stm, accessed September 1, 2005.

25. Von Hagens speaks from each perspective. When his London show opened, he told the BBC, "it's not dusty anatomy here—it's a kind of event anatomy—it's entertainment," but he went on, "[this space] was used for art and now it is used for anatomy." See previous note. The

audiotours for von Hagens's exhibits are similarly conflicted—and some dramatic displays bear the anatomist's signature as artist.

26. Dolan Cummings, "Corpus," *CultureWars*. Online, available at culturewars.org.uk/edinburgh 2003/morbid/corpus.htm, accessed March 29, 2008.

27. Angie Brown, "Over Our Dead Body," *Edinburgh Evening News* July 29, 2003. Online, available at news.scotsman.com/print.cfm?id=818992003, accessed September 1, 2005.

28. Jeanette Oldham, "Body Blow," *Scotsman* July 31, 2003. Online, available at news.scotsman.com/topics.cfm?tid=943&id=823382003, accessed September 1, 2005.

29. See http://www.the-dungeons.co.uk/edinburgh/en/attractions/burkehare.htm. The slogan is repeated at numerous tourist websites, for instance lastminute.com, 365tickets.com, easykidsshopping.co.uk.

30. "Nurses Bequeath Skeletons to Tourist Attraction to Highlight Shortage of Bodies for Trainee Doctors," *Daily Record* February 26, 2010. Online, available at http://www.dailyrecord.co.uk/news/weird-news/2010/02/26/nurses-bequeath-skeletons-to-tourist-attraction-to-highlight-shortage-of-bodies-for-trainee-doctors-86908-22071825/, accessed July 6, 2010.

31. See the coffins at the National Museums of Scotland website: http://www.nms.ac.uk/our_collections/collection_highlights/arthurs_seat_coffins.aspx, accessed July 6, 2010.

32. *The Meat Trade* has been "in production" for some time. See the IMDb website imdb.com/title/tt0466235/, accessed May 2, 2009. In 2009, Irvine Welsh reported filming about to commence (e-mail to Caroline McCracken-Flesher, May 4, 2009). Robert Carlyle's opposing manifestations come in *Trainspotting*, from Welsh's novel, dir. Danny Boyle (1996), and *Hamish Macbeth*, the BBC Scotland TV series about a local policeman (1995–97).

BIBLIOGRAPHY

ARCHIVES

British Library
Dundee Central Library (Local History Centre)
Edinburgh Central Library
Mitchell Library, Glasgow
National Library of Scotland
Pae family papers (Judith and Anthony Cooke)
Royal College of Physicians of Edinburgh
Royal College of Surgeons of Edinburgh
Royal Society of Edinburgh
Rylands Library Manchester
University of Bristol Theatre Collection
University of Edinburgh Centre for Research Collections
University of Glasgow Special Collections
University of Stirling Library
Wellcome Library, Wellcome Institute London

NEWSPAPERS AND JOURNALS

Aberdeen Press and Journal
Blackwood's Edinburgh Magazine
Caledonian Mercury
Courant

Curtain
Daily Telegraph
Dundee... People's Journal
Edinburgh Evening Courant
Edinburgh Evening Dispatch
Edinburgh Evening News
Edinburgh Weekly Chronicle
Edinburgh Weekly Journal
Era
Evening News
Evening Standard
Glasgow Bulletin
Glasgow Evening News
Glasgow Herald
Illustrated Sporting and Dramatic News
Lady
Lancet
Liverpool Post
Manchester Guardian
Medical Times and Gazette
Morning Post
News of the World
New Statesman and Nation
New York World Telegraph
Pall Mall Gazette
Saturday Review
Scotsman
Sheffield Daily Telegraph
Sphere
Stage
Star
Sunday Times
Times
Time and Tide
Worlds Fair

REFERENCE TEXTS

Dictionary of National Biography

PRIMARY BIBLIOGRAPHY: SOURCES AND HISTORIES

Academy of Death. Musical. *Audacious Productions*. Edinburgh Fringe, 2009.
Adam, H. L. *Burke and Hare, The Story of a Terrible Partnership*. London: C. Arthur Pearson, 1913; rpt. Mellifont Press, n.d.

Adams, Norman. *Dead and Buried? The Horrible History of Bodysnatching*. Aberdeen: Impulse Books, 1972.

———. *Scottish Bodysnatchers*. Musselburgh, Scotland: Goblinshead, 2002.

Anatomist, The. Dir. Dennis Vance. Writers James Bridie and Leonard William. With Alastair Sim. British International Pictures, 1961. DVD I.S. Filmworks, n.d.

Anatomist, The. Westminster Theatre Program. n.p: n.p., [1931].

"Apparent and Real Death." *Hogg's Weekly Instructor* NS 3 (1849): 307–8.

Atkinson, Kate. *One Good Turn*. 2006; rpt. New York: Little, Brown, 2007.

Authentic Confessions of William Burk, in the Jail. January 2, 1829; rpt Barzun: 230–36.

Bagby, Elizabeth. "Practical Anatomy." Perf. Storefront Theater Chicago, 2006. MS.

Bailey, Brian. *Burke and Hare: The Year of the Ghouls*. Edinburgh: Mainstream, 2002.

Bailey, James Blake. *The Diary of a Resurrectionist 1811–1812*. London: Swan Sonnenschein, 1896.

Baird, Donald. *Scottish Traveller Tales: Lives Shaped through Stories*. Jackson: University Press of Mississippi, 2002.

Ball, James Moores. *The Sack-'Em-Up Men: An Account of the Rise and Fall of the Modern Resurrectionists*. Edinburgh: Oliver & Boyd, 1928.

Ballance, Chris. *Water of Life*. 1989. MS GLA STA Js 9/3 and 9/5.

[Barclay, Dr. John]. *The Medical School of Edinburgh*. Edinburgh: Adam Black & David Brown, 1819.

Barzun, Jacques, ed. *Burke and Hare: The Resurrection Men*, subtitled *A Collection of Contemporary Documents Including Broadsides, Occasional Verses, Illustrations, Polemics, and a Complete Transcript of the Testimony at the Trial*. Metuchen, NJ: Scarecrow Press, 1974.

Bates, A. W. *The Anatomy of Robert Knox: Murder, Mad Science and Medical Regulation in Nineteenth-Century Edinburgh*. Brighton: Sussex Academic Press, 2010.

Berliner, Jonny, and Fintan O'Higgins. *Corpus*. Perf. Edinburgh Fringe, 2003. MS.

Bertram, James G. *The Story of a Stolen Heir*. 3 vols. London: T. C. Newby, 1858.

Bianchi, Dan. *The Burke and Hare Company*. Perf. Threepenny Theatre Company, New York, 1980. MS New York Public Library.

Blake, William. "An Island in the Moon." [1784–85]. In *Blake: Complete Writings with Variant Readings*. Oxford: Oxford University Press, 1966: 44–63.

Body Snatcher, The. Prod. Val Lewton. Dir. Robert Wise. Writers Philip MacDonald and Carlos Keith. With Boris Karloff and Bela Lugosi. RKO, 1945. DVD Warner Video, 2005.

Body Snatchers, The. UK/US crossover band. Singers 30H2 and BAOBINGA. Album *Feeling Good, Looking Nice, Smelling Right*. Passenger UK, 2008.

"Bodysnatching and Burking." *Once A Week* 10 (1863–64): 261–66.

Bodyworlds: The Anatomical Exhibition of Real Human Bodies. With Gunther von Hagens. DVD Heidelberg: Institute for Plastination, 2006.

Bolitho, William [Charles Ryall]. *Murder for Profit*. 1926; rpt. Marlboro, VT: The Marlboro Press, 1982.

Bonar, Horatius. *Edinburgh Tracts no.1: Christian Witness-Bearing Against the Sin of Intemperance*. Pamphlet. N.p.: n.p., n.d; rpt. *The Christian Repository* vol. 13 (1854): 425–26.

Bradley, James. *The Resurrectionist*. 2006; London: Faber and Faber, 2007.

Bridie, James. *The Anatomist*. Perf. July 6, 1930. *The Anatomist and Other Plays*. New York: Richard R. Smith, 1931.

———. "The Blighted Flyting of James Bridie and Hugh M'Diarmid." Handprinted. Bridie Published Speeches, etc., NLS Acc11309/18.

———. *Dramaturgy in Scotland*. Proceedings of the Royal Philosophical Society of Scotland 74.1 (1949).

———. *One Way of Living*. London: Constable, 1939.

———. *The Scottish Character As It Was Viewed by Scottish Authors from Galt to Barrie*. The John Galt Lecture for 1937. Papers of the Greenock Philosophical Society. Greenock, Scotland: Telegraph, 1937.

———. *The Switchback*. Perf. March 9, 1929. 2nd ed. London: Constable, 1932.

Bryson, Hector. *Doctors, Bodies and Snatchers*. Edinburgh: Canongate, 1978.

Bulwer Lytton, Sir Edward. *Lucretia or the Children of the Night*. London: Saunders and Otley, 1846.

Burke and Hare. Dir. John Landis. With Simon Pegg and Andy Serkis. Ealing Studios, 2010.

Burke and Hare. Radio program in series *The Secrets of Scotland Yard*, 22:33 minutes. Prod. Towers of London, [c. 1949–51]. Rebroadcast Mutual Broadcasting Group, America. Online, available at archive.org/details/OTRR_Secrets_Of_Scotland_Yard_Singles. Accessed May 21, 2009.

"Burke and Hare." Song. *The Sugar Puff Demons*. On *Falling From Grace*. 1989.

Burke and Hare: A Musical Play. Dir. George Young. Perf. Lochaber Onstage! Edinburgh Festival, August 11, 2009.

Burke and Hare: The Body Snatchers. (Inside title *Burke and Hare: Their True Lives, with Lives of the Resurrectionists*.) Glasgow: D. R. Burnside, [1910].

Burke and Hare: The Business of Murder. Edinburgh Dungeon show. Advertised online at the-dungeons.co.uk/edinburgh/en/attractions/burkehare.htm. Accessed July 6, 2010.

"Burke and Hare: The Musical." 2 parts. Dir. Stephen Murphy. With Sandy Nelson and Ricky Callan. Online, *Shadowplay*. Available at dcairns.wordpress.com/2008/09/30/edinburgh-1928/. Accessed April 27, 2009.

Burke, Raymond. *The Return of Burke and Hare*. Perf. Edinburgh Fringe, 1991. Glasgow: Dualchas, 1994.

"Burkism!" Broadsheet. Edinburgh: John Murray, [1831].

Byrd, Elizabeth. *Rest Without Peace*. 1974; New York: Avon, 1975.

———. *The Search for Maggie Hare*. 1976; New York: Avon, 1977.

Christison, Robert. *The Life of Sir Robert Christison, Bart*. Ed. by his Sons. 2 vols. Edinburgh: William Blackwood and Sons, 1885 and 1886.

Cockburn, Henry. *Memorials of his Time*. Edinburgh: Adam and Charles Black, 1856.

Cole, Hubert. *Things for the Surgeon: A History of the Resurrection Men*. London: William Heinemann, 1964.

Combe, George. *Answer to "Observations on the Phrenological Development of Burke, Hare, and Other Atrocious Murderers, &C" by Thomas Stone, Esq*. Edinburgh: John Anderson, 1829.

Conaghan, Martin, and Will Pickering. *Burke and Hare*. Comic Book. Edinburgh: Insomnia, 2009.

Corridors of Blood. Dir. Robert Day. Screenplay Jean Scott Rogers. With Boris Karloff. Producers Associates, 1958. DVD Image Entertainment, 1996.

Cowan, Charles. *The Danger, Irrationality, and Evils of Medical Quackery; Also, the Causes of Its Success; the Nature of Its Machinery; the Amount of Government Profits; with Reasons Why It Should Be Suppressed: and an Appendix Containing the Composition of Many Popular Quack Medicines: Addressed to All Classes*. London: Sherwood and Co., 1839.

Crane, Richard. "Burke and Hare." Perf. Tron Theatre Glasgow, 1983. Play not extant.
"Cure, The." *Smallville*. Episode 136 (Season 7: Episode 4, aired October 18, 2007 on The CW).
Currie, Andrew S. "Robert Knox, Anatomist, Scientist, and Martyr." *Proceedings of the Royal Society of Medicine* 26.1 (November 1, 1932): 177–87.
Day, Samuel Phillips. "Simple and Sanitary Burial." *Victoria Magazine* 32 (1879): 576–80; 33: 74–81; 163–67; 272–75.
de Quincey, "Second Paper on Murder Considered as One of the Fine Arts." *Blackwood's* 46.289 (November 1839): 661–68.
"Destiny," *Hamish Macbeth*. Writer Daniel Boyle. With Robert Carlyle. BBC Scotland, 1997. DVD *Hamish Macbeth* Series 3 Disk 2, BBC, 2006.
Dickens, Charles. *A Tale of Two Cities*. 1859; rpt. New York: Penguin, 2003.
Doctor and the Devils, The. Dir. Freddie Francis. Screenplay Ronald Harwood based on Dylan Thomas. With Timothy Dalton, Twiggy, Jonathan Pryce, Patrick Stewart, and Sian Phillips. Brooksfilms, 1985. DVD Twentieth Century Fox, 2005.
Doctor in Love. Dir. Ralph Thomas. With James Robertson Justice and Leslie Phillips. Rank, 1960. DVD Wham!USA, 2007.
Doctor Jekyll and Sister Hyde. Dir. Roy Ward Baker. With Ralph Bates and Martine Beswick. Hammer Film Productions, 1971. VHS Thorn Emi/HBO, n.d.
Doctor Who: Assassins in the Limelight. Audiobook. Dir. Barnaby Edwards. Writer Robert Ross. With Colin Baker and Leslie Phillips. N.p.: Big Finish Productions, 2008.
Doctor Who: Medicinal Purposes. Audiobook. Dir. Gary Russell. Writer Robert Ross. With Colin Baker and Leslie Phillips. Big Finish Productions, 2004.
Doherty, Karen. *Murderers! A Story of Burke and Hare*. Dunfermline, Scotland: Gallus, 2004.
Douglas, Hugh. *Burke and Hare: The True Story*. London: Robert Hale and Company, 1973.
Douglas, Sheila, ed. and intro. *The King of the Black Art and Other Folk Tales*. Aberdeen: Aberdeen University Press, 1987.
Dr. Bell and Mr. Doyle: The Dark Beginnings of Sherlock Holmes. Pilot for *Murder Rooms: Mysteries of the Real Sherlock Holmes*. Dir. Paul Seed. Writer David Pirie. BBC 2000. DVD BFS, 2003.
"Dr. K—Project, The." Designer Brandon Rickman. Videogame, n.d. Described at aaai.org/Papers/Symposia/Fall/1999/FS-99-01/FS99-01-021.pdf. Accessed July 5, 2010.
DR. Knox. UK hip-hop band. Singers Malakai and Wisdomtooth. Album *IEGO*. Rough Records UK, 2006.
Drummond, Andrew. *Elephantina: A Huge Misunderstanding*. Edinburgh: Polygon, 2008.
Edwards, Owen Dudley. *Burke and Hare*. 1980. 2nd. ed. Edinburgh: Mercat Press, 1993.
———. *Hare and Burke*. Dir. Ben Harrison. Perf. Edinburgh Fringe Festival, 1994. Edinburgh: Diehard, 1994.
"Elegiac Lines on the Tragical Murder of Poor Daft Jamie." Ballad. Edinburgh: Willie Smith, [1829].
Extreme Measures. Dir. Michael Apted. With Gene Hackman and Hugh Grant. Castle Rock, 1996. DVD Warner Brothers, 1999.
Finnemore, John, and Owen Powell. "Burke and Hare." Perf. Ophaboom, Unity Theatre Liverpool, 2004. MS not accessed.
Flesh and the Fiends, The. Aka *Mania* and *Psychokillers*. Dir. and written John Gilling. With Peter Cushing. Independent International Pictures, 1960. USA aka *The Fiendish Ghouls*, 1965 (cut 23 minutes). DVD Image Entertainment, 2000.

Forster, Joseph. *Studies in Black and Red*. London: Ward and Downey, 1896.
"Full and Particular Account of the Riot Which Took Place in Edinburgh on Thursday Last; Also of the Hoax Played Off on a Celebrated *Doctor*." Broadsheet. RCPEd R14988.
Fullmetal Alchemist. Manga. *Shōnen Gangan* magazine. Tokyo: Square Enix, August 2001–.
Galt, John. "The Buried Alive." *Blackwood's* 10.56 (October 1821): 262–64; rpt. *The Steam Boat*. New York: S. Campbell & Son, 1823: 169–73.
Gerritsen, Tess. *The Bone Garden*. New York: Ballantine, 2008.
Ghoul's Gold. Crime Does NOT Pay 43. Comic. Text Robert Bernstein. Illus. Jack Alderman. [New York]: Lev Gleason Publications, 1946. Online, available at pappysgoldenage.blogspot.com/2008/03/number-282-burke-and-hare-to-burke-is.html. Accessed May 30, 2008.
Goodsir, [Joseph]. Letter to *PMG*. "Linked Memories. Fife Coast, etc." NLS MS170 ff. 48–67.
Goodwin, I. *Bury Me in Lead*. London: Allan Wingate, 1952.
Graham, Mark. *The Resurrectionist: A Mystery of Old Philadelphia*. New York: Harper Collins, 1999.
"Grand Exhibition of the Effects Produced by Inhaling Nitrous Oxide, Exhilarating, or Laughing Gas, A." 1845.
Grant, David. "The Resurrectionists." *Scotch Stories or The Chronicles of Keckleton*. Edinburgh: E. and S. Livingstone, 1888: 27–52.
Grant, James. *Old and New Edinburgh*. 6 vols. London: Cassell, Petter, Galpin & Co., 1880s.
Gray, Alasdair. *Poor Things: Episodes from the Early Life of Archibald McCandless M.D. Scottish Public Health Officer*. London: Harcourt Brace Jovanovich, 1992.
Greed of William Hart, The. See *Horror Maniacs*.
Greg, W. R. *Observations on a Late Pamphlet by Mr Stone, on the Phrenological Development of Burke, Hare, &c*. Edinburgh: John Anderson, 1829.
Greyfriars Twisted Tales. With "The Martians." Perf. Bridewell Theatre Company and City of the Dead Walking Tours, Edinburgh Fringe, 2008. MS not accessed.
Guthrie, G. J. *Remarks on the Anatomy Bill Now Before Parliament*. London: Wm. Sams, 1832.
"Haddington Cobbler Defended, or the Doctors Dissected! Being a Reply to Three Poems Published by the Resurrection Men." By an East Linton Gravedigger. Scotland: n.p., n.d. Bound with Dr. Barclay, *The Medical School of Edinburgh*. UE.
"Haddington Cobbler Dissected Alive, in Answer to His Objections against Dissecting the Dead, The." Scotland: n.p., n.d. Bound with Dr. Barclay, *The Medical School of Edinburgh*. UE.
Hannibal. Dir. Ridley Scott. With Anthony Hopkins. MGM 2001. DVD MGM 2001.
Harris, Thomas. *Hannibal*. New York: Dell, 2000.
Hastings, N. *Burke & Hare*. Lord Chamberlain's Pamphlets, BL LCP 1947/8.
Hastings, Neil. *Burke & Hare*. Lord Chamberlain's Pamphlets, BL LCP 1966/20.
Henley, William Ernest. *In Hospital*. Portland, ME: Thomas B. Mosher, 1908. Many poems first published in *Cornhill*, 1875.
———. *The Selected Letters of W. E. Henley*. Ed. Damian Atkinson. Aldershot, England: Ashgate, 2000.
Hogg, James. *The Private Memoirs and Confessions of a Justified Sinner*. 1824. Ed. P. D. Garside. Edinburgh: Edinburgh University Press, 2001.
Holman, Sheri. *The Dress Lodger*. New York: Random House, 2000.
Hood, Evelyn. *A Wake for Donald*. Studio City, CA: Players Press, 1996.
Hood, Thomas. "Mary's Ghost." *The Complete Thomas Hood*. Ed. Walter Jerrold. London: Henry Frowde, 1906: 77.

Hooper, Mary. *Bodies for Sale*. London: Franklin Watts, 1999.

Horrible Histories Bus Tour (Edinburgh). Scripted and read Terry Deary. Online marykingsghostfest.com/calendar#1. Accessed July 6, 2010.

Horrible Histories "Vile Victorians." Season 1 Episode 13. Dir. Steve Connelly. BBC, screened July 9, 2009. Video online at Rosner, *Burke and Hare* website.

Horror Maniacs, aka The Greed of William Hart. Dir. Oswald Mitchell. Writer John Gilling. With Tod Slaughter. Bushey Studios/Gilbert Church Productions, 1948. DVD Alpha Video Productions, 2004.

Horrors of Burke and Hare, The. Dir. Vernon Sewell. Screenplay Ernle Bradford. Kenneth Shipman Productions, 1971. VHS New World Video, 1986.

House, Jack. *The Heart of Glasgow*. Rev. ed. London: Hutchinson, 1972.

If a Body Need a Body, Just Call Burke and Hare. Audio. Host, Thomas Highland. CBS Crime Classics. Broadcast December 2, 1952. Online, available at mediafire.com/?izdvoxztmjl. Accessed September 4, 2010.

I Sell the Dead! Dir. Glenn McQuaid. Glass Eye Pix, 2008. DVD with comic MPI, 2010.

"Jamie Wilson's Mother's Dream." Ballad. Edinburgh: W. Smith, [1829].

Johnson, A. "My Friend Dr Knox: A Pupil Writes about the Anatomist." *Surgeon* 3.6 (2005): 407–10.

Johnston, Paul. *Body Politic*. 1997; New York: St. Martin's, 1999.

"Key to Mr. Stevenson's 'Body-Snatcher,' A." *Pall Mall Gazette*, February 3, 1885: 6.

King, David. "A Glance at the History and Mystery of Christadelphianism." *Ecclesiastical Observer*, 1881. Online, available at members.aol.com/eusebos/zpayne1/christad.htm. Accessed August 21, 2008.

Kneale, Matthew. *English Passengers*. 2000; rpt. London: Penguin, 2001.

Knight, Alanna. *Burke and Hare*. Richmond, England: The National Archives, 2007.

Knox, Robert. "Anatomical Museums; Their Objects and Present Condition." *Medical Times* 14 (1846): 307–9 and 327–30.

———. *Fish and Fishing in the Lone Glens of Scotland*. London: G. Routledge & Co., 1854.

———. *Great Artists and Great Anatomists: A Biographical and Philosophical Study*. London: John Van Voorst, 1852.

———. "Inquiry into the Structure and Probable Functions of the Capsules Forming the Canal of PETIT, and of the Marsupium Nigrum, or the Peculiar Vascular Tissue Traversing the Vitreous Humour in the Eyes of Birds, Reptiles, and Fishes." Read March 15, 1824. *Transactions of the Royal Society of Edinburgh*, 10. Edinburgh: William Tait, 1826: 231–51.

———. *Letter to the Right Honourable the Lord Provost and Town-Council of Edinburgh*. July 6, 1837. Wellcome Medical Pamphlets 186 T.334.

———. *A Manual of Artistic Anatomy for the Use of Sculptors, Painters, and Amateurs*. London: Henry Renshaw, 1852.

———. *The Races of Men: A Fragment*. Philadelphia: Lea and Blanchard, 1850.

———. *Second Letter to the Right Honourable Lord Provost and Town-Council of Edinburgh*. July 15, 1837. Wellcome Medical Pamphlets 186. T.334.

Laconic Narrative of the Life and Death of James Wilson, Known by the Name of Daft Jamie. To Which Is Added a Few Anecdotes Relative to Him and His Old Friend Boby Awl, an Idiot Who Strolled about Edinburgh for Many Years, A. Edinburgh: W. Smith, 1829.

Lacroix, Jules. *L'Etouffer d'Edimbourg*. 2 vols. Paris: Cadot, 1844. (Not sourced.)

"Late Dr. Knox, The." Obit. *Medical Times and Gazette.* December 27, 1862: 683–85.

Leighton, Alexander. *The Court of Cacus; The Story of Burke and Hare.* London: Houlston and Wright, 1861.

———. "Mrs Corbet's Amputated Toe." *Mysterious Legends of Edinburgh.* Edinburgh: William P. Nimmo, 1864: 30–56.

Life and Times of Burke and Hare. Unacknowledged copy from Leighton's *Court.* Edinburgh: Hugh Jamieson, [1900].

"Lines Supposed to Have Been Written by Mrs. Wilson, Daft Jamie's Mother." Broadside Ballad. 1829. NLS RyIII.a.6(022).

Lonsdale, Henry. *A Sketch of the Life and Writings of Robert Knox the Anatomist.* London: Macmillan, 1870.

"Lost Will, The." *The Buchan Clown* 1.5 (July 1, 1838): 43–47.

MacDonald, Ross. *Famous Edinburgh Crimes.* 1953; Newtowngrange, Scotland: Lang Syne, 1987.

McDonald, Hal. *The Anatomists.* New York: HarperCollins, 2008.

MacGregor, George. *The History of Burke and Hare and of the Resurrectionist Times.* Glasgow: Thomas D. Morison, 1884.

MacKay, G. Eric. "Premature Burials" *Belgravia* 35 (1878): 95–103.

Mania. See *The Flesh and the Fiends.*

Marshall, Alice J. *Catalogue of the Anatomical Preparations of Dr. William Hunter.* Glasgow: University of Glasgow, 1970.

Marshall, Tim. *Murdering to Dissect: Grave-Robbing,* Frankenstein *and the Anatomy Literature.* Manchester: Manchester University Press, 1995.

Matania, F., writer and illustrator. "Old Tales Revived: Murder in Auld Reekie. The Crimes of Burke and Hare." *Britannia and Eve* August 1939: 32–37.

McGee, James. *Resurrectionist.* London: HarperCollins, 2007.

"McGregor Affair, The." *The Alfred Hitchcock Hour.* Season 3, Episode 7. Aired 23 November 1964. Dir. David Friedkin. Writers Morton S. Fine and David Friedkin. Alfred J. Hitchcock Productions. Online, available Flixster streaming video at flixster.com/watch-tv/alfred-hitchcock-hour--the-mcgregor-affair. Accessed September 4, 2010.

McNaughton, Douglas. "The Resurrectionists by Walter Scott." Edinburgh University Press Publicity Leaflet Spoof. March 2001.

Mercy/Mercey, Frédéric [de]. "Burk L'Etouffeur." Episodes in *Revue de Paris* NS 4- (1845); rpt. Paris: Hachette, 1858.

Miller, Leslie Adrienne. *The Resurrection Trade.* Saint Paul, MN: Graywolf, 2007.

Milton, Dick. "Theatre Rural, Dairy Lane: A Record of 'Portable' Performances, Consisting of Crimson Crimes, Dreadful Dramas, and Popular Plays of the Past." *World's Fair* June 30, 1962.

"Mind's Eye." Designer Shane Stevens. Videogame, 2005. Described at gamesolutions.efzeven.nl/minds-eye-walkthrough-shane-stevens2005/. Accessed July 5, 2010. Referenced at AGS wiki americangirlscouts.org/agswiki/Mind's_Eye. Accessed January 28, 2009.

Mitchell, Robin. *Grave Robbers.* Edinburgh: Luath, 1999.

———. [pseud. Adam Lyal]. *Witchery Tales: The Darker Side of Old Edinburgh.* 1988; rpt. Edinburgh: The Cadies, 1999.

Moir, David Macbeth. *The Life of Mansie Wauch, Tailor in Dalkeith.* 1828; Edinburgh: William Blackwood, 1905.

———. "Mansie Wauch's Dream." Broadside. 2 parts. 1829. NLS Ry.III.a.6.025.

Morgan, Edwin. "Caledonian Antisyzygy." In *Edwin Morgan Collected Poems*. Manchester: Carcanet, 1990: 446–47.

Morgan, Nicola. *Fleshmarket*. London: Hodder, 2003.

Murderers of the Close; A Tragedy of Real Life. London: Cowie and Strange, 1829.

Necessary Evil, A. Dir. Natalie Mains. Screened September 21, 2009, BBC 1 Northern Ireland and BBC HD; 28 September, BBC 2 Scotland. Information at bbc.co.uk/programmes/boon1lkj.

"Newgate Annual, The." *New Monthly Magazine* 58.229 (January 1840): 112–25.

Newman, Terry. *Burke and Hare*. With Rob Crouch. Perf. Skullduggery Theatre Company, Edinburgh Fringe, 2003. MS not accessed.

Nightmare in Blood. Dir. John Stanley. Writer Kenn Davis. With Kerwin Mathews. Xeromega, 1976. DVD Image Entertainment, n.d.

Norwood, Allan. *The Flesh and the Fiends*. Book from the movie. London: Corgi, 1960.

Noxiana. Edinburgh: Nimmo, 1829.

"On the Pleasures of 'Body-Snatching.'" [By L. R.]. *Monthly Magazine* NS 3 (April 1827): 355–65.

Pae, David. *The Coming Struggle Among the Nations of the Earth: or, The Political Events of the Next Fifteen Years Described in Accordance with Prophecies in Ezekiel, Daniel, and the Apocalypse. Showing Also the Important Position Britain Will Occupy during and at the End of, the Awful Conflict*. London: Houlston and Stoneman, 1853; rpt. in *Lucy*, ed. Law, 2001: 307–30.

———. *Lucy, the Factory Girl; or, The Secrets of the Tontine Close*. Newspaper serial, *North Briton* November 20, 1858–April 13, 1859; rpt. Graham Law ed., Hastings, England: Sensation Press, 2001.

———. *Mary Paterson; or, The Fatal Error*. Newspaper Serial *Dundee, Perth, Forfar, and Fife People's Journal* July 9, 1864–April 22, 1865; rpt. Dundee: John Leng, [1865].

[Paterson, David]. *Letter to the Lord Advocate, Disclosing the Accomplices, Secrets, and Other Facts Relative to the Late Murders; with a Correct Account of the Manner in Which the Anatomical Schools Are Supplied with Subjects, by the Echo of Surgeons Square*. Edinburgh: n.p., 1829.

Pelham, Camden, esq. "William Burke." *The Chronicles of Crime; or The New Newgate Calendar*. London: Thomas Tegg, 1841, vol. 2: 166–85.

Rae, Isobel. *Knox the Anatomist*. Edinburgh: Oliver and Boyd, 1964.

Rankin, Ian. *The Falls*. 2000; New York: St. Martins, 2003.

———. *Resurrection Men*. 2001; London: Orion, 2002.

———. *Set in Darkness*. 2000; New York: St. Martins, 2001.

Ranking, B. Montgomerie. "A Night in a Dissecting Room." *Belgravia* 32 (1878–79): 122–26.

Ravenous. Dir. Antonia Bird. With Guy Pearce, Robert Carlyle, David Arquette. Twentieth-Century Fox, 1999. DVD 2005.

Reece, Richard. *A Correct Statement of the Circumstances That Attended the Last Illness and Death of Mrs. Southcott, With an Account of the Appearances Exhibited on Dissection: and the Artifices That Were Employed to Deceive Her Medical Attendants*. London: n.p., 1815.

"Reflections Suggested by the Murders Recently Committed in Edinburgh, &c. Being an Epistle to the Right Hon Robert Peel, M.P.... in Which, Burke's Iniquitous Practices Are Traced to Their Real Source, and an Attempt Made to Indicate Measures Whereby the Recurrence of Similar Enormities May Be for Ever Prevented." By A Medical Officer in the Royal Navy. Glasgow: W. R. M'Phun., 1829.

Report from the Select Committee on Anatomy. London: House of Commons, 1828.

Richardson, Ruth. *Death, Dissection and the Destitute*. 1987. 2nd ed. Chicago: University of Chicago Press, 2000.

Rickman, Brandon. "The Dr. K——Project." Michael Mateas and Phoebe Sengers, eds., *Narrative Intelligence*. Philadelphia: John Benjamins, 2002: 131–42.

Robinson, J. H. *Marietta, or the Two Students: A Tale of the Dissecting Room and "Body Snatchers."* Boston: Jordan & Wiley, 1846. (Incomplete).

Robinson, Peter. "Blood on the Stones." Perf. Carpe Diem, Edinburgh Fringe, 2003. No MS extant. Information at carpe-diem-productions.com/Blood.html. Accessed June 10, 2008.

Robison, Sir John. Inventor. Material Relating to Papers Received by the RSE, 1828–31. NLS Acc. 10000/328.

———. Robison Correspondence. NLS Acc 10000/352.

Rodger, Johnny, and K. D. Farquharson. *(g) haun(s) Q*. Glasgow: Dualchas, 1996.

Rosner, Lisa. *The Anatomy Murders: Being the True yet Spectacular History of Edinburgh's Notorious Burke and Hare and of the Man of Science Who Abetted Them in the Commission of Their Most Heinous Crimes*. Philadelphia: University of Pennsylvania Press, 2010.

———. BurkeandHare.com. Website.

Ross, James A. and Hugh W. Y. Taylor. "Robert Knox's Catalogue." *Journal of the History of Medicine and Allied Sciences* 10 (1955): 269–76.

Roughead, William. *Burke and Hare*. Toronto: Canada Law Book Company, 1921.

———. *Knave's Looking-Glass*. London: Cassell, 1935.

———. "The Wolves of the West Port." 1938. *The Murderer's Companion*. New York: The Press of the Readers Club, [1941]: 115–74.

Rowland, Sidney. "The McGregor Affair." *Ellery Queen's Mystery Magazine* 22.116 (July 1953): 81–88.

Royal Society of Edinburgh General Minute Book. January 1824–May 1843. NLS Acc. 10000/5.

Sadducee, or, a Review of Some Pamphlets Lately Published on Important Subjects, by Mr Yorick, The. Edinburgh: Printed for the Booksellers, 1819. Wellcome, *Medical Pamphlets* 186, pamphlet 11.

"Sanctity of the Dead—Dissection." *Metropolitan* 3 (1832): 131–37.

Scarborough, Elizabeth Ann. *The Lady in the Loch*. 1998; rpt. New York: Ace, 1999.

Schwob, Marcel. "Messrs. Burke and Hare—Assassins." *Imaginary Lives*. Trans. Harry Hives. Wakefield, NH: Longwood Academic, 87–90.

Scott, Walter. *Disputatio Juridica, Ad Tit. XXIV. Lib. XLVIII. Pand. De Cadaveribus Damnatorum*. Edinburgh: Balfour & Smellie, 1792.

———. *The Journal of Sir Walter Scott*. Ed. W. E. K. Anderson. 1972; Edinburgh: Canongate, 1998.

———. *The Letters of Sir Walter Scott*. 12 vols. Ed. H. J. C. Grierson. 1936–1937 ; rpt. New York: AMS Press, 1971.

———. ["Malachi Malagrowther" Letters]. *Thoughts on the Proposed Change of Currency*. Intro. David Simpson and Alastair Wood. New York: Barnes & Noble, 1972.

"Search for Burke and Hare, The." Aka. "In Search of Burke and Hare." With David Hayman. History Channel (UK.). Scheduled October 29, 2010. Online, excerpts the historychannel. co.uk/videos.html?bctid=619562595001&In-Search-of-Burke-and-Hare: Skeletons.

Sergeant, Adeline. *Dr. Endicott's Experiment*. New York: The Mershon Company, 1894.
See, William. "The Extreme Rarity of Premature Burials." *Popular Science Monthly* 17 (1880): 526–30.
Sharpe, Charles Kirkpatrick. West Port Murders. MS Collection, ECL.
Smith, Adam. *The Theory of Moral Sentiments*. 1759. Ed. D. D. Raphael and A. L. Macfie. Oxford: Clarendon Press, 1976.
[Smith, Thomas Southwood]. *Use of the Dead to the Living*. *Westminster Review* 1824; rpt. London: Baldwin and Cradock, 1828.
Smith, W. Gordon. *Mister Jock*. Edinburgh Festival, 1987. Online, available at arts.gla.ac.uk/STELLA/STARN/scotplay/SMITH/MRJOCK/intro.htm. Accessed March 28, 2008.
Smith, William. [The Haddington Shoemaker]. *A Collection of Original Poems, Moral, Instructive, and Entertaining*. Edinburgh: Printed for the author by Balfour and Clarke, 1821.
Spoliation of the Grave: The Trial of John Eaton, Sexton of "St. George's Chapel," Manchester, Convicted of Felony, On Friday, May 11 1827 … Considerations in Reference to the Safest Mode of Interment, and Cases of Body-Stealing in Manchester, Liverpool and Nottingham. Manchester: J. Pratt, n.d.
Stephen, Kathy. *Scottish Men of Medicine: Robert Knox M.D., F.R.S.E. (1791–1862)*. Edinburgh: n.p., 1981).
Stephenson, Shelagh. *An Experiment with an Air Pump*. Perf. Manchester, February 12, 1998. New York: Dramatists Play Service, 2000.
Stevenson, Robert Louis. "The Body Snatcher." *Pall Mall Gazette* Christmas "Extra." 1884: 3–12.
———. "A Chapter on Dreams." *Scribner's Magazine* 3 (January 1888): 122–28; rpt. Glenda Norquay, ed. *R. L. Stevenson on Fiction: An Anthology of Literary and Critical Essays*. Edinburgh: Edinburgh University Press, 1999: 136–38.
———. *Deacon Brodie: Or the Double Life*. Prod. 1882. *The Works of Robert Louis Stevenson* vol. 24. London: William Heinemann, 1924: 1–82.
———. *The Letters of Robert Louis Stevenson*. Ed. Bradford A. Booth and Ernest Mehew. 8 vols. New Haven, CT: Yale University Press, 1994–95.
———. *Strange Case of Dr Jekyll and Mr Hyde*. 1886. Ed. Richard Dury. Edinburgh: University of Edinburgh Press, 2004.
———, and Lloyd Osborne. *The Wrong Box*. 1889; rpt. New York: Dover, 1985.
"Stitch, Cut & Dye." Videogame, 2007. Developer Heidi J. Boisvert. Referenced at City Without Walls website: cwow.org/see/feature.php?f_id=142&s_id=2&c_id=5. Accessed April 24, 2009.
Stocks, Robert, and Tommy Luther. "The Butcher and the Thief." Perf. CAA, Covent Garden, 2005; Edinburgh Fringe, 2005. MS.
Stone, Thomas. *Observations on the Phrenological Development of Burke, Hare, and Other Atrocious Murderers; Measurements of the Heads of the Most Notorious Thieves Confined in the Edinburgh Jail and Bridewell, and of Various Individuals, English, Scotch, and Irish, Presenting an Extensive Series of Facts Subversive of Phrenology*. Edinburgh: Robert Buchanan, 1829.
Symonds, Deborah A. *Notorious Murders, Black Lanterns, & Moveable Goods: The Transformation of Edinburgh's Underworld in the Early Nineteenth Century*. Akron, OH: University of Akron Press, 2006.
Taylor, Joseph. *The Danger of Premature Interment, Proved from Many Remarkable Instances*. London: n.p. 1816.

Taylor, Rev. Robert. "Christianity, the Cause of Crime." *The Lion* 3.2 (January 9, 1829): 49–54.

Thomas, Dylan. *The Doctor and the Devils*. Screenplay 1953; n.p.: New Directions, 1970. See also *Doctor and the Devils, The*.

Thomas, Dr. [John]. *The Coming Struggle among the Nations of the Earth: or The Political Events of the Next Thirteen Years, Described in Accordance with Prophecies in Ezekiel, Daniel, and the Apocalypse. Shewing Also the Important Position Britain Will Occupy during, and at the End of, the Awful Conflict*. A New Edition, Revised and Corrected by the Original Author, Dr. Thomas. Toronto: Thomas MacLear, 1853.

"Timely Hint to Anatomical Practitioners and Their Associates—the Resurrectionists, A." Ballad. Edinburgh: W. Smith, [1829].

Tobar an Dualchais/Kist o Riches. Website. Oral Narratives 22503/1, 4314/3, 55955/3, 2836/3, 2833/3, 44611/3, 14364/3.

Townsend, John. *Burke and Hare: The Body Snatchers*. Cheltenham: Nelson Thornes, 2001.

———. *A Painful History of Medicine: Scalpels, Stitches, and Scars*. Chicago: Raintree, 2005: 24 ff.

Trial of William Burke and Helen M'Dougal Before the High Court of Justiciary at Edinburgh on Wednesday, December 24, 1828 for the Murder of Margery Campbell or Docherty. Edinburgh: Robert Buchanan, William Hunter, John Stevenson, Baldwin & Cradock, 1829.

Turner, Cecil Howard. *The Inhumanists*. London: Alexander Ouseley, 1932.

Turner, John, ed. *The Anatomical Memoirs of John Goodsir, with a Biographical Memoir by Henry Lonsdale, M. D*. Edinburgh: Adam and Charles Black, 1868.

"Up the Close and Down the Stair." Cache GPS tour. Available at geocaching.com/seek/cache_details.aspx?guid=5cefffb3-27ee-4f40-9e27-bca37faa3821. Accessed June 11, 2009.

Ure, Andrew. "An Account of Some Experiments Made on the Body of a Criminal Immediately after Execution, with Physiological and Practical Observations." Read at the Glasgow Literary Society, December 10, 1818. *Journal of Science and the Arts*, 6 (1819): 283–94.

Wallace, Christopher. *The Resurrection Club*. 1999; rpt. London: HarperCollins, 2000.

Walton, Gladys Hastings. *The Wolves of Tanner's Close*. Also known as *The Crimes of Burke and Hare*. BL Lord Chamberlain's Pamphlets, 1930/54. Promptbook, BTA EJE/000607; partbook, BTA EJE/001473.

Warner, Alan. *The Man Who Walks*. London: Jonathan Cape, 2002.

Warren, Samuel. "The Resurrectionist," aka "Grave Doings." *Affecting Scenes: Being Passages from the Diary of a Late Physician*. Vol. 2. New York: J and J Harper, 1833: 94–109.

West Port Murders: or an Authentic Account of the Atrocious Murders Committed by Burke and His Associates; Containing a Full Account of all the Extraordinary Circumstances Connected with Them. Also, a Report of the Trial of Burke and M'Dougal. With a Description of the Execution of Burke, His Confessions, and Memoirs of His Accomplices, Including the Proceedings against Hare, &c. Illustrated by Portraits and Views. Edinburgh: Thomas Ireland, Junior, 1829.

Whiter, Walter. *A Dissertation on the Disorder of Death; Or That State of the Frame under the Signs of Death Called Suspended Animation; to Which Remedies Have Been Sometimes Successfully Applied, as in Other Disorders, in Which It Is Recommended, That the Same Remedies of the Resuscitative Process Should Be Applied to Cases of NATURAL DEATH, As They Are to Cases of Violent Death, Drowning, &c. under the Same Hope of Sometimes Succeeding in the Attempt*. London: n.p., 1819.

Winslow, J. B. *The Uncertainty of the Signs of Death and the Danger of Precipitate Interments and Dissections, Demonstrated*. 1740; 1742 trans. and expanded, Jean Bruhier; 1746 ed. and expanded M. Cooper. London: M. Cooper, 1746.

Worthington, Edward, M. D. "Reminiscences of Medical Student Life Fifty Years Ago—in Edinburgh." *The Medical Age* 12.13 (1894): 385–91.

Wretch's Illustrations of Shakespeare. Edinburgh: Nimmo, 1829.

Zaillian, Steven. *Hannibal*. Movie Script. Online, available at sfy.ru/?script=hannibal2001. Accessed October 16, 2010.

SECONDARY BIBLIOGRAPHY: CRITICISM AND THEORY

Allard, James Robert. *Romanticism, Medicine, and the Poet's Body*. Aldershot, England: Ashgate, 2007.

Anderson, Benedict. *Imagined Communities: Reflections on the Origin and Spread of Nationalism*. 1983; rpt. London: Verso, 1991.

Ashcroft, Bill, Gareth Griffiths, and Helen Tiffin. *The Postcolonial Studies Reader*. 2nd ed. London: Routledge, 2006.

Balfour, Graham. *The Life of Robert Louis Stevenson*. 2 vols. New York: Charles Scribner's Sons, 1901.

Bannister, Winifred. *James Bridie and His Theatre*. London: Rockliff, 1955.

Barker, Francis. *The Tremulous Private Body: Essays on Subjection*. Ann Arbor: University of Michigan Press, 1995.

Behlmer, George K. "Grave Doubts: Victorian Medicine, Moral Panic, and the Signs of Death." *Journal of British Studies* 42 (April 2003): 206–35.

Benjamin, Walter. "The Storyteller." *Illuminations*. N.p.: Schocken, 1969.

Bhabha, Homi K. "DissemiNation." Homi K. Bhabha, ed., *Nation and Narration*. London: Routledge, 1990: 291–322.

Bernstein, Stephen. *Alasdair Gray*. Lewisburg, PA: Bucknell University Press, 1999.

Bishop, William John. *The Early History of Surgery*. New York: Barnes & Noble, 1995.

Bondeson, Jan. *Buried Alive: The Terrifying History of Our Most Primal Fear*. New York: Barnes & Noble, 2001.

Bradley, James, Marguerite Dupree, and Alastair Durie. "Taking the Water Cure: The Hydropathic Movement in Scotland, 1840–1940." *Business and Economic History* 26.2 (Winter 1997): 426–37.

Brake, Laurel, Bill Bell, and David Finkelstein. *Nineteenth-Century Media and the Construction of Identities*. Houndsmills, England: Palgrave, 2000.

Brown, Stewart J. *Thomas Chalmers and the Godly Commonwealth in Scotland*. Oxford: Oxford University Press, 1982.

Browner, Stephanie P. *Profound Science and Elegant Literature: Imagining Doctors in Nineteenth-Century America*. Philadelphia: University of Pennsylvania Press, 2005.

Bruhm, Steven. *Gothic Bodies: The Politics of Pain in Romantic Fiction*. Philadelphia: University of Pennsylvania Press, 1994.

Burgh, Druin. *Digging up the Dead: Uncovering the Life and Times of Astley Cooper, an Extraordinary Surgeon*. London: Vintage, 2008.

Burney, Ian A. *Bodies of Evidence: Medicine and the Politics of the English Inquest 1830–1926*. Baltimore: Johns Hopkins University Press, 2000.

Bynum, W. F. et al. eds. *Medical Journals and Medical Knowledge*. London: Routledge, 1992.

Bynum, W. F., and Roy Porter, eds. *Medical Fringe and Medical Orthodoxy 1750–1850*. London: Croom Helm, 1987.

———. *William Hunter and the Eighteenth-Century Medical World*. Cambridge: Cambridge University Press, 1985.

Campbell, Neil, and R. Martin S. Smellie. *The Royal Society of Edinburgh (1783–1983)*. Edinburgh: The Royal Society of Edinburgh, 1983.

Canuel, Mark. *The Shadow of Death: Literature, Romanticism, and the Subject of Punishment*. Princeton, NJ: Princeton University Press, 2007.

Carruthers, Gerard, ed., *The Devil to Stage: Five Plays by James Bridie*. Glasgow: Association for Scottish Literary Studies, 2007.

Caruth, Cathy, ed. *Trauma: Explorations in Memory*. Baltimore, MD: Johns Hopkins University Press, 1995.

Cixous, Hélène. "The Laugh of the Medusa." 1975. Trans Keith and Paula Cohen. *Signs* 1.4 (Summer 1976): 875–93.

Clarke, J. F. *Autobiographical Recollections of the Medical Profession*. London: J. & A. Churchill, 1874.

Connolly, Tristianne, and Steven Clark, eds. *Liberating Medicine, 1720–1835*. London: Pickering and Chatto, 2009.

Cooter, Roger. *The Cultural Meaning of Popular Science: Phrenology and the Organization of Consent in Nineteenth Century Britain*. Cambridge: Cambridge University Press, 1984.

———. *Phrenology in the British Isles: An Annotated Historical Biobibliography and Index*. Metuchen, NJ: Scarecrow Press, 1989.

Craig, Cairns. *The Modern Scottish Novel: Narrative and the National Imagination*. Edinburgh: Edinburgh University Press, 1999.

———. *Out of History: Narrative Paradigms in Scottish and English Culture*. Edinburgh: Polygon, 1996.

———. "Recovering History." Caroline McCracken-Flesher, ed., *Culture, Nation, and the New Scottish Parliament*. Lewisburg, PA: Bucknell, 2007: 23–43.

Crawford, Robert. *Devolving English Literature*. Rev. ed. Edinburgh University Press, 2000.

Crawford, Robert, and Thom Nairn. *The Arts of Alasdair Gray*. Edinburgh: Edinburgh University Press, 1991.

Curtis, L. Perry. *Jack the Ripper and the London Press*. New Haven, CT: Yale University Press, 2001.

Danahay, Martin. Intro. *The Strange Case of Dr Jekyll and Mr Hyde*. 2nd ed. N.p.: Broadview Press, 2005.

Danahay, Martin, and Alexander Chisholm. *Jekyll and Hyde Dramatized*. Jefferson, NC: McFarland, 2004.

Devlin-Thorp, Sheila, ed. *One Hundred Medical and Scientific Fellows of the Royal Society of Edinburgh*. Vols. 1–3. Edinburgh: Royal Society of Edinburgh, 1981–82.

Dickey, Colin. *Cranioklepty: Grave Robbing and the Search for Genius*. [Lakewood, CO]: Unbridled Books, 2009.

Digby, Anne. *Making a Medical Living: Doctors and Patients in the English Market for Medicine, 1720–1911*. Cambridge: Cambridge University Press, 1994.

"Doctors Say 'I'm Sorry' Before 'See You in Court.'" *New York Times*, May 18, 2008. Online, available at nytimes.com/2008/05/18/us/18apology.html?em&ex=1211256000&en=0022f0dd55 09455e&ei=5087%0A. Accessed May 18, 2008.

Donaldson, William. *Popular Literature in Victorian Scotland: Language, Fiction and the Press*. Aberdeen: Aberdeen University Press, 1986.

Edwards, Owen Dudley. *City of a Thousand Worlds: Edinburgh in Festival.* Edinburgh: Mainstream, 1991.
———. *The Quest for Sherlock Holmes.* Totowa, NJ: Barnes and Noble, 1983.
Erving, Henry Wood. "The Discoverer of Anaesthesia: Dr. Horace Wells of Hartford." 1933; rpt. *Connecticut Tercentenary Commission* 1.29.
Fanon, Frantz. *The Wretched of the Earth.* 1961. Trans. Constance Farrington. New York: Grove Weidenfeld, 1963.
Ferris, Paul. *Dylan Thomas: The Biography.* Berkeley: Counterpoint, 2000.
Fido, Martin. *Bodysnatchers: A History of the Resurrectionists 1742–1832.* London: Weidenfield and Nicolson, 1988.
Foucault, Michel. *The Birth of the Clinic: An Archaeology of Medical Perception.* 1963. Trans. A. M. Sheridan Smith. New York: Vintage, 1994.
———. *Discipline and Punish: The Birth of the Prison.* 1975. Trans. Alan Sheridan. New York: Vintage, 1979.
Frank, Mortimer. "Resurrection Days." *Interstate Medical Journal* 3 (1907): 293–310.
Fullmer, June Z. *Young Humphry Davy: The Making of an Experimental Chemist.* Philadelphia: American Philosophical Society, 2000.
Gilbert, Pamela K. *The Citizen's Body: Desire, Health, and the Social in Victorian England.* Columbus: Ohio State University Press, 2007.
Glass, Rodge. *Alasdair Gray: A Secretary's Biography.* London: Bloomsbury, 2008.
Gray, Alasdair. *1982 Janine.* New York: Viking Penguin, 1984.
———. *Lanark: A Life in Four Books.* Edinburgh: Canongate, 1981.
———. *Why Scots Should Rule Scotland.* Edinburgh: Canongate, 1997.
"Greed of William Hart, The." *Classic Horror* website. Online, available at classichorror.free-online.co.uk/greed.htm. Accessed May 21, 2009.
Green, Richard, and K. Silem Mohammed, eds. *The Undead and Philosophy: Chicken Soup for the Soulless.* Chicago: Open Court, 2006.
Guthrie, Douglas, and Charles D. Waterston. *The Royal Society Club of Edinburgh 1820–2000.* Edinburgh: RSE Foundation, 1999.
Guttmacher, Alan F. "Bootlegging Bodies: A History of Body-Snatching." *Bulletin of the Society of Medical History of Chicago* 4.4 (January 1935): 353–402.
Hansen, Julie V. "Resurrecting Death: Anatomical Art in the Cabinet of Dr. Frederik Ruysch." *The Art Bulletin* 78.4 (December 1996): 663–79.
Harrington, Anne. *Medicine, Mind, and the Double Brain: A Study in Nineteenth-Century Thought.* Princeton, NJ: Princeton University Press, 1987.
Haslam, Fiona. *From Hogarth to Rowlandson: Medicine in Art in Eighteenth-Century Britain.* Liverpool: Liverpool University Press, 1996.
Hay, Douglas et al. *Albion's Fatal Tree: Crime and Society in Eighteenth-Century England.* New York: Pantheon, 1975.
Hayot, Eric. *The Hypothetical Mandarin: Sympathy, Modernity, and Chinese Pain.* Oxford: Oxford University Press, 2009.
Hilton, Boyd. *The Age of Atonement: The Influence of Evangelicism on Social and Economic Thought, 1795–1865.* Oxford: Clarendon Press, 1988.
Holmes, Oliver Wendell (Senior). *Our Hundred Days in Europe.* London: Sampson Low, Marston, 1895.

Hume, David. *Dialogues Concerning Natural Religion.* 2nd ed. London: n.p., 1779.
Kaufman, M. H. "Another Look at Burke and Hare: The Last Day of Mary Paterson—a Medical Cover-Up?" *Journal of the Royal College of Physicians of Edinburgh* 27.1 (1997): 78–88.
———. "Frederick Knox, Younger Brother and Assistant of Dr Robert Knox: His Contribution to Knox's Catalogues." *Journal of the College of Surgeons of Edinburgh* 46 (February 2001): 44–56. Online, available at rcsed.ac.uk/journal/vol46_1/4610008.htm. Accessed July 25, 2008.
Kelly, Veronica, and Dorothea Von Mücke. *Body and Text in the Eighteenth Century.* Stanford, CA: Stanford University Press, 1994.
Kemp, Martin, and Marina Wallace. *Spectacular Bodies: The Art and Science of the Human Body from Leonardo to Now.* Berkeley: University of California Press, 2000.
Kidd, Colin. "Race, Empire, and the Limits of Nineteenth-Century Scottish Nationhood." *Historical Journal* 46.4 (December 2003): 873–92.
Kristeva, Julia. *Powers of Horror: An Essay on Abjection.* New York: Columbia University Press, 1982.
LaCapra, Dominick. *History and Memory after Auschwitz.* Ithaca, NY: Cornell University Press, 1998.
———. *Writing History, Writing Trauma.* Baltimore, MD: Johns Hopkins University Press, 2001.
Laing, R. D. *The Facts of Life: An Essay in Feelings, Facts, and Fantasy.* New York: Pantheon Books, 1976.
———. "Notes" in "Bibliography." *R. D. Laing Society* website. Online, available at laingsociety, org/biblio/factsolife.htm. Accessed January 14, 2009.
———. *The Politics of Experience.* London: Routledge and Kegan Paul, 1967.
———. *The Self and Others: Further Studies in Sanity and Madness.* London: Tavistock, 1961.
Lakoff, George, and Mark Johnson. *Metaphors We Live By.* Chicago: University of Chicago Press, 1980.
Law, Graham. *Serializing Fiction in the Victorian Press.* Houndsmills, England: Palgrave, 2000.
Lawrence, Christopher. "Alexander Monro *Primus* and the Edinburgh Manner of Anatomy." *Bulletin of Medical History* 62 (1988): 193–214.
Lazare, Aaron. *On Apology.* New York: Oxford University Press, 2004.
Levine, George. *Dying to Know: Scientific Epistemology and Narrative in Victorian Britain.* Chicago: University of Chicago Press, 2002.
Loudon, Irvine. *Medical Care and the General Practitioner 1750–1850.* Oxford: Clarendon Press, 1986.
Low, John Thomas. *Doctors Devils Saints and Sinners.* Edinburgh: Ramsay Head, 1980.
Luyben, Helen L. *James Bridie: Clown and Philosopher.* Philadelphia: University of Philadelphia Press, 1965.
MacDiarmid, Hugh. *Hugh MacDiarmid, The Raucle Tongue: Hitherto Uncollected Prose.* Vol. 3. Ed. Angus Calder, Glen Murray, and Alan Riach. Manchester: Carcanet, 1998.
———. *Hugh MacDiarmid: Selected Prose.* Ed. Alan Riach. Manchester: Carcanet, 1992.
———. "Scotland and the Arts." *Bookman* 1934 (September): 285.
MacDonald, Helen. *Human Remains: Dissection and its Histories.* New Haven, CT: Yale University Press, 2005.
Mack, Douglas S. *Scottish Fiction and the British Empire.* Edinburgh: Edinburgh University Press, 2006.

Mack, Robert L. *The Wonderful and Surprising History of Sweeney Todd: The Life and Times of an Urban Legend*. London: Continuum, 2007.

Maixner, Paul. *Robert Louis Stevenson: The Critical Heritage*. London: Routledge & Kegan Paul, 1981.

Manning, Susan. "A View from David Hume's Tower." *Culture, Nation, and the New Scottish Parliament*. Ed. Caroline McCracken-Flesher. Lewisburg, PA: Bucknell University Press, 2007: 76–94.

Marland, Hilary. "The Medical Activities of Mid-Nineteenth-Century Chemists and Druggists, with Special Reference to Wakefield and Huddersfield." *Medical History* 31 (1987): 415–39.

Marmoy, C. F. A. "The 'Auto-Icon' of Jeremy Bentham at University College, London." *Medical History* 2.2 (April 1958): 77–86.

Maulitz, Russell C. *Morbid Appearances: The Anatomy of Pathology in the Early Nineteenth Century*. Cambridge: Cambridge University Press, 1987.

Maunder, Andrew, and Grace Moore, eds. *Victorian Crime, Madness and Sensation*. Aldershot, England: Ashgate, 2004.

Mavor, Ronald. *Dr. Mavor and Mr. Bridie*. Edinburgh: Canongate, 1988.

McCracken-Flesher. *Possible Scotlands: Walter Scott and the Story of Tomorrow*. Oxford: Oxford University Press, 2007.

———. "Speaking the Colonized Subject in Walter Scott's *Malachi Malagrowther* Letters." *Studies in Scottish Literature* 29: 73–84.

McGuirk, Carol. "Burns and Nostalgia." *Burns Now*. Ed. Kenneth Simpson. Edinburgh: Canongate, 1994: 31–69.

McManners, John. *Death and the Enlightenment: Changing Attitudes to Death Among Christians and Unbelievers in Eighteenth-Century France*. Oxford: Clarendon Press, 1981.

Menikoff, Barry. *Narrating Scotland: The Imagination of Robert Louis Stevenson*. Columbia: University of South Carolina Press, 2005.

Mergenthal, Silvia. "An Anatomy of Edinburgh: The Case of Burke and Hare." Unpublished paper. Technische Universität Chemnitz, 2003.

Metcalf, Peter, and Richard Huntington. *Celebrations of Death: The Anthropology of Mortuary Ritual*. 2nd. ed. Cambridge: Cambridge University Press, 1991.

Mighall, Robert. "Diagnosing Jekyll: The Scientific Context to Dr Jekyll's Experiment and Mr Hyde's Embodiment." *Strange Case of Dr. Jekyll and Mr. Hyde*, ed. Mighall. East Rutherford, NJ: Viking Penguin, 2002: 145–61.

Miller, Gavin. *Alasdair Gray: The Fiction of Communion*. Amsterdam: Rodopi, 2005.

Mitchell, G. A. G. "Anatomical and Resurrectionist Activities in Northern Scotland." *Journal of the History of Medicine* 4 (Autumn 1949): 417–30.

Mitton, Lavinia. *The Victorian Hospital*. Botley, England: Shire, 2008.

Moore, Wendy. *The Knife Man: Blood, Body-Snatching and the Birth of Modern Surgery*. 2005; London: Bantam, 2006.

Moores, Phil. *Alasdair Gray: Critical Appreciations and a Bibliography*. Boston Spa, England: British Library, 2002.

Nairn, Tom. *The Break-Up of Britain*. 1977; rev. ed. Victoria: Common Ground, 2003.

———. *Faces of Nationalism: Janus Revisited*. London: Verso, 1998.

———. "The Three Dreams of Scottish Nationalism." 1970; rpt. Lindsay Paterson, ed. *A Diverse Assembly: The Debate on a Scottish Parliament*. Edinburgh: Edinburgh University Press, 1998: 31–39.

Nancy, Jean-Luc. *Corpus*. Trans. Richard A. Rand. New York: Fordham, 2008.

Naugrette, Jean-Pierre. "The Strange Cases of Doctors Haeckel and Jekels: Fake Onomastic European Associations as Interpretation." Paper delivered at *RLS 2008: European Stevenson*, 5th biennial Stevenson conference, Universita di Bergamo June 30–July 3, 2008.

Neuberger, Max. "Sir James Young Simpson." Wellcome MS 8289.

Nochlin, Linda. *The Body in Pieces: The Fragment as a Metaphor of Modernity*. 1995; rpt. London: Thames and Hudson, 2001.

Packard, Francis R. "The Resurrectionists of London and Edinburgh" *Medical News* 81.2 (July 12, 1902): 64–73.

Paris, John Ayrton. *The Life of Sir Humphry Davy*. London: Henry Colburn and Richard Bently, 1831.

Park, Katharine. "The Criminal and the Saintly Body: Autopsy and Dissection in Renaissance Italy." *Renaissance Quarterly* 47.1 (Spring 1994): 1–33.

———. "The Life of the Corpse: Division and Dissection in Late Medieval Europe." *Journal of the History of Medicine and Allied Sciences* 50 (1995): 111–32.

Parry, Noel and José. *The Rise of the Medical Profession*. London: Croom Helm, 1976.

Patrizio, Andrew, and Dawn Kemp. *Anatomy Acts: How We Come to Know Ourselves*. Edinburgh: Birlinn, 2006.

Pernick, Martin S. "Back from the Grave: Recurring Controversies over Defining and Diagnosing Death in History." *Death: Beyond Whole-Brain Criteria*. Ed. Richard M. Zaner. Dordrecht, Netherlands: Kluwer Academic Publishers, 1988: 17–74.

Peterson, M. Jeanne. *The Medical Profession in Mid-Victorian London*. Berkeley: University of California Press, 1978.

Pilbeam, Pamela. *Madame Tussaud and the History of Waxworks*. London: Hambledon and London, 2003.

Porter, Roy. *Bodies Politic: Disease, Death and Doctors in Britain 1650–1900*. Ithaca, NY: Cornell University Press, 2001.

———. *Flesh in the Age of Reason*. New York: Norton, 2003.

Quigley, Christine. *The Corpse: A History*. Jefferson, NC: McFarland, 1996.

Reid, Julia. *Robert Louis Stevenson, Science, and the Fin de Siecle*. Houndsmills, England: Palgrave, 2006.

Richards, Evelleen. "The 'Moral Anatomy' of Robert Knox." *Journal of the History of Biology* 22.3 (Fall 1989): 373–436.

Richardson, Alan. *British Romanticism and the Science of the Mind*. Cambridge: Cambridge University Press, 2001.

Ritchie, Murray. *Scotland Reclaimed: The Inside Story of Scotland's First Democratic Parliamentary Election*. Edinburgh: The Saltire Society, 2000.

Rivington, Walter. *The Medical Profession*. Dublin: Fannin, 1879.

Roach, Mary. *Stiff: The Curious Lives of Human Cadavers*. New York: Norton, 2003.

Rosenthal, Laura J. and Mita Choudhury, eds. *Monstrous Dreams of Reason: Body, Self, and Other in the Enlightenment*. Lewisburg, PA: Bucknell University Press, 2002.

Rosner, Lisa. *Medical Education in the Age of Improvement: Edinburgh Students and Apprentices 1760–1826*. Edinburgh: Edinburgh University Press, 1991.

Rossington, Michael, and Anne Whitehead, eds. *Theories of Memory: A Reader*. Edinburgh: Edinburgh University Press, 2007.

Roth, Michael S. *The Ironist's Cage: Memory, Trauma, and the Construction of History*. New York: Columbia University Press, 1995.
Rudolph, Julia, ed. *History and Nation*. Lewisburg, PA: Bucknell University Press, 2006.
Sawday, Jonathan. *The Body Emblazoned: Dissection and the Human Body in Renaissance Culture*. London: Routledge, 1995.
Scarry, Elaine. *The Body in Pain: The Making and Unmaking of the World*. New York: Oxford University Press, 1985.
Schultz, Suzanne M. *Body Snatching: The Robbing of Graves for the Education of Physicians in Early Nineteenth Century America*. Jefferson, NC: McFarland, 1992.
Scott, Andrew Murray. *Dundee's Literary Lives* 1. Dundee: Abertay Historical Society, 2003.
Searle, G. R. *Morality and the Market in Victorian Britain*. Oxford: Clarendon Press, 1998.
Siegel, Jonah. *The Emergence of the Modern Museum: An Anthology of Nineteenth-Century Sources*. Oxford: Oxford University Press, 2008.
Smout, C. F. V. "The Story of the Resurrectionists." *Cambridge University Medical Journal* 23 (1946): 76–83.
Spence, Donald P. *Narrative Truth and Historical Truth: Meaning and Interpretation in Psychoanalysis*. 1982; rpt. New York: W. W. Norton, 1984.
Stacey, Margaret. *Regulating British Medicine: The General Medical Council*. Chichester, England: John Wiley & Sons, 1992.
Stafford, Barbara Marie. *Body Criticism: Imagining the Unseen in Enlightenment Art and Medicine*. Cambridge, MA: MIT Press, 1993.
Stevenson, Robert Benjamin III. "Stevenson's Dentist: An Unsung Hero." *Journal of Stevenson Studies* 4 (2007): 43–51.
Stiles, Anne. *Neurology and Literature, 1860–1920*. Houndsmills, England: Palgrave, 2007.
Strong, Roy. *Bodies Politic: Disease, Death and Doctors in Britain, 1650–1900*. Ithaca, NY: Cornell University Press, 2001.
Sugg, Richard. *Murder after Death: Literature and Anatomy in Early Modern England*. Ithaca, NY: Cornell University Press, 2007.
Swearingen, Roger. *The Prose Writings of Robert Louis Stevenson*. Hamden, CT: Archon Books, 1980.
Tait, H. P. "Some Edinburgh Medical Men at the Time of the Resurrectionists." *Edinburgh Medical Journal* 55 (February 1948): 116–23.
Taylor, D. W. "The Manuscript Lecture-Notes of Alexander Monro *Primus* (1697–1767)." *Medical History* 30 (1986): 444–67.
Ticktin, Stephen. "Biography." *R. D. Laing Society* website. Online, available at laingsociety.org/biograph.htm. Accessed January 14, 2009.
Tobin, Terence. *James Bridie*. Boston: Twayne, 1980.
Turner, Terence D. "'Secret Nostrums': Aspects of the Development of Patent and Proprietary Medicines." *A Pox on the Provinces: Proceedings of the 12th Congress of the British Society for the History of Medicine*. Ed. Roger Rolls and Jean and John R. Guy. Bath: Bath University Press, 1990: 159–68.
Veeder, William, and Gordon Hirsch, eds. *Dr Jekyll and Mr Hyde after One Hundred Years*. Chicago: University of Chicago Press, 1988.
Waddington, Ivan. "The Development of Medical Ethics—A Sociological Analysis." *Medical History* 19 (1975): 36–51.

Warner, Marina. *Phantasmagoria: Spirit Visions, Metaphors, and Media into the Twenty-First Century*. Oxford: Oxford University Press, 2008.

Warwick, Alexandra, and Martin Willis, eds. *Jack the Ripper: Media, Culture, History*. Manchester: Manchester University Press, 2007.

Whaley, Joachim, ed. *Mirrors of Mortality: Studies in the Social History of Death*. New York: St. Martin's, Press, 1981.

Wilde, Oscar. "The Decay of Lying." 1889. *Complete Works of Oscar Wilde*. London: Collins, 1977: 970–92.

Wise, Sarah. *The Italian Boy: Murder and Grave-Robbery in 1830s London*. London: Jonathan Cape, 2004.

Wootton, David. *Bad Medicine: Doctors Doing Harm Since Hippocrates*. Oxford: Oxford University Press, 2006.

Young, James E. *The Texture of Memory: Holocaust Memorials and Meaning*. New Haven, CT: Yale, 1993.

Youngquist, Paul. *Monstrosities: Bodies and British Romanticism* Minneapolis: University of Minnesota Press, 2003.

Zimmerman, Susan. *The Early Modern Corpse and Shakespeare's Theatre*. Edinburgh: Edinburgh University Press, 2005.

INDEX

Aberdeen, 11, 38
"An Account of the Most Horrid and Unchristian Actions of the Grave Makers," 10
Adam, Hargrave L., 119
Adams, Norman, 165
alcohol, 28, 78. *See* Pae, David
Allan, Thomas, 37, 42
The Anatomist. *See* Bridie, James
anatomists, 9. See also *by name*
   as a community, 35, 36, 89, 92
   English, 4
   fictionalized, 78
   as heroes, 12, 26, 91–92
   response, 31, 53, 61
anatomy
   British, 10–11
   comparative, 5
   and criminality, 12, 57
   curricula, 6 (*see also* Edinburgh University)
   French, 13
   pathological, 48, 63, 235n12
   study of, 4–5, 13
   subjects, 7, 10–11
   supply of subjects, 11–16
   transcendental, 56
Anatomy Act, 12, 15, 16, 66, 98, 120, 236n1
anesthesia, 93, *109*, *111*. *See also* Stevenson, Robert Louis, *Jekyll and Hyde*
anime, 19, 197
anthropology, 62, 63, 105. *See also* anatomy, transcendental
antiseptics, 93, 106
anxiety, 9, 19, 26, 33–34
   Scottish, 10, 16, 30, 35, 47, 54, 59, 70
apology, 35
assistants to Knox, 46, 75, 235n9. *See also* Fergusson, William; Lonsdale, Henry
   fictive, 131–33
audiodrama, 9, 19, 119. *See also* Doctor Who
autopsy, 46–47

Bagby, Elizabeth, 19, 228
Baker, Roy Ward, 19, 178–79
Ball, Doctor James Moores, 39, 122
ballads, 17, 73, 78, 101, 160
Ballance, Chris, 171
Barclay, Doctor John, 5, 12–13, 14
Barzun, Jacques, 164

Bates, A. W., 23, 165
Bell, Doctor, 233n5
Berliner, Jonny, and Fintan O'Higgins, 207, 212–14
Bertram, J. G., 72, 78. See also North Briton
Bianchi, Dan, 19, 171, 239n4
Big-Nose George, 234n2
Bishop and Williams (the London Burkers), 16, 28
Black, Doctor, 53
Blackwood's Edinburgh Magazine, 28, 33, 38, 54, 87, 234n1
body politic, 27, 47, 126, 159. See also Gray, Alasdair
The Body Snatcher (1945 film), 145, 151
The Body Snatchers (rock band), 197
bodysnatchers, 3, 11, 16, 19, 20, 74. See also by name
bodysnatching, 10–15. See also Hood, Thomas
   British, 10–11
   English, 120
   Irish, 11
   locations, 11
   motivation, 69
   parodies about, 15, 181
   poetry about, 10, 14
   Scottish, 165
Bodyworlds. See von Hagens, Gunther
Bolitho, William (Charles William Ryall), 164
Bradley, James, 197
Bridie, James (Doctor Osborne Henry Mavor), 18, 21, 123–39. See also Hitchcock, Alfred
   The Anatomist, 18, 19, 26, 123–35, 130, 139, 152–54, 160, 167
   and film, 145–51
   and MacDiarmid, 135–38, 150, 238n8
broadsheets, 17, 58, 59–60
Brookes, Doctor Joshua, 11
Bryson, Doctor Hector, 26, 161, 163–64
burial grounds, 11
burke (as verb), 28–29, 35, 38, 98
Burke and Hare, 8, 193
   class, 10
   history, 7–8, 10, 15, 16–17, 173
   and hospitality, 19
   as Irish, 28, 41, 100, 234n1 (see also Edwards, Owen Dudley)
   with Knox, Robert, 4, 8, 64, 161, 164

   medical assistance, 36, 61, 83
   outside Scotland, 9
   parodies of, 16, 17, 163
   technique, 8, 16, 83
   as theatre, 67, 133
Burke and Hare—The Musical, 231
"The Burke Mania," 85
Burke, Raymond, 166, 171–72
Burke, William. See also Burke and Hare
   appearance, 8, 30, 33, 33, 58, 121, 221, 235n14
   as character, 78–79, 81, 85–86, 140, 145, 149, 152, 167, 175
   confession, 17, 34, 36
   execution and dissection, 16, 28–29, 29, 40, 69, 235n8
   fictionalized, 79, 157
   on Knox, 36
   as procurer, 8
   as souvenirs, 24, 29–30, 234n2
   trial, 40, 58, 159
Burns, Robert, 47
Burnside, D. R., 118–119
Byrd, Elizabeth, 26, 173–78, 179
Byron, Lord George Gordon, 12

Caledonian Mercury, 36, 42, 58. See also Allan, Thomas
caricatures
   Noxiana, 17, 45, 60
   Wretch's Illustrations of Shakespeare, 17
Carlyle, Robert, 20, 234n14, 234n16
Carpue, Doctor, 3, 233n5
cause of death, 53–54
Chalmers, Thomas, 72
cheap editions. See Adams, Hargrave L.; Jamieson, Hugh; Burnside, D. R.
children's literature, 18, 19, 27, 201–6
Christison, Doctor Robert, 53, 122, 159
Christmas story, 44, 61, 236n1. See also Stevenson, Robert Louis, "The Body Snatcher"
chronicle, 120–22. See also, historicism; Leighton, Alexander; Trial of William Burke; West Port Murders
Clarke, William, 11
class, 10, 12, 42, 77, 78, 100. See also victims
   and literacy, 15
   in retellings, 71
   upper, 27, 35
Clydesdale, Matthew, 50, 51, 53

Index

Cobbe, Francis Power, 52
Cockburn, Henry (advocate for the defense), 30–31, 53, 122
coffins, 11, 52
Cole, Hubert, 164
comedy, 16, 20, 27, 141, 143, 145, 152–53, 196. *See also* Bryson, Hector; Burke, Raymond
commerce, 4, 9, 13, 27, 107, 171–72, 195. *See also* Burke, Raymond; Edinburgh Festival; Edwards, Owen Dudley; Leighton, Alexander; Pae, David
Communist Party, 26
community
   response, 31–42
   in retellings, 122 (*see* Bridie, James; Byrd, Elizabeth; Leighton, Alexander; Pae, David)
   at risk, 58
   theory of, 20–22, 47, 227
Conaghan, Martin, and Will Pickering, 228, *229, 232*
Cooper, Sir Astley, 4, 15, 233n5
copycat crime, 38–39; *see also* Bishop and Williams; Ross, Elizabeth
Corridors of Blood, 18, 237n14
Craig, Cairns, 20–21
Crane, Richard, 171, 239n5
Crawford, Robert, 21
Crime Does NOT Pay. See *Ghoul's Gold*
crime fiction, 17, 24, 119–20
criminality, 12, 13–14, 57, 58, 69
criminology, 24
Cullen, Doctor William, 13
cultural studies, 166–71
The Cure. See *Smallville*
Cuvier, Georges, 5

Daft Jamie, 8, 17, 17, 43, 58, 73. *See also* Mrs. Wilson
   as character, 73–74, 140–43, 144–45, 149, 159, 162, 168–69, 202, 203–4, 211, 219
   dissection of, 36, 97
   images of, *141, 169*

Darwin, Charles, 5, 62, 68, 105, 163, 168, 233n2
Darwin, Erasmus, 50
Deacon Brodie, 102, 219
de Quincey, 139, 235n7
dialogue (as philosophical practice), 57–58, 64, 75, 88

Diary of a Resurrectionist, 120, 238n3
Dickens, Charles, 16
Dickson, Margaret, 52–53, 235n15
dissection, 13
   of criminals, 13
   curriculum, 6, 48
   of Lord Byron, 12
   as metaphor, 47–48, 51, 53, 54, 112–15, 159, 182, 193–94
   parodies about, 3, 13–15
   poetry about, 3
   public attitudes, 12–15, 52
   and secrecy, 35
   stories about, 39
Docherty, Mrs., 8, 16, 17, 91, 122, 159, 160
   as character, 119, 151
   images of, *159*
doctor, 122–23. See also *by name*
   as audience, 134
   as disease, 19
   as hero, 92–93
   fictional, 83–85 (*see also* Bryson, Hector; Goodwin, I.; Gray, Alasdair; Knox as character, Scarborough, Elizabeth Ann)
   as murderer, 110
   nature of, 62, 92–93, 102–103, 107–108
   professionalism of, 93, 107–108, 122 (*see also* ethics)
   as writer (*see* Bridie, James; Bryson, Hector; Leighton, Alexander; Warren)
The Doctor and the Devils, 18
Doctor in Love, 19, 151, 239n17
Doctor Jekyll and Sister Hyde. See Baker, Roy Ward
Doctor Who, 9, 19, 210–12
Doherty, Karen, 203–4
double brain, 104
Douglas, Hugh, 160
Doyle, Doctor Arthur Conan, 119–20
"The Dr. K—Project," 197, 198
DR Knox (hip-hop band), 197
Drummond, Andrew, 230
Dundee ... People's Journal, 76, 77–78. *See also* Pae, David

Ealing Studios, 20
"The East Linton Gravedigger," *see* "The Haddington Cobbler Defended"
"The Echo of Surgeons Square," *see* David Paterson

economics, *see* class, and commerce
Edgeworth, Maria, 28, 41, 234n1
Edinburgh
  and anatomists, 4, 8, 13
  Dungeon, 9, 220
  as enlightened, 32, 34, 37, 57, 215
  Festival, 9, 18, 27, 124, 171, 193, 201, 206–220
  as location for retelling, 20, 103–104, 206–26
  medical schools, 13–14
  police, 8, 70, 97–98
    as characters, 70, 82, 204
  response, 29–46, 54–55, 58–59, 63–64, 234n1
  University of, 4–6, 63, 69, 165, 166, 233n4
    curricula, 6, 63, 90
    professors, 35, 57, 63, 89–91 (*see also* Monro, Alexander)
Edinburgh Evening Courant, 34, 37
Edinburgh Weekly Journal, 36
Edwards, Owen Dudley, 18, 19, 27, 32, 119, 239n3
  and Irishness, 165–171, 172, 234n1
"Elegiac Lines on the Tragical Murder of Poor Daft Jamie," 17
encyclopedism, 156–81
Enlightenment, 4, 9
  end of, 25, 35–36, 42, 56–64 (*see also* Pae, David; system)
Erskine, Gary (illustrator), *see* Conaghan, Martin
"The Ettrick Shepherd," 38
exhibit. *See* von Hagens, Gunther; Edinburgh Dungeon
"An Expostulation," 59–60
Extreme Measures, 19

feminism. *See* gender concerns
Fergusson, Doctor William, 96–98, 224, 236–37n3
film, 18–20, 145–52
The Flesh and the Fiends, 18, 149, 151, 234n9
folk narratives, 17, 118
Forster, Joseph, 139
Fullmetal Alchemist, 19, 197, 200

Galt, John, 53, 98
galvanism, 50, *51*
gender concerns, 18, 26–27, 172–92
generational change. *See* Pae, David
Ghoul's Gold, 19, *151*
Glasgow, 11, 12, 32, 38, 124, 125
  in retellings, 71, 74–75, 142 (*see also* Bridie, James; Gray, Alasdair)
Goodsir, Joseph, 99–100, 237nn4–5
Goodwin, I., 161–62
gothic, 9, 19–20, 39, 99. *See also* Stevenson, Robert Louis; Adam, Hargrave L.
  literature, 53, 65, 101
  medicine as, 50
Graham, Mark, 197
Grant, James, 167
Gray, Alasdair, 21, 156
  Poor Things, 4, 18, 27, 158 181–92, *184*
Gray, Mr. and Mrs., 8
  as characters, 79, 82, 95–96, 146, 175
The Greed of William Hart. See Horror Maniacs
Greyfriars Twisted Tales, 209
Guthrie, Doctor G. J., 15
Guy's Hospital, 3
"The Haddington Cobbler Defended," 14
"The Haddington Cobbler Dissected Alive," 14
"The Haddington Shoemaker." *See* Smith, William

Haeckel, Ernst, 104
Hagens, Gunther von, 27, 200, 212–14, 241n25
Mrs. Haldane and daughter, 8
  as characters, 83
Hamish Macbeth, 228
Hannibal, 197
Hare, Margaret, 7, 31, 32
  appearance, *174*
  as character, 27, 79, 170, 172–77
  her child (*see* Byrd, Elizabeth)
  testimony, 58
Hare, William. *See also* Burke and Hare
  appearance, *8*, 30, *59*, 68
  Catholicism, 234n1
  as character, 84–85, 145, 149, 175–78
  history, 28, 31, 32
  mistaken identity, 39
  testimony, 58
Harrison, Ben, 207
Hastings, N. 144
Henley, W. E., 95, 102, 105
historicism, 19, 21, 76, 93, 118, 157, 165, 195, 201
  in Bridie, 124
  in Leighton, 24, 64–70
  and Scott, 40
  in Stevenson, 89–91

Hitchcock, Alfred, 9, 19, 147–48, 150, 151
Hogg, James, 47
Hollywood, 26, 150
Holman, Sheri, *The Dress Lodger*, 19, 197–98
Holmes, Doctor Oliver Wendell, 119
Honeyman, William Crawford, 119
Hood, Evelyn, 128
Hood, Thomas, 233n1, 233n5
   "Mary's Ghost," 3–4
Hooper, Mary, 202
Horrible Histories, 202, 203
Horror Maniacs, 18, 143–45, 151
The Horrors of Burke and Hare, 18, 148, 151
houses of refuge, 39
Hunter, Doctor John, 48, 50, 125, 185
Hunter, Doctor William, 47, 185
hypocrisy, 114–15
If a Body Needs a Body, 119

internet, 27
investigatory committee, 37, 42, 45
Ireland, 11, 32, 195
   in plot, 85
Ireland, Thomas, 40. See also *West Port Murders*
Irish. See also; Edwards, Owen Dudley; retellings, Irish
   context, 17, 18, 195
   immigration, 28, 42, 167
   perpetrators, 28
   victims, 8
irony, 27, 215. See also Berliner
   theory, 23, 46
Irving, Edward, 71, 72
I Sell the Dead, 19, 197–98, 200

Jack the Ripper, 117, 178–79
Jamieson, Hugh (publ. *Life and Times*), 118
Joe the Miller (character), 78
Johnston, George, 64
Johnston, Paul, 18, 215–6

kailyard, 78–79. See also Pae, David
Kneale, Matthew, *English Passengers*, 19, 197
Knight, Alanna, 17, 24
Knox, Doctor Robert
   actors as, 128, 138, 139, 152, 238n5
   advertisements, 6, 7, 62
   in Africa, 5, 91

   appearance, 5, *6*, 24, *60*, 70, 91, 97–98, 128, 194
   autobiography, 114
   biography, 4–10, 35–39, 48, 53–54, 56, 58–64, 75, 89, 91–93, 160, 241n23
   blame, 10, 28–29, 34, 36, 61, 81, 97, 127, 162, 237n17
   and Burke and Hare, 10, 15, 44, 56, 64, 70
   candidacy for Chair of General Pathology, 63
   as character, 26, 71–75, 81–84, 125–34, 143, 146–47, 149, 152–53, 160, 162, 171, 185, 197–200, 202, 205–6, 211–12
   and class, 35, 42, 77
   discoveries, 54, 56, 62, 105, 168
   as enlightened, 37, 45, 56, 63–64, 168, 235n3
   in London, 48, 63, 74
   and newspapers, 37–38, 61
   parodied, 17, 160, 162 (see *Noxiana*, *Wretch's Illustrations*)
   personality, 5, 37, 44, 52, 63–64, 108, 112
   race, theories of, 5, 62, 167–68, 237n9
   and Scott, 43–45, 53–55
   silence of, 25, 35, 36–37, 41, 59–63, 93, 104, 110–11
   slander, 38
   and students, 5–6, 25, 38, 45–46, 56, *60*, 62, 63, 77, 92, 161, 233n4, 235n5, 235n9 (*see also* Fergusson, William)
   as subject of "dissection" (*see* Stevenson, Robert Louis)
   trial, lack of, 30–31, 58
   and vivisection, 237n16
   works
      Fish and Fishing, 62
      Great Artists and Great Anatomists, 62–63
      Medical Times and Gazette, 62
      Races of Men, 62, 105
      thesis, 53–54

Lacroix, Jules, 139
Laing, R. D., 183, 187
Lancet, 16
Landis, John, 4, 19, 27, 220
Latto, William, 77. See also *Dundee... People's Journal*

lawyers, 122–23. *See also* Stevenson, Robert Louis; and by name
    as characters, 74, 169–70, 187
Leighton, Alexander, 85, 87, 89, 101, 112, 122
    The Court of Cacus, 18, 24, 25, 64–70, 99, 161
    "Mrs Corbet's Amputated Toe," 65
    on phrenology, 34, 68
Leng, John, 77. *See also* Dundee... *People's Journal*
Lister, Doctor Joseph, 93, 105, 185
Liston, Doctor Robert, 5, 11–12, 48, 92
lodger (victim), 10
London, 11
    as location, 26, 95, 101–102, 120, 148
    opinion, 16, 57, 117
Lonsdale, Doctor Henry, 5, 17, 24, 61, 100, 122, 124, 126
    interpretation by, 35, 52, 77, 91–92, 147
    on retellings, 87
Lord Advocate (William Rae), 30, 31, 32
Lord Justice-Clerk (David Boyle), 30
"The Lost Will," 98
Lytton, Bulwer, *Lucretia*, 16

MacDiarmid, Hugh (Christopher Murray Grieve), 26, 135–38, 150, 207–8
MacGregor, George, 17, 100–101
Maclaren, Charles, 37
Malthusian theory, 67, 170
manga, 19
Mania. See *The Flesh and the Fiends*
Mansfield, Richard, *116*, 117
Marshall, Tim, 164, 185
Matania, F., 150–51
McDonald, Hal, 197
McDougal, Helen, 7, 8, 31, 32, 53
    appearance, 30, *8*, *80*
    as character, 75, 79, 83, 173, 175–76
    trial, 58
McGee, James, 197
The McGregor Affair. See Hitchcock, Alfred
McLevy, James, 119
McNaughton, Douglas, 230
Meadowbank, Lord (Alexander Maconochie), 35, 56–57
    as character, 170
medical biography. *See* Bates, A.W.; Rae, Isobel; Richardson, Ruth; Rosner, Lisa

medical journals, 64
    Annals of Chemical Medicine, 106
    Medical Times and Gazette, 62
medicine
    chemical/pharmacological, 26, 237n11 (*see also* Stevenson, Robert Louis, *Jekyll and Hyde*)
    early twentieth-century (*see* Bridie, James; Bryson, Hector)
    eighteenth-century, 48–49
    ethics, 92
    field surgery, 5
    military hospitals, 5
    nineteenth-century, 48–49 (*see also* Bryson, Hector; Stevenson, Robert Louis)
melodrama, 9, 18, 26, 139–45
memory, 20, 21–23, 27, 182, 210, 213, 223, 226. See also *Doctor Who*
    authorial, 43, 102
    decline, 63, 75, 85, 93, 111, 123, 195–96
    narrative, 123, 206
Mercy, Frédéric, 139
metaphor, 16, 21, 68–70, 93. *See also* Stevenson, Robert Louis, *Jekyll and Hyde*
    national, 25, 46, 47–48, 51, 54, 66, 158, 189, 193–94
"Mind's Eye," 197, 198
Mitchell, Robin, 27, 215, 216–8
Monro, Doctor Alexander (*tertius*), 5, 10, 92
moral anatomy, 105
Morgan, Edwin, 231–32
Morgan, Nicola, 204
Morning Chronicle, 40
mort safe, 11
mortuary, 52
mortuary rituals, 156, 182
murder as means of anatomical supply, 15–16
Murderers of the Close (Rosner), 15, 38, 40, 57, 69, 77, 167, 236n1
museums
    anatomy, 5
    Royal College of Surgeons of Edinburgh, 13, 62–64, 92, 158
musicals and music hall, 18, 145. *See also* Berliner, Jonny; Bianchi, Dan; Burke, Raymond

Nairn, Tom, 182–83
narrative, 64

political, 9, 65–66
nation
   culture, 25, 66, 120, 226
   theories of, 20–21, 196–7 (*see also* Nairn, Tom)
"A Necessary Evil," 195
"The Newgate Annual," 16
Newgate Calendar, 16, 117
Newman, Terry, 208–9
newspapers, 9, 17, 23–24, 25, 31–40, 46. *See also* Pae, David; and by name
   Knox's relations with, 37–38
newspaper serials. *See* Pae, David
"A Night in a Dissecting Room," 98
Nightmare in Blood, 18, 148–49, 151
North, Christopher (John Wilson), 38, 90
North Briton, 71, 72, 75, 78
nostalgia, 20–23
novel, 9, 19. *See also* by author
novelist, as subject, 87
Noxiana, 17, 45, *45*

"On the Pleasures of Body-Snatching," 12, 53, 112
Ophaboom, 241n17
Oracle of Health, Economy, and Good Living, 12

Pae, David, 18, 21, 25, 64, 70–88, 89, 120
   The Coming Struggle, 71, 86
   Lucy the Factory Girl, 18, 25, 71–75, 81, 87, 99, 236n4
   Mary Paterson, 18, 25, 75–86, 151, 173
Pall Mall Gazette. *See* Stevenson, Robert Louis, "The Body Snatcher"
Pasteur, Louis, 106, 109
Paterson, David ("The Echo of Surgeon's Square"), 36, 42, 235n9
   as character, 130, 152, 156–58
Paterson, Mary, 8, 75, 89, 96, 176, 236nn5–6, 236–37n3
   appearance, *76*, *82*
   as character, 126–27, 140, 149, 152, 159, 162, 163, 173 (*see* Pae, David)
Pattison, Doctor Granville Sharp, 12, 13
Peel, Robert (Home Secretary), 13, 32, 37
penny geggies, 140, 238n9
Phiz (Hablot Knight Browne), *80*
phrenology, 33–34, 58, 68, 235n3
physiognomy, 101

plaistering, 38
plays, 18, 206–214. *See also* Bridie, James
police, 11. *See also* Edinburgh police
Polidori, John, 38
political fiction, 18
politics, 9, 22, 26, 47. *See also* Ballance, Chris; Burke, Raymond; Clydeside, Red; Communist Party; Edwards, Owen Dudley; Gray, Alasdair; Scottish National Party; Tories
popular culture, 25, 27. *See also* ballads, broadsheets, Edinburgh Festival, film, Internet, newspapers
portable theater. *See* melodrama; penny geggies
postcolonialism, 20–21, 47. *See also* Gray Alasdair; Nairn, Tom
professionalism, 9
prophecy, 86. *See also* Irving, Edward; Pae, David; Thomas, John
psychology, 101, 123. *See* Laing, R.D. ; Leighton, Alexander
Punch, 115–16

quackery, 107–109

Rae, Isobel, 23, 24, 160
Rankin, Ian, 4, 21, 27, 221–26
   The Falls, 18, 223–25
   Resurrection Men, 18, 225–26
   Set in Darkness, 18, 221–23
Ravenous, 197
reanimation, 49–53, 54–55, *49*, *51*, 180, 182–92. *See also* Stevenson, Robert Louis, "The Body Snatcher"
religion, 9, 25, 61, 163. *See also* Gray, Alasdair; Leighton, Alexander; Pae, David; Stevenson, Robert Louis
   Calvinist, 12
   Catholic, 166, 234n1
   Irish Catholic, 13
religious response, 10, 12–13
responsibility, 26, 35
resurrection. *See* bodysnatching
   Christian, 13
resurrection men. *See* bodysnatchers
retelling, 9. *See also* trauma; theory; medical biography
   American, 18–19, 26, 147, 148, 151, 173–80, 197

retelling (*continued*)
  Australian, 197
  Darwinian, 68
  English, 15, 16, 18–19, 26, 77, 138, 139, 146–48, 151, 164, 197, 202–3, 206–9 (see also *Murderers of the Close*)
  enlightened, 66–70 (*see also* Leighton, Alexander; Pae, David)
  German (*see* Goodwin, I.; Wallace, Christopher)
  Indian (*see* Bryson, Hector)
  Irish, 27, 195 (*see also* Edwards, Owen Dudley)
  Japanese, 19
  legal, 29–34, 38, 39, 40
  in medical history, 120–21
  phrenological, 33–34, 68
  psychological, 68
  religious (*see* Leighton, Alexander; Pae, David)
  varieties of Scottish, 10, 16–18, 19–20, 25–27, 39 (*see also* Bridie, James; Doherty, Karen; Gray, Alasdair; Leighton, Alexander; melodrama; Mitchell, Robin; Morgan, Edwin; Morgan, Nicola; Pae, David; Rae, Isobel; Rankin, Ian; Stevenson, Robert Louis)
Richardson, Ruth, 23, 165
riots, 11, 15, 31, 38, 58, *60*, 69, 77, 153
Robinson, Peter, 209
Robison, John, 37, 44, 62
romance, 20–21, 23, 66, 70, 126. *See also* Pae, David
Rosner, Lisa, 23, 165
Ross, Elizabeth, 16, 28
Roughead, William (Writer to the Signet), 24, 122, 124
Rowland, Sidney, 147
Royal College of Physicians, Edinburgh, 30, 31, 158
Royal College of Surgeons of Edinburgh, 5, 13, 124
  curricula, 6, 48, 94
Royal College of Surgeons, London, 15
Royal Medical Society, 33
Royal Society of Edinburgh, 5, 37, 40, 42, 43, 44, 64, 235n3
rumor, 38–39
Rutherford, Doctor John (Walter Scott's grandfather), 42
Ruysch, Frederick, 50
"The Sadducee," 14–15

scandal,
  of bodysnatching, 11–12, 15
  and Knox, 9, 63
  medical, 21
Scarborough, Elizabeth Ann, 179–80
Schwob, Marcel, 139
Scotland, 9, 10, 15, 19
  lack of politics, 22
Scotsman, 32, 37. *See also* Maclaren, Charles
Scott, Walter, 39–46, 47–48, 51, 53–55, 120
  analysis of situation, 25, 42–44, 71, 88, 166
  and Burke's execution, 69, 157–58, 235n10
  as character, 180
  and Charles Kirkpatrick Sharpe, 24, 42
  and Enlightenment, 42–43
  on the Irish, 28, 41, 42
  Malachi Malagrowther Letters, 47
  and metaphor, 47–48, 51, 54
  and nostalgia, 22, 54
  opinion sought, 40–42
  portrait, *41*
  President of the Royal Society of Edinburgh, 40, 43, 44, 62
  refuses to tell tale, 4, 42, 44, 46, 87, 193
  and tartanry, 20–21, 40
  and thesis (Faculty of Advocates), 54
  works, 54, 65
Scottish
  devolution, 18, 26, 182–83, 189, 240n9
  guilt, 10, 57, 66, 68–70
  identity, 27, 28, 33–34, 40, 61, 196–97
Scottish National Party, 26
Scottish National Players, 26
Scottish National Theatre Society, 124, 135–6
Scottish Parliament, 10, 26, 182, 193–94
  retellings inflected by, 193–95, 201 (*see* Mitchell, Robin; Rankin, Ian; Wallace, Christopher)
Secrets of Scotland Yard, 119
Select Committee on Anatomy Report, 11
  testimony to, 12, 15
sensation writing, 24, 39. *See also* Leighton, Alexander; Pae, David
Seton, Robert, 235n10
Seymour, Robert, 155, *159*

Sharpe, Charles Kirkpatrick, 24, 39, 42, 235n10.
    See also *Trial of William Burke*
    (Buchanan)
Sheffield Daily Telegraph, 84, 236n7
Shelley, Mary, 9, 53, 164, 185–86
Simpson, Doctor James Young, 106, 109–10, 185
Slaughter, Tod, 143, 145, 151
Smallville, 19, 197–98
Smith, J., S. S. C. (confessor), 34
Smith, Doctor Thomas Southwood, 12,
    14, 233n7
    "Use of the Dead to the Living," 14, 48
Smith, W. Gordon, 156–58
Smith, William ("The Haddington
    Shoemaker"), 13, 14
Stephen, Kathy, 165
Stephenson, Shelagh, 197, 228
Stevenson, J., 40
Stevenson, Robert Louis, 21, 25–26, 89–117,
    121–22, 195
    and history, 89–91
    and medicine, 25, 89, 102–13
    as Scottish, 25, 100, 120
    works: 94, 99, 100
        "The Body Snatcher," 9, 18, 89, 94–101, 96
        "A Chapter on Dreams," 103–104
        Deacon Brodie, 102, 237n7
        Jekyll and Hyde, 4, 18, 26, 89, 101–17, 118
            (*see* Baker, Roy Ward)
        The Wrong Box, 26, 118, 121
"Stitch, Cut & Dye," 197, 198
Stocks, Robert, and Tommy Luther,
    206–7, 209
Stone, Doctor Thomas, 33–34, 235n3
students, 92
    as characters, 65, 95–100, 148, 149, 151,
        161–64
    as complicit, 38, 45–46, 56, 60, 61, 69, 75,
        235n5, 235n9
    in later life, 25, 92
Sun (newspaper), 32, 41, 235n7
suppression of the story, 30–32, 34, 54–55, 58
Surgeon's Square, 8, 10, 58, 69, 84
sympathy, 68–70
system, 41, 46, 61, 64, 66–68
    systematic thinking, 56–57

tartanry, 17–18, 20, 22
temperance campaigns, *see* Pae, David

Thomas, Dylan, 146–47, 151
Thomas, John, 86–87
Times, 40
Tories, 35
Torrence, Helen, 16, 28
Townsend, John, 203
transcriptions, 40 (see also *West Port
    Murders*)
trauma, 25
    Scottish, 10, 20, 24–27, 39, 65, 69
    exacerbation of, 44, 46, 58, 64, 68, 88
    progress of, 25, 40, 118, 120, 165, 190,
        194–95, 201, 204, 206, 220, 227–28
    theory, 21–23, 29, 46, 121, 183–84, 190,
        234n15
Trial of William Burke (publ. Buchanan), 24,
    65, 195
Turner, Cecil Howard, 120
Tussaud, Madame, 50, 235n14

Ure, Andrew, 50–51, *51*, 53

vampires, 38, 148
Vesalius, 52, 62
victims, 7–8, 10, 26–27, 155–92, *232*. See also
    under specific names or roles
    additional, 32, 34
    and alcohol, 28, 70
    as characters, 70 (see also *by name*)
    and class, 24, 77, 103–104, 165–73
    and "freshness," 8, 15, 36, 46
    and gender, 172–92 (*see also* Mrs. Docherty;
        Paterson, Mary)
    as Irish, 165–69, 173, 176, 189 (*see also*
        Byrd, Elizabeth; Edwards, Owen
        Dudley)
    tinkers, 180
Victoria Regina, 97
video games, 19, 197, 198–200
Vyse, Doctor, 3, 233n5

Wakley, Doctor Thomas (editor of the
    Lancet), 16
Waldie, Jean, 15, 28
Wallace, Christopher, 27, 218–220
Walton, Gladys Hastings, 142–43
Warner, Alan, 228
Warren, Doctor Samuel, 122
washerwoman (victim), 8

watch house, 11
Waterloo, 5
Wells, Doctor Horace, 110, 237n14–15
Welsh, Irvine
   "The Meat Trade," 4, 19, 27, 231, 242n32
   Trainspotting, 20
West Port, 167
West Port Murders, 17, 40, 119, 234n8
Whiter, Walter, 50, 53

Williams, Thomas (London Burker). *See* Bishop and Williams
Wilson, Mr. (turnkey), 34
Wilson, Mrs. (Daft Jamie's mother), 58
Winslow, J. B., 49–50, 51, 52
Wretch's Illustrations of Shakespeare, 17
Wright, Doctor Thomas Giordani, 5

Young, George, 209